University of London Library

Reference Only

THIS BOOK MUST NOT BE REMOVED
FROM THE LIBRARY

Neural Basis of Semantic Memory

The advent of modern investigative techniques to explore brain function has led to major advances in understanding the neural organization and mechanisms associated with semantic memory. This book presents current theories by leading experts in the field on how the human nervous system stores and recalls memory of objects, actions, words and events. Chapters range from models of a specific domain or memory system (e.g. lexical–semantic, sensorimotor, emotion) to multiple modality accounts; from encompassing memory representations, to processing modules, to network structures, focusing on studies of both normal individuals and those with brain disease.

Recent advances in neuro-exploratory techniques allow for investigation of semantic memory mechanisms noninvasively in both normal healthy individuals and patients with diffuse or focal brain damage. This has resulted in a significant increase in findings relevant to the localization and mechanistic function of brain regions engaged in semantic memory, leading to the neural models included here.

John Hart Jr. is Professor of Behavioral and Brain Sciences and Medical Science Director at The Center for BrainHealth, The University of Texas at Dallas.

Michael A. Kraut is Associate Professor of Radiology at Johns Hopkins University School of Medicine.

Neural Basis of Semantic Memory

Edited by

John Hart Jr.

Michael A. Kraut

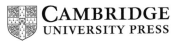

CAMBRIDGE
UNIVERSITY PRESS

CAMBRIDGE UNIVERSITY PRESS
Cambridge, New York, Melbourne, Madrid, Cape Town, Singapore, São Paulo

Cambridge University Press
The Edinburgh Building, Cambridge CB2 8RU, UK

Published in the United States of America by Cambridge University Press, New York

www.cambridge.org
Information on this title: www.cambridge.org/9780521848701

First published 2007

Printed in the United Kingdom at the University Press, Cambridge

A catalog record for this publication is available from the British Library

Library of Congress Cataloging in Publication data

Neural basis of sematic memory/[edited by] John Hart Jr. and Michael Kraut.
     p. ; cm.
   Includes bibliographical references.
   ISBN-13: 978-0-521-84870-1 (hardback)
   ISBN-10: 0-521-84870-9 (hardback)
1. Memory. 2. Memory disorders. 3. Language disorders. 4. Neurosychology.
5. Semantics. I. Hart, John, 1957– II. Kraut, Michael.
[DNLM: 1. Memory -- physiology. 2. Brain -- physiology. 3. Semantics.
WL 102 N49087 2007]   I. Title.

   QP406.N478 2007
   612.8′2--dc22

                                                    2006037299

ISBN-13   978-0521-84870-1 hardback

Contents

Contributors

Michal Assaf
Olin Neuropsychiatry Research Center
Institute of Living
Hartford CT 06106, USA

Michelle Benjamin
Brain Rehabilitation Research Center of
    Excellence
Malcolm Randall VA Medical Center
Gainesville FL, USA

Jeffrey Binder
Department of Neurology
Medical College of Wisconsin
9200 W Wisconsin Avenue
Milwaukee WI 53226, USA

Vince Calhoun
Olin Neuropsychiatry Research Center
Institute of Living
Hartford CT 06106, USA

Alfonso Caramazza
Department of Psychology
Harvard University
33 Kirkand Street
Cambridge MA 02138, USA

Bruce Crosson
Brain Rehabilitation Research Center of
    Excellence
Malcolm Randall VA Medical Center
Gainesville FL, USA

Sebastian Crutch
Division of Neuroscience and Mental Health
Imperial College London, UK

Guido Gainotti
Servizio de Neuropsicologia
Universita Cattolica/Policlinico Gemelli
Largo A. Gemelli 8
00168 Roma, Italy

Murray Grossman
Department of Neurology
University of Pennsylvania Medical Center
Philadelphia, PA., USA

Kerrie Elston-Güttler
Max-Planck-Institute for Human Cognitive
    and Brain Sciences
Stephanstraße 1A
04103 Leipzig, Germany

John Hart, Jr.
The Center for BrainHealth
University of Texas at Dallas
2200 Mockingbird Lane
Dallas TX 75235, USA

Argye Hillis
Department of Cognitive Science
Johns Hopkins University, Phipps
600 N Wolfe Street
Baltimore MD 21287, USA

Phyllis Koenig
Department of Neurology
University of Pennsylvania Medical Center
Philadelphia, PA., USA

Sonja Kotz
Max-Planck-Institute for Human Cognitive
  and Brain Sciences
Stephanstraße 1A
04103 Leipzig, Germany

John Kounios
Department of Psychology
Drexel University
Mail Stop 626, 245 N 15th Street
Philadelphia PA 19102-1192, USA

Michael A. Kraut
Department of Radiology
Johns Hopkins Hospital, Phipps 112
600 N Wolfe Street
Baltimore MD 21205, USA

Ilana Levy
Department of Clinical and Health
  Psychology
University of Florida
Gainesville FL, USA

Alex Martin
National Institute of Mental Health
Building 10, Room 4C-104
10 Center Drive MSC 1366
Bethesda MD 20892, USA

Helen Moss
Centre for Speech and Language
Department of Experimental Psychology
University of Cambridge, UK

Uta Noppeney
Max-Planck-Institute for Biological
  Cybernetics
Spemannstraße 38
72076 Tübingen, Germany

Godfrey Pearlson
Olin Neuropsychiatry Research Center
Institute of Living
Hartford CT 06106, USA

Paul Rivkin
Department of Psychiatry
Johns Hopkins University
Baltimore MD 21205, USA

Kevin Shapiro
Department of Psychology
Harvard University
33 Kirkand Street
Cambridge MA 02138, USA

Kirsten Taylor
Memory Clinic – Neuropsychology Center
University Hospital Basel
Schanzenstraße 55
4031 Basel, Switzerland

Lorraine Tyler
Centre for Speech and Language
Department of Experimental
    Psychology
University of Cambridge, UK

Elizabeth Warrington
Dementia Research Centre
Department of Neurodegeneration
Institute of Neurology
University College London, UK

Preface

As investigative techniques have advanced, there has also been a significant increase in information regarding the storage and access of semantic memory in the human brain. The initial investigations in this area were limited to lesion studies focusing on delineating the organization of the lexical–semantic system for categories of objects and entities. With the advent of modern neuroimaging and brain activation studies, investigations of semantic processing in normal, healthy individuals have resulted in the shaping of the functional–anatomic architecture of semantic memory for entities (e.g. object, animals, and actions) in the human brain. These advances have led to the maturation of the basic knowledge base to the point that a work dedicated to the neural organization of semantic memory was indicated.

Just as in any emerging field, there has been less agreement in some domains than in others, as is evidenced in this book by several alternative accounts for the same general neural instantiation for a specific aspect of semantic memory. It is our belief that we will continue to balance multiple accounts of neural mechanisms and localizations associated with semantic memory, even with refinement in experimental tools. The reasons for this may relate to difficulties inherent in establishing functional–anatomic consistencies in general for semantic memory, aside from broad regions associated with common semantic functions. These reasons include, but are not limited to, individual variations of the anatomic substrates that encode semantic memories, different and ever-changing life experiences (affecting salience for example), the likely existence of multiple neural mechanisms to perform certain semantic functions, variability in the extent of semantic memory recall engaged depending on the task to be performed, and likely a select set of semantic memory instantiations that are common to all humans.

The focus of this book is on current theories of components of semantic memory that also encompass the neural elements associated with these components. Other than a concentration on the memory of single entities (objects, animal, actions, etc.), the chapters range from being specific to a domain and/or memory system (e.g. lexical–semantic, sensorimotor, multiple modalities, etc.) or amodal; cover memory representations, processing, both, and/or parallel network structures; general storage principles of knowledge; and/or focused on studies of normal, healthy individuals as well as those with brain disease. The neural specification ranges from anatomic localizations, physiological accounts, mechanistic explanations, and in some instances extend to providing insights into pathophysiological disruptions of semantic memory.

The following chapters elucidate the leading theories of neural organization of semantic memory, with each extending from the unique approaches of the investigators. Investigators have focused on (i) performing extensive studies on patients with lesions and utilizing the inferences from their performance to inform models of neural function, (ii) insights from electrophysiological measurements of semantic operations, (iii) applying theoretical models to understanding the formal thought disorder in schizophrenia, (iv) the long-running debate in semantic memory over the representations of nouns and verbs and their semantic memory conceptual counterparts of objects and actions, (v) uncovering the essential role of subcortical nuclei in semantic memory, which had been obscure before the advent of current neuroinvestigative techniques, and (vi) overarching models of semantic memory stemming from a variety of investigative perspectives. As those of us investigating semantic memory have gleaned so much from these approaches, we are confident the readers of this book will, too.

John Hart, Jr.
Dallas
Michael A. Kraut
Baltimore

Part I

Semantic Memory: Building Models from Lesions

Semantic refractory access disorders

Elizabeth K. Warrington and Sebastian J. Crutch

University College London

Every individual has a vast thesaurus of conceptual knowledge. The cerebral organization of this knowledge base has intrigued philosophers for centuries and experimental psychologists for decades. By studying patients with brain lesions, neuropsychologists have been able to provide a powerful and direct source of evidence of the properties and organization of this conceptual knowledge base. This thesaurus is multifarious, encompassing words, objects, facts, people, places, and much more. In this chapter we will examine one particular neurological syndrome, "semantic refractory access dysphasia," and hope to demonstrate that patients with this disorder can provide a window on the organization of conceptual knowledge.

The original studies of semantic memory impairment were concerned to establish the selectivity of the deficit, especially with regard to the integrity of other cognitive systems. The boundaries with episodic memory, propositional language, and perceptual systems were all explored (Warrington, 1975). However, these early studies of semantic memory impairment did not attempt to differentiate between impairments of access to an intact knowledge base and damage to or loss of stored conceptual knowledge itself. "Storage" deficits are attributed to damage to the central representations of concepts, resulting in a static/stable, consistent, item-specific, loss of knowledge. Such storage deficits can be contrasted with what are termed "access" deficits, which reflect the temporary unavailability of stored representations. We wish to clarify at the outset that the term "access" is not used to refer to impairments of transmission of input between different cognitive domains but rather to the instability of activation within a system. The cardinal property of a semantic refractory access disorder (one subtype of access disorder) is sensitivity to temporal factors, resulting in an inconsistent performance. Response accuracy is improved when an interval is introduced between a response and the presentation of a subsequent stimulus. Such refractoriness has been defined as the reduction in the ability to use the system for a period of time following activation (Warrington & McCarthy, 1983, p. 874).

1.1   Description of the syndrome

The syndrome termed semantic refractory access dysphasia was first described in a patient (VER) who had sustained a major left hemisphere infarction (Warrington & McCarthy, 1983). Clinically this patient's propositional speech was gravely impaired and her comprehension of the simplest verbal instructions appeared to be all but absent. When asked to point to one of two objects she frequently succeeded with the first probe, only to make an error with the next. As a consequence, it was of interest to establish how long a delay was necessary between successive probes for VER's response accuracy to improve. The patient was tested on a picture vocabulary test (Dunn *et al.*, 1979) in which a series of words of increasing difficulty had to be matched to one of four pictures. The task was administered under both a fast (2 s) and a slow (30 s) presentation rate condition. Unexpectedly introducing a delay between making a response and presenting the next stimulus item (the response–stimulus interval, RSI) improved her performance significantly. This suggested that her comprehension vocabulary was much more extensive than was apparent clinically. In a series of further experiments using spoken word to picture matching it was shown that her performance with a 15 s RSI was consistently better than with a 3 s RSI. Furthermore, VER's performance on spoken word to written word matching tests was qualitatively very similar, suggesting again that under optimal conditions VER possessed a much more extensive written word vocabulary than might have been expected using standard assessment techniques. Although performance on word–picture matching tests comprising arrays of phonologically similar items (e.g. *cat, hat*) was no different than for random item arrays (e.g. *cat, leg*), her performance with arrays of semantically related items (e.g. *cat, dog*) was less accurate.

Despite subsequent single case studies reporting broadly congruent results on tests of spoken word, written word, and picture comprehension (e.g. Warrington & McCarthy, 1987; McNeil *et al.*, 1994), the theoretical validity of the distinction between refractory access and storage deficits was brought into question (Rapp & Caramazza, 1993). Such criticisms led to a more direct comparison of access dysphasics with patients with semantic storage deficits in an effort to provide a solid empirical base for the refractory access/storage distinction and, thereby, to delineate the criteria that identify a refractory semantic disorder (Warrington & Cipolotti, 1996). In this series of experiments word–picture matching tests were used to assess the residual comprehension skills of two patients with semantic refractory access deficits (consequent to either tumor or vascular damage) and four patients with semantic storage deficits (resulting from neurodegenerative disease). Typically the patients were presented with arrays of four or six items and asked to point to the named target. Each item in the array was probed repeatedly (three or four times) in a pseudorandom order. The performance of the two groups of patients gave rise to four factors which enable the delineation of refractory access and storage impairments of semantic processing.

1.1.1 Temporal factors

A sensitivity to temporal factors is a cardinal feature of refractory access syndromes. As noted above in the original description of patient VER, this can be demonstrated by varying the response–stimulus interval (RSI). It should be noted that an effect of temporal factors can be elicited without rushing the subject; typically a natural response pace is compared with longer delays. In Warrington and Cipolotti's study, a fast rate (1 s RSI) was compared with a slow rate (15 s RSI). Introducing this short interval between each response and the presentation of the next stimulus improved the accuracy of the access patients dramatically; however, no equivalent facilitation was observed for the degenerative cases (see Figure 1.1). This contrast, between the access cases and the degenerative cases, in their sensitivity to temporal factors was replicated in a subsequent investigation involving one access patient and three individuals with degenerative conditions (Crutch & Warrington, 2005).

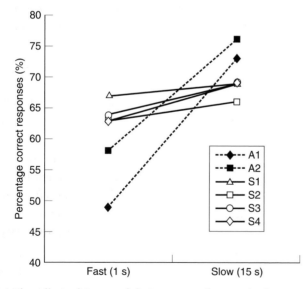

Figure 1.1.   The effect of temporal factors upon the word–picture matching response accuracy of patients with refractory access disorders (A1, A2) and static storage disorders (S1, S2, S3, and S4) of semantic processing (Warrington & Cipolotti, 1996; Experiment 2).

1.1.2 Response consistency

A second critical distinction between refractory access and storage deficits lies in the degree of response consistency which emerges when subjects attempt to comprehend stimuli which are presented repetitively (Warrington & Cipolotti, 1996; Crutch & Warrington, 2005). In refractory access patients, this behavioral characteristic is integrally linked to their sensitivity to temporal factors: the occurrence of refractoriness, which has been defined as the inability to utilize the system for a period of time following activation, inevitably results in inconsistency of response. Such patients respond inconsistently to specific items, whilst storage patients who appear to have an item-specific deficit do not. Furthermore, the accuracy of refractory access patients has been found to decline with repeated probes of the same items in an array, resulting in characteristic serial position curves. Serial position effects have not though been observed in patients with degenerative conditions, who tend to make consistent errors with each successive probe (see Figure 1.2).

1.1.3 Frequency

Stimulus frequency is a very powerful determinant of performance at all stages of cognition. In individuals with storage deficits of semantic knowledge (who comprise the majority of patients reported in the neuropsychological literature), massive word frequency effects are often observed. However, in refractory access cases frequency effects have been reported to be either minor or absent.

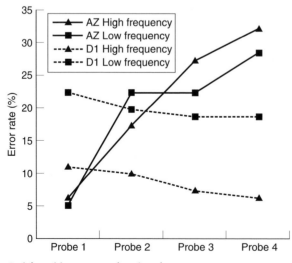

Figure 1.2.   Serial position curves showing the percentage error rates of a refractory access patient (AZ) and a static storage patient (D1) on each probe of stimuli in a spoken word–picture matching task (Crutch & Warrington, 2005; Experiment 1).

In the investigation that compared directly these two syndromes, the performance of the access patients was equally compromised for both a high- and a low-frequency vocabulary, whereas the expected robust frequency effects were observed in the degenerative patients. Indeed there was a cross-over in performance: the individuals with degenerative conditions were superior to the access cases with the high-frequency vocabulary but the converse held for the low-frequency vocabulary. This contrast was subsequently replicated in an experiment comparing an access patient with an Alzheimer's disease patient who had a storage deficit (Crutch & Warrington, 2005). These individuals were presented with high- and low-frequency three-item picture arrays, for which the identity of each item was probed four times in a pseudorandom order using a spoken word−picture matching technique. As in the Warrington and Cipolotti study, only the patient with a storage deficit showed any sensitivity to item frequency (also see Figure 1.2).

1.1.4   Semantic relatedness

The semantic relatedness of stimulus arrays can vary greatly, ranging from semantically very distant arrays containing items which cross broad category boundaries (e.g. *slipper, tiger, cherry*), to arrays with items from within a broad category (e.g. man-made artifacts: *slipper, knife, stool*), to arrays with items that are semantically closer in that they are drawn from a subordinate category (e.g. clothes: *slipper, pyjamas, socks*) or even a very narrow category (e.g. footwear: *slipper, sandal, stiletto*). By comparing "close" and "distant" within-category arrays, it was shown that semantic relatedness had a strong deleterious effect for the access cases but less so for the degenerative cases. However, when performance on close arrays was compared with performance on distant arrays containing items that crossed major category boundaries, a significant semantic distance effect was observed in the degenerative cases (Warrington and Cipolotti, 1996).

In a subsequent investigation by Crutch and Warrington (2005), the basis of the semantic relatedness effect was explored in more detail by contrasting the effects of semantic similarity in the two types of patient. Specifically, we observed an interaction of word frequency with semantic relatedness in the degenerative cases such that a semantic similarity effect was observed with middle-frequency items but not with the high- or low-frequency items. By contrast, the access patient tested showed clear semantic distance effects with high-, medium- and low-frequency stimuli (see Figure 1.3). It was suggested that the weak semantic relatedness effect observed in the degenerative patients could be accounted for by relative preservation of superordinate information which could serve to mediate responses in the semantically distant arrays but would be ineffective in the semantically close arrays. By contrast, we attributed the semantic relatedness in

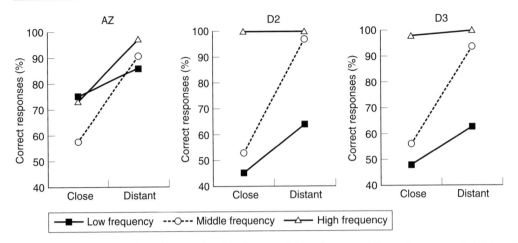

Figure 1.3.   The interaction of semantic relatedness and item frequency. Percentage correct responses are shown for the performance of one refractory access patient (AZ) and two static storage patients (D2 and D3) on a spoken word–picture matching task involving semantically close and distant arrays comprising low-, middle- and high-frequency man-made artifact stimuli (Crutch & Warrington, in press; Experiment 2).

the access patient to refractoriness that affects not only the repeated items but also other concepts whose representations partly share semantic space. Indeed, refractoriness has been shown to spread not only between target items and distractors but also to previously untested items (Forde & Humphreys, 1995).

Thus the concept of semantic refractory access disorders was evoked to unify these four identifying criteria. All four characteristics are held to reflect a semantic system in which there is a reduction in the ability to access concepts for a period of time following activation. More specifically, response inconsistency and serial position effects are considered to be direct consequence of such refractoriness, whereas semantic relatedness effects are held to reflect the spread of refractoriness between items that share semantic space. Furthermore, a number of empirical investigations suggest that low- and high-frequency semantic concepts become equally refractory. Having established the criterion by which semantic refractory deficits may be identified, we now move on to consider how such deficits have been harnessed to investigate the organization of semantic knowledge in more depth than can be achieved by investigating patients with static category-specific deficits.

1.2   Semantic refractory access category dissociations

The categorical organization of an individual's semantic knowledge base is well established for broad classes of information. The evidence for the most part rests on the documentation of category-specific impairments and category-specific preservations observed in patients with cerebral structural damage. The double dissociations between knowledge of abstract and concrete concepts (e.g. Warrington, 1975; Sirigu *et al.*, 1991; Breedin *et al.*, 1994), animate and inanimate stimuli (e.g. Warrington & Shallice, 1984; Caramazza & Shelton, 1998; Capitani *et al.*, 2003 [review]), and proper nouns and common nouns (e.g. Semenza & Zettin, 1988, 1989; Miceli *et al.*, 2000; Lyons *et al.*, 2002) have been replicated in many centers. Refractory access deficits also have the potential to reflect dissociations if refractoriness can be shown to affect or spare a particular semantic category. In such cases we would suppose there was a degree of independence of the neural structures supporting those respective semantic fields. By contrast, evidence of semantic distance effects would be considered to indicate the organization of concepts within a semantic field.

In the original semantic refractory access patient described above (VER; Warrington & McCarthy, 1983), an artifacts deficit was observed. Comparing word–picture matching performance on two- and five- item arrays of food items with man-made artifacts at two presentation rates, VER's performance on comparable conditions was shown to be impaired for the nonliving items. In a further experiment that compared her ability to identify items within picture arrays of flowers, animals and man-made artifacts, her performance was significantly worse with the artifacts than with the other two categories. Thus it appeared that the activation of nonliving object conceptual representations was more likely to elicit a refractory state than the activation of concepts supported by other areas of semantic space.

This dissociation between living and nonliving items was replicated in a second case (YOT; Warrington & McCarthy, 1987). This patient was unable to speak and had very limited comprehension after suffering an occlusion of the left middle cerebral artery. Apart from establishing a living/nonliving dissociation, YOT's comprehension of multiple categories was explored using spoken word–written word and spoken word–picture matching procedures. These investigations yielded several findings. First, a dissociation was demonstrated *within* the broad category of inanimate objects. YOT had significantly more difficulty with arrays of manipulable objects than with arrays of large man-made artifacts. Secondly, her comprehension of proper nouns was remarkably well preserved. This contrasted with her exceptionally poor comprehension of common Christian names. Thirdly, YOT's comprehension of certain abstract concepts was explored and these items appeared to be of middling difficulty for her. This pattern of preserved and impaired categories was subsequently replicated by Forde and Humphreys (1995, 1997) in a patient who also showed a greater build-up of refractoriness for nonliving than living items and for common proper names than famous proper names. Furthermore, McNeil *et al.* (1994) described a global dysphasic patient with the defining characteristics of a semantic refractory access deficit who appeared to have the selective preservation of famous person names.

The first attempt to give a principled account of semantic category dissociations was by the contrast of sensory and functional attributes within the domain of animate and inanimate stimuli. However, there were a number of anomalies that were difficult to encompass by this simple dichotomy: the selective impairment of action verbs, the isolated preservation of maps, and evidence of more fine-grain impairments such as fruits and vegetables. Indeed, it was the evidence of multiple selective impairments and dissociations observed in a semantic refractory access case that motivated the initial elaboration of the original sensory–functional framework (Warrington & McCarthy, 1987). It was proposed instead that there are multiple channels of processing within both the motor and sensory input systems. Differential activation or weightings of these channels during acquisition were held to provide the basis for a fine-grain categorical organization of semantic knowledge in the adult (see also Crutch & Warrington, 2003a).

1.3   Evidence for fine-grain semantic organization within broad categories

The evidence of categorical dissociations derived from refractory access patients must be interpreted with caution. Semantic relatedness effects are so robust that it is possible that an apparent category dissociation could be reduced to unequal semantic relatedness within an array. For example, it would not be appropriate to claim a living/nonliving dissociation if a patient's identification performance with arrays of five very distant animals were to be compared to performance with arrays of five semantically similar man-made artifacts. Nevertheless semantic refractory access deficits have proved to be most illuminating with regard to the organization of conceptual knowledge in the brain. Not only do specific items become refractory, but semantically related items also become refractory. For example, with repeated probes in a word–picture matching task there will be a higher error rate with a semantically related array than with a semantically more distant array. It is the ubiquity of semantic distance effects that provides the opportunity to observe the organization of an intact knowledge base or at least one that can be accessed under favorable conditions.

Before discussing the evidence for fine-grain organization of the semantic knowledge base, one procedural point will be described. Despite the relative insensitivity of patients with refractory access deficits to item frequency, it is important in assessing semantic similarity that the frequency of items being probed in each condition is carefully balanced. One procedure whereby this is achieved is to probe the same items both in a semantically close array and in a semantically distant array. This technique was first used in the investigation of YOT (Warrington & McCarthy, 1987), the patient whose comprehension of nonliving concepts was more impaired than comprehension of living concepts. Six pictures from each of six close semantic categories were selected. Each of these items was probed in a semantically close array containing items from the same category. These same items were then rearranged into semantically distant arrays each containing one item from each category. Thus by equating the array size to the number of categories or subcategories it is possible to explore semantic relatedness in depth (i.e. four categories in arrays of four items, three categories in arrays of three items, etc). Indeed, this procedure can be extended to more levels of semantic similarity by dividing each of the broad categories into subcategories (i.e. *pigeon, crow, sparrow*; *pigeon, goldfish, cow*; *pigeon, leek, shirt*). By using this procedure for constructing semantic relatedness experiments, not only item frequency but many other relevant variables such as concreteness, familiarity, and visual complexity are controlled because exactly the same stimulus items are examined under each semantic distance condition.

In our extensive series of experiments with our patient AZ we used this procedure to assess her comprehension of a very broad range of concepts within the domains of proper nouns, common nouns, parts of speech, abstract knowledge, and concrete knowledge. AZ had sustained a major left hemisphere stroke in the territory of the middle cerebral artery. Clinically, she was globally and severely dysphasic, dysgraphic, and dyslexic. However, our investigations focused upon her comprehension skills because AZ demonstrated all the core features of a semantic refractory access disorder. These characteristics can be illustrated by her performance on a "levels of semantic similarity" experiment conducted using spoken word—picture matching (Crutch & Warrington, 2005). The test stimuli were high- and low-frequency concrete items from the broad categories of animals, plants, and man-made artifacts which were arranged into three-item semantically close (e.g. *crow, pigeon, sparrow*), medium (e.g. *crow, dolphin, sheep*) and distant arrays (e.g. *crow, potato, jumper*; see Figure 1.4 for examples of low frequency items). It was observed that AZ's response accuracy was a function of semantic relatedness for both high- and low-frequency set items. Her error rate on the first probe of a stimulus item in a given array was also found to be negligible but to increase with successive probes (see Figure 1.2). Furthermore, there was no significant difference in response accuracy with high- and low-frequency stimuli. In a similar experiment, arrays containing matched sets of semantically close,

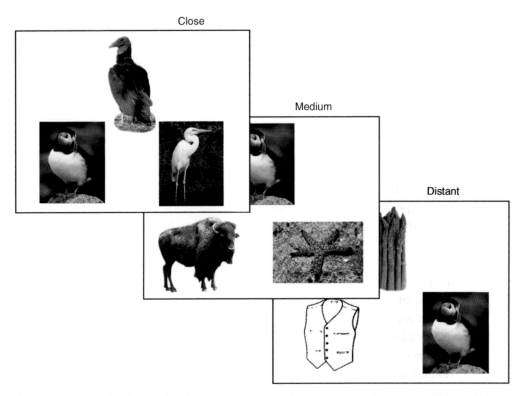

Figure 1.4.   Example picture stimulus arrays employed in the semantically close, middle and distant conditions of variable distance spoken word–picture matching tasks.

medium, and distant stimulus items were selected not from across broad domains but entirely from within a single domain, namely man-made artefacts (e.g. close: *sandal, Wellington, clog, slipper*; middle: *sandal, cap, clog, top hat*; distant: *sandal, speedboat, tankard, golf ball*). Again performance was found to alter as a function of semantic relatedness. Taken together, these experimental findings were held to indicate that semantic relatedness can be considered as a continuous rather than discrete variable which forms a gradient across semantic space.

The next issue to be examined was whether semantic relatedness constitutes a general property of the organization of conceptual space or whether this property is restricted to certain semantic domains. Consequently the effect of semantic distance upon response accuracy was tested within a proper-noun vocabulary (Crutch & Warrington, 2004). Arrays representing three levels of semantic relatedness were constructed by selecting stimuli from three broad proper-noun categories: people, places, and brand names (e.g. close: *Monet, Van Gogh, Rembrandt*; middle: *Monet, Nixon, Chaucer*; distant: *Monet, Manchester, Kelloggs*). Consistent with the findings in the man-made artifact domain, a gradient of semantic relatedness was observed across AZ's comprehension of proper nouns. For example, there was a higher error rate with arrays containing the names of three famous people with the same occupation (close condition) than different occupations (middle condition), which in turn elicited a higher error rate than arrays containing a person name, a place name, and a brand name (distant condition). These results lend weight to the notion that semantic relatedness effects in the context of refractory access disorders reflect a spread of refractoriness between concepts whose representations share semantic space.

There does, however, appear to be a limit to such fine-grain organization. In an experiment that explored AZ's comprehension of mass nouns, no semantic similarity effects were found for subcategories of drinks (e.g. arrays containing spirits [e.g. rum, brandy, vodka, whisky], long drinks, hot drinks, or mixers, as compared with distant arrays containing one item for each category) or materials (Crutch & Warrington, in press). However, such effects were quite robust for other mass nouns such as foods (e.g. close array [cheeses]: *Stilton, Brie, Cheddar, Edam*; distant array: *Stilton, custard, pork, vinegar*). Similarly in the plant domain, fruits, vegetables, and flowers were clearly categorically organized whereas different types of vegetables (salad, root, brassica) were not (Crutch & Warrington, 2005, Exp 5). Here we suppose that for this particular patient we had reached the limit of the categorical organization of her knowledge base. It is of interest to consider whether for an individual with very developed specialist knowledge, such as a gardener in the case of plant life and vegetables, there would be empirical evidence of categorical organization even at this subordinate level.

Investigations of semantic similarity have revealed that gradients of semantic relatedness are a general feature of the conceptual knowledge base. These gradients of semantic relatedness suggest that there must be multiple levels of semantic superordinates. We would suggest that such a conceptual framework is to be preferred to a simple dichotomous division of superordinate and subordinate information. These robust effects of semantic relatedness provide the opportunity to investigate categorical organization within the context of a relatively intact conceptual knowledge base. While some fine-grain category-specific deficits have been documented, we have been able to demonstrate that a more fine-grain semantic organization can be revealed in patients with a semantic refractory dysphasia. However, we do not wish to claim that semantic distance effects are in any way analogous to the evidence of a selective category impairment or preservation. Although we have demonstrated a semantic relatedness effect for example in the plant domain, we would not consequently anticipate the possibility of a selective impairment for fruit but not vegetables.

1.4 The organization of geographical knowledge

Neuropsychological studies of the nature and organization of conceptual knowledge have tended to concentrate upon certain semantic domains more than for others. One area of our understanding which has received relatively little attention is geographical knowledge. Previous studies in patients with storage deficits of comprehension and naming have revealed category-specific impairments and preservations of geographical terms (e.g. McKenna & Warrington, 1978; Warrington & Clegg, 1993; Incisa della Rocchetta et al., 1996, 1998; Incisa della Rocchetta & Cipolotti, 2004). Patients with a global comprehension deficit may have an isolated ability to name maps and to point to named maps. However, our patient AZ provided an opportunity to make a more detailed assessment of geographical knowledge by examining refractory effects of her comprehension of country and city names (Crutch & Warrington, 2003b). First, an effort was made to establish that her performance for this class of stimuli was indeed affected by temporal factors. On a spoken word—written word matching task with arrays each containing four country names, her score improved from 59 percent correct with a natural presentation rate (1 s RSI) to 84 percent correct with a long delay (10 s RSI). Secondly, the influence of geographical proximity was considered using a series of semantic relatedness experiments similar in methodology to those described above. The names of countries from four different geographical regions (Southern Europe, Scandinavia, Asia, South America) were arranged into both geographically close (all countries from the same area) and geographically distant arrays (one item from each area). With the usual repetitive probing procedure, performance levels were observed to be significantly worse for close than distant arrays. Geographical proximity also affected AZ's performance on arrays of close and distant world cities. Even more fine-grain organization was observed by comparing AZ's ability to identify the names of British towns using arrays containing either four towns located in the same country (e.g. Edinburgh, Glasgow, Aberdeen, Inverness) or one town from each of the four countries (e.g. Edinburgh, Dublin, Swansea, Newcastle). Once again, response accuracy was significantly higher for geographically distant than close city names. More unexpected was the effect of geographical proximity on English city name identification. The geographically close city name arrays represented the rough compass groupings of north (e.g. Bradford, Manchester, Liverpool, Sheffield), south, east, and west, and could not in any direct way be classified by county (see Figure 1.5). Nevertheless, AZ's performance was significantly worse on the close arrays than on the distant arrays. Thus it was claimed that the semantic distance effects observed reflect the subject's knowledge of the actual geographical location of the cities/ towns and not only their superordinate category membership. Furthermore,

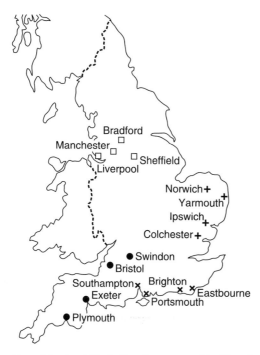

Figure 1.5.   Map of England illustrating the geographical location of the northern, southern, western and eastern cities whose names were included in the spoken word–written word matching task used to investigate the influence of real-world spatial proximity upon the identification skills of a refractory access patient (AZ; Crutch & Warrington, 2005).

in relation to the earlier claim that the extent of fine-grain semantic organization in a given domain may vary from individual to individual, it was possible to demonstrate in the geographical domain that an individual's knowledge base is shaped by experience. AZ claimed to know by name the American states but, not having visited the country, to have only a very hazy notion of their relative geographical position. Arrays of geographically close states (e.g. Wisconsin, Michigan, Illinois, Indiana) and geographically distant states (e.g. Wisconsin, Georgia, Oklahoma, Kentucky) were arranged. Although a typical refractory response was recorded, with an increasing error rate over successive trials, absolutely no effect of geographical distance was observed.

This series of experiments concerned with geographical information has brought to light an unexpected principle of the organization of semantic knowledge. By establishing that AZ's ability to identify accurately the names of national and international countries and cities was significantly influenced by their real-world proximity to one another, it has been suggested that a much more fine-grain organization of geographical knowledge exists than had been anticipated previously. Although knowledge about many place names can be represented relative to a series of superordinate categories (e.g. Norwich is in Norfolk [county], England [country] and Europe [continent]), it is difficult for such a classification to account for the experimental performance of AZ. In particular, the greater build-up of refractoriness among geographically close than distant English towns (groupings which did not correspond to any common or formal classification such as county membership) suggests an organizational principle which can cut across categories that could possibly be verbally or visually encoded. Consequently, it is proposed that a distinct spatial code or framework is available for encoding and storing geographical knowledge. The existence of this type of spatial coding of semantic information would go some way to understanding the evidence of highly selective sparing of geographical place names (Gipolitti, 2000; Mckenna & Warrington, 1978).

1.5 Modality specificity

Refractory access disorders may be highly selective, affecting one cognitive system while sparing another. For example, a refractory access anomia has been described in a patient whose verbal comprehension was intact (McCarthy & Kartsounis, 2000). Alternatively, in patients who have multiple cognitive deficits, one impaired function may meet the criteria of a refractory disorder whereas a co-occurring deficit may not. Thus a refractory access speech production deficit that was selective for reading has been documented (Crutch & Warrington, 2001). This patient's naming skills were also compromised but his performance on naming tasks was not affected by temporal factors. It is analogous dissociations within the semantic system that have been harnessed in the context of semantic refractory disorders to address the issue of multiple semantics: is information from verbal and visual domains integrated within a unified representational system (e.g. Caramazza et al., 1990)? Or alternatively, do verbal and visual semantic processing operate in parallel or have a degree of autonomy (e.g. Shallice, 1993)?

In this context, Forde and Humphreys (1995) were the first to recognize the potential of semantic refractory access dysphasic patients. They described a patient who demonstrated strong serial position effects with repeated probes of the same items in a spoken word–written word matching test. On the fourth and final probe they introduced a switch to spoken word–picture matching without any reduction in refractoriness. On this basis they favored the amodal, unitary model of semantic knowledge. However, it should be noted that the category switch was not complete as the stimulus item was a spoken word in both conditions.

Visual–visual matching tests which require matching by functional equivalence are held to access object identification at the level of semantic processing, a level at which a structural description will not suffice. In the original investigation of a semantic access dysphasic (VER) it was shown that the patient's performance on a test of visual–visual matching of object photographs was superior (but by no means intact) to her performance on a comparable spoken word–picture matching condition.

Following on from this work, a series of experiments has been conducted with our refractory patient (AZ) to compare and contrast her performance on verbal–visual and visual–visual matching tasks (Warrington & Crutch, 2004). In each of these experiments, two structurally dissimilar pictorial representations were assembled for each test stimulus. One of the two pictures was arranged in an array of semantically similar items. The identity of each item in the array was then probed either by the spoken name or the alternate picture. Clear-cut results were obtained: in the verbal–visual condition, AZ reliably became refractory as demonstrated by an increase in the error rate with successive probes of each target. By contrast, in the visual–visual condition, her performance remained at or close to ceiling with successive probes (see Figure 1.6). This result was replicated four times with different stimulus items. Thus both qualitative and quantitative differences between the tasks were demonstrated: qualitative in the sense that inconsistency and serial position effects were

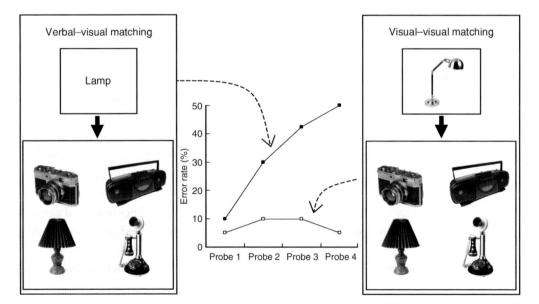

Figure 1.6.   Modality-specific refractory deficits. Serial position curves showing the percentage error rates of the verbal–visual (■–■) and visual–visual (□–□) matching performance of a patient with a semantic refractory access deficit (AZ; Crutch & Warrington, 2004; Experiments 5 and 6 combined).

only present in the task with a verbal component, and quantitative in that the overall error rate was higher in the verbal condition. The implication of these findings is that in this patient the processes by which verbal semantic representations are activated become refractory, whereas access to visual semantics does not. This pattern of results has been interpreted as providing evidence that converges with the findings of studies of patients with modality-specific semantic storage deficits (e.g. McCarthy & Warrington, 1986, 1988) in favor of the multiple semantics position.

1.6   Principles of semantic organization

Studies of semantic knowledge have for the most part focused on an individual's concrete word vocabulary despite the fact that in normal propositional speech an abstract word vocabulary is the more high frequent (e.g. Crutch & Warrington, 2003c). In the literature on semantic storage impairments, category-specific deficits are most common; however, a reversal of this concreteness effect has been documented in several patients (e.g. Warrington, 1975; Warrington & Shallice, 1984; Sirigu *et al.*, 1991; Breedin *et al.*, 1994). It is commonly assumed that any differences between the use of concrete and abstract concepts can be accounted for by quantitative rather than qualitative factors (e.g. Schwanenflugel & Shoben, 1983; Paivio, 1986; Plaut & Shallice, 1993). As with storage disorders, very few studies of refractoriness have considered the status of abstract concepts. However, the repeated observations of robust effects of semantic relatedness in refractory access dysphasic patients have motivated a detailed investigation of the organizational principles underlying the concrete and abstract components of our vocabulary.

Within the concrete word vocabulary, semantic similarity is typically defined by category membership. Indeed, the majority of the semantic relatedness experiments described in the current chapter consist of comparing response accuracy levels when items have to be identified from among distractor items drawn from the same category or a different category. Abstract words by contrast rarely have an obvious category membership. Such words do though often have multiple semantic coordinates, or synonyms, which convey a near identical or very similar meaning. Thus, in a further series of experiments with patient AZ, an attempt was made to compare directly the influence of semantic similarity upon concrete and abstract word comprehension skills (Crutch & Warrington, 2005). Semantic close and distant effects within the abstract word domain were achieved by comparing arrays of synonyms (e.g. *divine, religious, sacred, holy*) with the same words rearranged into arrays of non-synonymous words (e.g. *divine, rash, furious, deficient*). Unexpectedly, the semantic relatedness effects which were so ubiquitous in the experiments with concrete word comprehension were not observed in abstract spoken word—written word matching tasks (see Figure 1.7). This null result was replicated repeatedly using arrays of abstract adjectives, verbs, nouns, and even prepositions. Yet analogous arrays of concrete nouns, for which semantic similarity was defined by category membership, continued to yield strong semantic distance effects.

Consequently, an alternative principle of organization was considered: similarity by semantic association. Association here was defined as concepts which could occur in the same real-world or sentential context. Analogous to the semantic similarity tasks, semantic association tasks compared AZ's ability to identify words in contextually associated arrays with words in arrays of non-associated items. Associatively "close" arrays were assembled for both abstract words (e.g. *fight, punch, violent, struggle*) and concrete words (e.g. *farm, cow, tractor, barn*). The distant arrays were again constructed by reallocating the items in the close abstract word arrays (e.g. *fight, healthy, past, casino*) and concrete word arrays (e.g. *farm, shelf, sailor, oven*). Our patient AZ was significantly less accurate at identifying items on the close associative arrays than the distant associative arrays of abstract words. Importantly, though, she appeared to be totally impervious to the influence of semantic association when identifying concrete words (see Figure 1.7). This result was replicated with a different vocabulary and, more recently, in a second semantic refractory access dysphasic (Crutch *et al.*, 2006).

In these two groups of experiments we observed a double dissociation that points to qualitatively different principles of organization within the abstract and concrete word vocabulary. There appears to be a fundamental difference in the architecture of their representations. Abstract concepts appear to be linked to other contextually associated concepts rather than to semantically similar items. By contrast, concrete concepts appear to be linked more strongly to other concepts which are semantically similar rather than semantically associated. Consequently, we have proposed that abstract words are organized in an associative network. Such an organizational principle has often been proposed to account for the representations of a concrete word knowledge base (e.g. Allport, 1985; Hodges *et al.*, 1995; McClelland & Rogers, 2003). Not only have we found no evidence for such an organization, but also, given our present data, the representational framework of the concrete word vocabulary appears to be structurally different. Indeed, the abstract and concrete word findings in this refractory access patient perhaps bear out Warrington's (1975) original prediction that in the domain of concrete concepts, the primary organizational principle is categorical and not associative. This difference perhaps goes some

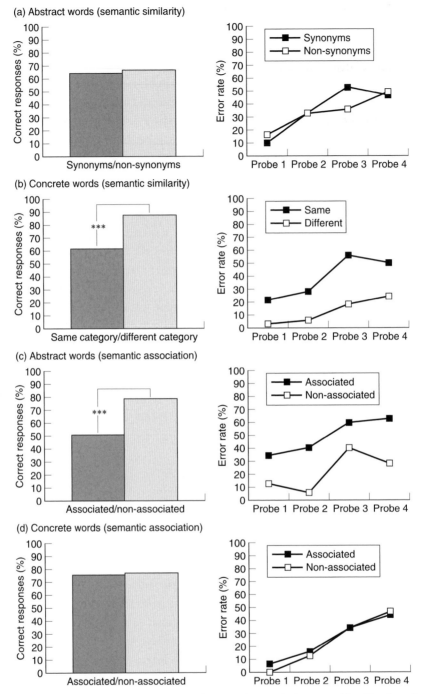

Figure 1.7. The influence of semantic similarity and semantic association upon identification of abstract and concrete words. Percentage correct responses are shown for spoken word–written word matching performance with similar/dissimilar and associated/non-associated arrays of abstract and concrete words. Serial position curves showing the percentage error rate under each semantic condition (close ■; distant □) are also provided (Crutch & Warrington, 2005; Experiments 4 and 5).

way to providing a principled account of the double dissociation between knowledge of abstract and concrete concepts.

1.7 The neurophysiological basis of semantic refractory access disorders

Establishing the empirical base for the refractory access/storage distinction motivated the notion that storage and refractory access disorders might be underpinned by different neurophysiological phenomena (Warrington & Cipolotti, 1996). It was suggested that refractoriness might result from reduced neural conductivity whilst storage deficits reflected damage or loss of the neural structures themselves. Subsequent cognitive neuropsychological studies of refractoriness have not attempted to elucidate further the mechanism by which refractoriness affects the semantic processing abilities of given individuals. However, a recent computational modeling study into the refractory access/storage distinction has provided a more detailed account of the physiological damage which may result in the two subtypes of semantic impairment (Gotts & Plaut, 2002). This model suggests that different behavioral phenotypes of semantic impairment may be understood in relation to damage to two neurological systems: refractory access deficits are held to arise following damage to neuromodulatory systems whereas storage deficits arise following damage to neurons which encode semantic information.

The physiological account of semantic refractory deficits is based on the observation of a naturally occurring form of refractoriness called synaptic depression (see Tsodyks & Markram, 1997, for an account of short-term synaptic depression). Synaptic depression refers to the decrease in effect which a pre-synaptic neuron has upon a post-synaptic neuron when it fires repetitively. As Gotts and Plaut (2002) point out, the fact that synaptic depression occurs at the level of individual synapses makes it a particularly appropriate model for explaining a number of aspects of the semantic refractory access syndrome such as serial position and semantic relatedness effects; stimulus repetition will only trigger synaptic depression at synapses which were activated recently by a previous stimulus. In the normal healthy brain, this down-regulation of neural firing rates following stimulus repetition is counterbalanced by neuromodulators such as acetylcholine and noradrenaline which act in part to reduce synaptic depression and block firing rate adaptation effects (e.g. Gil *et al.*, 1997; Barkai & Hasselmo, 1994). Therefore damage to the pathways by which such neuromodulators address the cerebral cortex lead to an excess of synaptic depression and an abnormally prolonged suppression of post-synaptic activity. An additional relevant property of synaptic depression is that the size of the down-regulation effect is related to the firing rate of the pre-synaptic neuron (Tsodyks & Markram, 1997; Varela *et al.*, 1997). As a consequence, the common behavioral phenomenon of frequency effects is counteracted in patients with refractory disorders because synaptic depression is stronger when pre-synaptic activity is higher, as in the case of high-frequency items.

By contrast, the physiological account of storage deficits assumes a relative intactness of neuromodulatory systems, attributing the syndrome instead to damage to connections between groups of neurons that encode semantic information. The consequence of such damage is a storage pattern with strong frequency effects because the damaged connections are sensitive to the frequency of particular words. Meanwhile, the preserved neuromodulation reduces synaptic depression in a relatively normal fashion such that responses to repeatedly presented stimuli are consistent and unaffected by presentation rate.

This dual pattern of physiologically motivated impairments has been instantiated with a connectionist model which learned to map spoken word input to semantic representations. In doing so, Gotts and Plaut (2002) were able to simulate the pattern of performance shown by the refractory access and storage patients described in Warrington and Cipolotti (1996; Experiment 2). In addition to providing a hypothetical mechanism by which classical refractory access and storage deficits may arise, the authors have also demonstrated that a partial impairment of both neuromodulatory and neural encoding systems can account for patients in the literature who do not fulfill all the main criteria for either type of disorder. For example, the performance of individuals who show response consistency without any evidence of frequency effects (e.g. Howard, 1985; Hillis *et al.*, 1990) can be produced under network conditions of moderate damage to connections and moderate to severe damage to neuromodulatory systems. Understanding of the biological mechanisms underlying refractory phenomenon affecting not only semantic processing but also other areas of cognition will be furthered by increased appreciation of the pathways which link the origins of neuromodulatory projections with their target cortical areas (as described in the case of cholinergic pathways by Selden *et al.*, 1998). However, further specification of the exact neuromodulatory system impairments which give rise to refractory deficits will have to be elucidated in the context of the intricate and complex interactions which exist between neuromodulators and the neurotransmitters whose effects they influence (see Hasselmo, 1995, for a review of relevant issues).

Further evidence in favor of a neuromodulatory explanation of refractoriness comes from consideration of the etiology of the brain damage sustained by refractory access and storage patients. The projection of neuromodulators to the cortex tends to be dependent upon the integrity of specific subcortical structures and fiber pathways. Consistent with this fact, the influence of temporal factors has, to date, only been documented in patients with lesions extending beyond the neocortex. Most typically this damage is of vascular origin, with the commonest neurological diagnosis being left hemisphere stroke, and more specifically left middle cerebral artery stroke. However, refractoriness has also been observed in a patient with multifocal cerebral tumors (A2; Warrington & Cipolotti, 1996). By contrast, all the patients with a semantic storage impairment who have been tested for their sensitivity to temporal factors have neurological and neuroradiological evidence of progressive cerebral atrophy consistent with the degenerative processes of either Alzheimer's disease or semantic dementia (Warrington & Cipolotti, 1996; Crutch & Warrington, 2005). Notably, both the patients who exhibit what Gotts and Plaut (2002) have referred to as a "mixed pattern" of access and storage deficits (PW and KE; Howard, 1985 and Hillis *et al.*, 1990) sustained left hemisphere strokes. This indicates that damage both to neurons which encode information directly and to neuromodulatory systems may occur following cerebrovascular injuries. However, it remains unclear whether any of the behavioral symptoms which are peculiar to semantic refractory access disorders may be observed in individuals with degenerative disease.

1.8   Conclusions

In this chapter, an attempt has been made to outline the core characteristics of the semantic refractory access syndrome and to highlight the insight which studying patients with this condition can offer into the fine-grain organization of many aspects of conceptual knowledge. The examination of individuals with semantic refractory access disorders has not in fact yielded much evidence of category-specific dissociations. Investigations have nevertheless revealed a remarkable degree of organization within the conceptual system. For example, such studies have demonstrated a semantic organization within brand names, people's occupations, and types of plant life, to list but a few. Whilst it may seem obvious that such organizational principles apply to our psychological space, the point is that investigation of a neurophysiologically based syndrome has shown that this organization of psychological space is mirrored in neurological space. Repetitive probe experiments have also led to the proposal of information within conceptual knowledge which is spatially encoded rather than verbally or visually encoded to support geographical knowledge. However, perhaps most significant is the discovery that different domains of conceptual knowledge are supported by different representational frameworks. This claim has implications for research into not only abstract and concrete semantics but all aspects of our knowledge, because it suggests that attempting to model or explain the organization of conceptual knowledge with a single set of network principles is overly simplistic. We hope this short account of semantic refractory access disorders will motivate more detailed studies of conceptual knowledge, particularly in patients who have suffered damage to subcortical structures and pathways.

REFERENCES

Allport, D. A. (1985). Distributed memory, modular systems and dysphasia. In S. K. Newman and R. Epstein (eds.), *Current Perspectives on Dysphasia* Edinburgh: Churchill Livingstone.

Barkai, E. and Hasselmo, M. E. (1994). Modulation of the input/output function of rat piriform cortex pyramidal cells. *Journal of Neurophysiology*, **72**: 644–58.

Breedin, S. D., Saffran, E. M., and Coslett, H. B. (1994). Reversal of the concreteness effect in a patient with semantic dementia. *Cognitive Neuropsychology*, **11**: 617–60.

Capitani, E., Laiacona, M., Mahon, B., and Caramazza, A. (2003). What are the facts of semantic category-specific deficits? A critical review of the clinical evidence. *Cognitive Neuropsychology*, **20**: 213–61.

Caramazza, A., Hillis, A. E., Rapp, B. C., and Romani, C. (1990). Multiple semantics or multiple confusions? *Cognitive Neuropsychology*, **7**: 161–8.

Caramazza, A. and Shelton, J. R. (1998). Domain-specific knowledge systems in the brain: the animate–inanimate distinction. *Journal of Cognitive Neuroscience*, **10**: 1–34.

Cipolotti, L. (2000). Sparing of country and nationality names in a case of modality-specific oral output impairment: implications for theories of speech production. *Cognitive Neuropsychology*, **17**: 709–29.

Crutch, S. J. and Warrington, E. K. (2001). Refractory dyslexia: evidence of multiple task-specific phonological output stores. *Brain*, **124**: 1533–43.

Crutch, S. J. and Warrington, E. K. (2003a). The selective impairment of fruit and vegetable knowledge: a multiple processing channels account of fine-grain category specificity. *Cognitive Neuropsychology*, **20**: 355–72.

Crutch, S. J. and Warrington, E. K. (2003b). Spatial coding of semantic information: knowledge of country and city names depends upon their geographical proximity. *Brain*, **126**: 1821–9.

Crutch, S. J. and Warrington, E. K. (2003c). Preservation of propositional speech in a pure anomic: the importance of an abstract vocabulary. *Neurocase*, **9**: 465–81.

Crutch, S. J. and Warrington, E. K. (2004). The semantic organisation of proper nouns: the case of people and brand names. *Neuropsychologia*, **42**: 584–96.

Crutch, S. J. and Warrington, E. K. (2005). Abstract and concrete concepts have structurally different representational frameworks. *Brain*, **128**: 615–27.

Crutch, S. J. and Warrington, E. K. (2005). Gradients of semantic relatedness and their contrasting explanations in refractory access and storage semantic impairments. *Cognitive Neuropsychology*, **22**: 815–76.

Crutch, S. J. and Warrington, E. K. (in press). The semantic organisation of mass nouns: evidence from semantic refractory access dysphasia, *Cortex*.

Crutch, S. J., Ridha, B. H., and Warrington, E. K. (2006). The different frameworks underlying abstract and concrete knowledge: evidence from a bilingual patient with a semantic refractory access dysphasia. *Neurocase*, **12**: 1–13.

Dunn, L. M., Dunn, L. M., Robertson, G. J., and Eisenberg, J. L. (1979). *Peabody Picture Vocabulary Test – Revised*, American Guidance Centre, MN, USA.

Forde, E. M. E. and Humphreys, G. W. (1995). Refractory semantics in global aphasia: on semantic organisation and the access–storage distinction in neuropsychology. *Memory*, **3**: 265–307.

Forde, E. M. E. and Humphreys, G. W. (1997). A semantic locus for refractory behaviour: implications for access–storage distinctions and the nature of semantic memory. *Cognitive Neuropsychology*, **14**: 367–402.

Gil, Z., Connors, B. W., and Amital, Y. (1997). Differential regulation of neocortical synapses by neuromodulators and activity. *Neuron*, **19**: 679–86.

Gotts, S. J. and Plaut, D. C. (2002). The impact of synaptic depression following brain damage: a connectionist account of "access/refractory" and "degraded store" semantic impairments. *Cognitive, Affective and Behavioral Neuroscience*, **2**: 187–213.

Hasselmo, M. E. (1995). Neuromodulation and cortical function: modelling the physiological basis of behavior. *Behavioural Brain Research*, **67**: 1–27.

Hillis, A. E., Rapp, B. C., Romani, C., and Caramazza, A. (1990). Selective impairment of semantics in lexical processing. *Cognitive Neuropsychology*, **7**: 191–243.

Hodges, J. R., Graham, N., and Patterson, K. (1995). Charting the progression in semantic dementia: implications for the organisation of semantic memory. *Memory*, **3**: 463–95.

Howard, D. (1985). The semantic organisation of the lexicon: evidence from aphasia. Unpublished Ph.D. thesis: University of London.

Incisa della Rocchetta, A. and Cipolotti, L. (2004). Preserved knowledge of maps of countries: implications for the organisation of semantic memory. *Neurocase*, **10**: 249–64.

Incisa della Rocchetta, A., Cipolotti, L., and Warrington, E. K. (1996). Topographical disorientation: selective impairment of locomotor space? *Cortex*, **32**: 727–35.

Incisa della Rocchetta, A., Cipolotti, L., and Warrington, E. K. (1998). Countries: their selective impairment and selective preservation. *Neurocase*, **4**: 99–109.

Lyons, F., Hanley, J. R., and Kay, J. (2002). Anomia for common names and geographical names with preserved retrieval of names of people: a semantic memory disorder. *Cortex*, **38**: 23–35.

McCarthy, R. A. and Kartsounis, L. D. (2000). Wobbly words: refractory anomia with preserved semantics. *Neurocase*, **6**: 487–97.

McCarthy, R. A. and Warrington, E. K. (1986). Visual associative agnosia: a clinico-anatomical study of a single case. *Journal of Neurology, Neurosurgery & Psychiatry*, **49**: 1233–40.

McCarthy, R. A. and Warrington, E. K. (1988). Evidence for modality-specific meaning systems in the brain. *Nature*, **334**: 428–30.

McClelland, J. L. and Rogers, T. T. (2003). The parallel distributed processing approach to semantic cognition. *Nature Reviews Neuroscience*, **4**: 310–22.

McKenna, P. and Warrington, E. K. (1978). Category-specific naming preservation: a single case study. *Journal of Neurology, Neurosurgery & Psychiatry*, **41**: 571–4.

McNeil, J. E., Cipolotti, L., and Warrington, E. K. (1994). The accessibility of proper names. *Neuropsychologia*, **32**: 193–208.

Miceli, G., Capasso, R., Daniele, A., Esposito, T., Magarelli, M., and Tomaiuolo, F. (2000). Selective deficit for people's names following left temporal damage: an impairment of domain-specific conceptual knowledge. *Cognitive Neuropsychology*, **17**: 489–516.

Paivio, A. (1986). *Mental Representations: a dual coding approach*. Oxford: Oxford University Press.

Plaut, D. C. and Shallice, T. (1993). Deep dyslexia: a case study of connectionist neuropsychology. *Cognitive Neuropsychology*, **10**: 377–500.

Rapp, B. C. and Caramazza, A. (1993). On the distinction between deficits on access and deficits of storage: a question of theory. *Cognitive Neuropsychology*, **10**: 113–41.

Schwanenflugel, P. J. and Shoben, E. J. (1983). Differential context effects in the comprehension of abstract and concrete verbal materials. *Journal of Experimental Psychology: Learning, Memory and Cognition*, **9**: 82–102.

Selden, N. R., Gitelman, D. R., Salamon-Murayama, N., Parrish, T. B., and Mesulam, M. M. (1998). Trajectories of cholinergic pathways within the cerebral hemispheres of the human brain. *Brain*, **121**: 2249–57.

Semenza, C. and Zettin, M. (1988). Generating proper names: a case of selective inability. *Cognitive Neuropsychology*, **5**: 711–21.

Semenza, C. and Zettin, M. (1989). Evidence from aphasia for the role of proper names as pure referring expressions. *Nature*, **342**: 678–9.

Shallice, T. (1993). Multiple semantics: whose confusions? *Cognitive Neuropsychology*, **10**: 251–61.

Sirigu, A., Duhamel, J. R., and Poncet, M. (1991). The role of sensorimotor experience in object recognition. A case of multimodal agnosia. *Brain*, **114**: 2555–73.

Tsodyks, M. V. and Markram, H. (1997). The neural code between neocortical pyramidal neurons depends on neurotransmitter release probability. *Proceedings of the National Academy of Sciences USA*, **94**: 719–23.

Varela, J. A., Sen, K., Gibson, J., Fost, F., Abbott, L. F., and Nelson, S. B. (1997). A quantitative description of short-term plasticity at excitatory synapses in layer 2/3 of rat primary visual cortex. *Journal of Neuroscience*, **17**: 7926–40.

Warrington, E. K. (1975). The selective impairment of semantic memory. *Quarterly Journal of Experiment Psychology*, **27**: 635–57.

Warrington, E. K. and Cipolotti, L. (1996). Word comprehension. The distinction between refractory and storage impairments. *Brain*, **119**: 611–25.

Warrington, E. K. and Clegg, F. (1993). Selective preservation of place names in an aphasic patient: a short report. *Memory*, **1**: 281–8.

Warrington, E. K. and Crutch, S. J. (2004). A circumscribed refractory access disorder: a verbal semantic impairment sparing visual semantics. *Cognitive Neuropsychology*, **21**: 299–315.

Warrington, E. K. and McCarthy, R. A. (1983). Category specific access dysphasia. *Brain*, **106**: 859–78.

Warrington, E. K. and McCarthy, R. A. (1987). Categories of knowledge. Further fractionations and an attempted integration. *Brain*, **110**: 1273–96.

Warrington, E. K. and Shallice, T. (1984). Category specific semantic impairments. *Brain*, **107**: 829–54.

2

The anatomical locus of lesion in category-specific semantic disorders and the format of the underlying conceptual representations

Guido Gainotti

Catholic University of Rome

Our knowledge of the world is based upon two main kinds of cognitive processes: perceptual activities, which continuously give us information about external objects and actions performed with these objects; and conceptual activities, which allow us to have stable internal representations of objects, actions, and more abstract entities. However, in spite of the complementary nature of these two kinds of cognitive activities, and of the fact that sensory—motor functions certainly play a preliminary role in the acquisition of conceptual knowledge, there is a discrepancy between the large amount of information available about the nature, mechanisms, and neural basis of perceptual activities and the very poor and controversial knowledge that we still have about the nature and the neural substrates of conceptual representations. This lack of solidly established knowledge concerns two main aspects of the semantic—conceptual activities, namely the format of the semantic representations and the neuroanatomical substrates of concepts. On the contrary, there is general agreement that concepts are categorically organized in the brain. The aim of the present chapter is to show that format and categorical organization of semantic representations are strictly intermingled and that the study of the anatomical lesions underlying category-specific semantic disorders can contribute to clarifying the nature of these intimate relationships.

The plan that I intend to follow in the development of this chapter will, therefore, consist of the following steps: (i) I shall discuss the problem of the format of the semantic representations and of their relationships with the underlying sensory—motor activities; (ii) I shall, then, take into account the question of the categorical organization of semantic knowledge, focusing on the most relevant and debated dichotomies, namely on the distinction between category-specific disorders for actions (verbs) and for objects (nouns) and, within the latter, on the distinction between living things and artifacts. In the discussion of these category-specific semantic disorders, I shall consider in turn: their clinical and cognitive aspects; the most relevant pathophysiological interpretations; the predictions that these interpretations make as to the corresponding neuroanatomical lesions; and the consistency between neuroanatomical data and predictions based on the various theoretical models. Overall, the outcome of this complex review will be consistent with a model of semantic representation assuming that various categories of knowledge bear the stamp of the sensory–motor activities which have mainly contributed to their acquisition. (iii) I will, finally, take into account the main objections that have been raised to this general model and discuss the possibility that these objections may not be necessarily inconsistent with the "sensory–motor model of semantic knowledge".

2.1 The format of conceptual representations and their relationships with the underlying perceptual activities

Persistent controversies exist about the relationships between semantic representations and sensory–motor processes preliminary to the acquisition of these representations. As a matter of fact, even if a clear distinction is usually made between perceptual processes and conceptual–semantic representations, the format of the conceptual representations and their relationships with the sensory–motor activities involved in their acquisition remains very controversial. Two main lines of thought exist on this subject.

The first is supported by authors who consider perceptual and conceptual functions as resulting from the activity of interrelated, but completely independent, systems. According to this view, the hierarchical stages of perceptual analysis proceed up to the level of a three-dimensional structural description, which includes a complete perceptual specification of objects prior to their meaningful recognition. At this stage, according to most authors (e.g. Anderson & Bower, 1973; Moran, 1973; Pylyshyn, 1973; Kieras, 1978; Seymour, 1979; Warren & Morton, 1982; Chambers & Reisberg, 1985 and, more recently, Humphreys & Riddoch, 1988; Riddoch *et al.*, 1988 and Caramazza *et al.*, 1990), no trace of the previous sensory–motor mechanisms should persist, since the format of semantic representations, accessed through these structural descriptions, is deemed to be symbolic, abstract, amodal, and propositional. The Organized Unitary Content Hypothesis (OUCH) put forward by Caramazza *et al.* (1990) is the most authoritative and influential contemporary model of this kind. This model assumes that the meaning of a term consists of a set of semantic predicates, represented in an amodal format. These predicates can be organized in subsystems, concerning: the perceptual features of objects; the action patterns associated with them; the context in which an object is found; and its relations with other objects and concepts, but all these subsystems share the same amodal format. Accordingly, even the subsystem storing the visual–perceptual properties of objects keeps no physical trace of the channel through which it was acquired, since it is stored in a propositional, symbolic, abstract format.

The second line of thought is defended by authors who refute the hypothesis of a central, amodal, abstract semantic system and assume that the semantic representations might be stored in the same format in which they have been perceived, or, in any case, bear the stamp of the perceptual mechanisms through which they have been formed. From the historical point of view, these positions can be traced back to the classical associationistic views, which maintained that sensory–motor activities are followed by "images", specific for each sensory modality, and that these "images" tend to be associated, due to the co-occurrence of the excitation provoked by the same object in different sensory modalities. According to these classic views, which have been more recently revisited by Geschwind (1965, 1967), conceptual representations of objects result from the convergence (in the posterior multimodal association areas) of the visual, auditory, somatosensory, and kinesthetic images that constitute the basic attributes on which the core conceptual representation is constructed.

Cognitive models consistent with this line of thought have been proposed in recent years by several cognitive psychologists, such as Kolers and Brison (1984), Allport (1985), Jackendoff (1987), and Shanon (1988). All these models, reacting against the notion of abstract, modality-independent conceptual representations, envisaged concepts as activity patterns, distributed across different perceptual and motor attribute domains, and predicated that the organization of semantic representations reflects the manner in which information most relevant for their development has been acquired. In particular, Allport's (1985) model seems to reframe, in terms of a distributed network, the main assumptions of the associationistic models. According to Allport (1985), each object-concept is represented as a pattern of activation over featural units in different attribute domains that have become "auto-associated" (that is interconnected) so that partial activation will recreate the whole pattern. The object concept of *telephone*, for example, must involve visual, tactile, auditory, and action-coding domains of representation, including manipulation and speech. Individual units within the attribute domains participate in many different patterns, representing different objects, and the same neural elements that are involved in coding the attributes of an object presented in a sensory modality also make up the elements of the auto-associated activity patterns that represent familiar object-concepts in semantic memory. Allport (1985) concludes that his model is "in radical opposition to the view that semantic memory is represented in some abstract, modality-independent conceptual domain, remote from the mechanisms of perception and of motor organization." Very consistent with this theoretical construct are the connectionistic models (e.g. Ballard, 1986; Churchland & Sejnowski, 1988; Farah & McClelland, 1991), which maintain that, since information is stored as a pattern of activity in the connections between the units of the net processing a given type of information, processing and storage must be closely intertwined.

It should be acknowledged, however, that two different positions must be distinguished within those that maintain that information stored in semantic memory bears the stamp of the perceptual activities through which it was acquired. The more radical of these views, defended by Warrington, Shallice, and co-workers (Warrington, 1975; Warrington & McCarthy, 1994; Shallice, 1988; McKenna & Warrington, 2000), postulates the existence of multiple modality-specific semantic systems, in which objects are represented in the same format in which they have been perceived. A less strong view is proposed by authors (e.g. Lauro-Grotto *et al.*, 1997) who, for parsimony reasons, do not accept the hypothesis of multiple modality-specific semantic systems, but view semantic memory as an unintegrated multimodal network, in which different subsystems are accessed by different channels, storing modality-specific information. In keeping with Allport's (1985) model, these authors assume that under normal circumstances the various components of the net are interconnected, allowing retrieval of the entire representation from any input channel, but that in pathological conditions one or more components of the net could be preferentially damaged, giving rise to dissociations in performance. A detailed discussion of the empirical data supporting or weakening the unitary amodal abstract model (Caramazza *et al.*, 1990), the multiple modality-specific semantic systems hypothesis (Warrington & McCarthy, 1994; Shallice, 1988; McKenna & Warrington, 2000) and the multimodal network model (Lauro-Grotto *et al.*, 1997) clearly exceeds the scope of the present chapter. The interested reader is, therefore, referred to Shallice (1988), Caramazza *et al.* (1990), Hillis and Caramazza (1995), Patterson and Hodges (2000), McKenna and Warrington (2000), Coccia *et al.* (2004), Snowden *et al.* (2004), and Gainotti (2006) for different viewpoints on this subject.

From the theoretical point of view, it could, however, be argued that both the "unitary amodal" and the "multiple modality-specific semantic systems" hypothesis raise some problems with respect to the "parsimony principle." The "multiple modality-specific semantic systems" hypothesis is obviously not parsimonious, since it postulates a duplication of information across different semantic subsystems. On the other hand, the unitary abstract model is only apparently more parsimonious, since, as Jackendoff (1987) had already noticed, it implies a translation process, devised to transform information coming from different sensory modalities into a uniform propositional format. This problem becomes even more relevant if we accept Damasio's (1989, 1990) model, suggesting that semantic representations must not be conceived as structures localized in a static store, but as a process of recollection of fragmented features, inscribed in multiple sensory and motor cortices. In this case, it would be necessary to evaluate the costs for the brain of this bidirectional translation mechanism, or, in any case, to acknowledge that an abstract, amodal system is not necessarily very parsimonious.

Furthermore, making reference to the general problem of the relationships between semantic representations and underlying perceptual activities, I think it useful to recall some data recently obtained by Rogers *et al.* (2004) that cast some doubt on the assumption of a complete independence between the last stages of the perceptual processing (structural description) and the corresponding semantic representations. These authors tried to investigate the impact of semantic degradation on object decision tasks, i.e. on tasks that are currently used to assess the integrity of the corresponding structural description. Results showed that object decision tasks are impaired in semantic dementia patients and this impairment mainly concerns atypical and less familiar objects, and increasingly so in patients with greater semantic deterioration. These data are not surprising, since Patterson *et al.* (1994) and Gainotti *et al.* (1995) had already shown that within the language domain a severe semantic impairment can have a deleterious influence upon (presemantic) purely lexical tasks. Anyway, the disruptive influence of a severe semantic defect upon the structural description, shown by this study, obviously points to a continuous interaction between perceptual and semantic representations, rather than stressing the independence between modality-specific perceptual channels and a unitary, amodal semantic system.

2.2 The categorical organization of conceptual knowledge

A very influential seminal role in the identification of selective defects of semantic memory was played by Warrington (1975), who in a highly influential series of papers opened a most fruitful area of inquiry in the field of semantic memory and proposed that this field be categorically organized. This proposal stemmed from the detailed description of patients showing different kinds of category-specific disorders, as a consequence of different kinds of brain lesions. To be sure, Warrington and co-workers contrasted disorders selectively affecting abstract vs. concrete words (Warrington, 1975, 1981), action names/verbs vs. object names/nouns (Baxter & Warrington, 1985; McCarthy & Warrington, 1985), and, within the general category of concrete entities, contrasted the impairment of living beings with that of man-made artifacts (Warrington & McCarthy, 1983, 1987; Warrington & Shallice, 1984; McCarthy & Warrington, 1991).

But the contribution of Warrington and co-workers to the exploration of this field was not limited to the identification of different kinds of category-specific semantic disorders and to the consequent proposal that semantic knowledge be categorically organized in the brain. On the contrary, Warrington and McCarthy (1983) and Warrington and Shallice (1984), while discussing the contrast between category-specific disorders for biological entities and artifacts, also advanced a general hypothesis about the brain representation of semantic knowledge. This general hypothesis, which challenged the traditional views about the cortical representation of concepts and offered a general key to understanding the basic mechanisms subserving category-specific semantic disorders was labeled the "differential weighting hypothesis" and added an important source of specificity to the associationistic views, which generically assumed that concepts result from the linkage of multiple perceptual information in cortical association areas. As a matter of fact, the "differential weighting hypothesis" acknowledged that, even if each concept is based upon the convergence of the output of various perceptual systems, the weights that these sensory modalities have in the acquisition of different semantic categories may be very different. Within this context, the distinction between disorders selectively affecting living beings and artifacts was viewed as the consequence of the different weighting that visuoperceptual and functional attributes have in the identification of members of these different categories of knowledge. The "differential weighting hypothesis" has important implications from both the cognitive and the anatomical viewpoint. From the cognitive point of view, it assumes that different categories should be characterized by a different pattern of underlying sensory–motor activities. From the anatomical point of view, it predicts a close relationship between cortical areas crucially involved in storing (or recollecting the fragmented features forming) a given category and the localization of sensory–motor mechanisms that have mainly contributed to the development of that category.

In the present discussion of the categorical organization of semantic memory, I will focus on the two main dissociations that have been identified within the field of category-specific semantic disorders and which refer respectively to the contrast between the semantic–lexical representations of actions/verbs and objects/nouns and, within the latter, to the contrast between living beings and artifacts. In both domains, I will first report some clinical data that have supported the dissociation and discuss the principal interpretations that have been advanced to explain these data. I will then take into account the neuroanatomical lesions underlying these category-specific semantic disorders, discussing their consistency with a set of predictions based on "the sensory—motor model of semantic knowledge" (Gainotti, 1990, 2000, 2006; Gainotti *et al.*, 1995; Saffran & Schwartz, 1994; Martin, 1998; Martin *et al.*, 2000; Martin & Chao, 2001), which can be considered as an extension of the "differential weighting hypothesis." The results of a recent review (Gainotti, 2004) in which this set of predictions has been used to foresee the patterns of naming impairment for different categories of knowledge in patients with a visuoverbal disconnection will also be shortly discussed.

2.2.1   Disorders in production and comprehension of nouns and verbs in brain-damaged patients

The first data suggesting a differential impairment of nouns and verbs in aphasic patients were reported by Goodglass *et al.* (1966), who observed that patients with fluent aphasia are more impaired in naming objects (producing nouns), whereas nonfluent aphasics are more impaired in naming actions (producing verbs). These observations prompted a series of investigations conducted both in single cases (e.g. Marin *et al.*, 1976; McCarthy & Warrington, 1985; Zingeser & Berndt, 1988; Caramazza & Hillis, 1991; Breedin *et al.*, 1994; Daniele *et al.*, 1994; Marshall *et al.*, 1996a, 1996b; Hillis *et al.*, 2002a) and in groups of patients (e.g. Miceli *et al.*, 1984, 1988; Zingeser & Berndt, 1990; Tranel *et al.*, 2001; Hillis *et al.*, 2002b), focusing attention on agrammatic patients, within nonfluent aphasics and on anomic patients within fluent aphasics. In particular, these studies showed that: (a) agrammatic patients are more impaired in naming actions than objects, whereas anomic patients show the opposite pattern of impairment (Miceli *et al.*, 1984; McCarthy & Warrington, 1985; Zingeser & Berndt, 1988, 1990; Breedin *et al.*, 1994; Hillis *et al.*, 2002a); (b) an analogous dissociation can be observed in comprehension of nouns and verbs (McCarthy & Warrington, 1985; Miceli *et al.*, 1988; Breedin *et al.*, 1994). These investigations also showed that some anomic and agrammatic patients present a selective disorder only in production (but not in comprehension) of nouns and respectively of verbs (Miceli *et al.*, 1988; Zingeser & Berndt, 1988, 1990; Caramazza & Hillis, 1991; Silveri & Di Betta, 1997; Shapiro *et al.*, 2000; Tranel *et al.*, 2001; Hillis *et al.*, 2002a), whereas other anomic and agrammatic patients show a selective disorder both in production and in comprehension of nouns and respectively of verbs (McCarthy & Warrington, 1985; Miceli *et al.*, 1988; Damasio & Tranel, 1993; Breedin *et al.*, 1994; Daniele *et al.*, 1994; Breedin & Martin, 1996).

The cognitive defects underlying these category-specific disorders for nouns and verbs were interpreted in different manners by various authors. Thus, Miceli *et al.* (1984, 1988) claimed that the association between agrammatism and verb retrieval pointed to a defect located at the syntactic level. On the other hand, Caramazza and co-workers, having described patients with a modality-specific defect in verb production restricted to the oral (Caramazza & Hillis, 1991) or to the written modality (Caramazza & Hillis, 1991; Rapp & Caramazza, 1998), suggested that the cognitive defect should concern the lexical level, selectively affecting verbs as a specific grammatical category. Finally, Gainotti *et al.* (1995), Breedin and Martin (1996), Bird *et al.* (2000) and Marshall (2003) reasoned that, at least in patients who show a selective impairment for nouns or verbs both in production and in comprehension, the defect should be located at the semantic level.

As the previous paragraphs exemplify, the greatest uncertainties about the cognitive defects subserving category-specific disorders for nouns and verbs mainly concern verbs. This is due to theoretical reasons, concerning: (a) the complex relationships between semantic and syntactic aspects of verb representations (Pinker, 1989; Jackendoff, 1990); (b) the fact that verbs have an argument structure, whereas nouns (and especially those referring to concrete objects) have not; (c) the different learning style needed to acquire nouns and verbs (see Marshall, 2003 for review). A consequence of all these properties of verbs is that a very heterogeneous set of disturbances is usually grouped under the heading "category-specific impairments for verbs" (see Breedin & Martin, 1996; Marshall *et al.*, 1996b; Bird *et al.*, 2000; Marshall, 2003; and Shapiro & Caramazza, 2003 for different viewpoints on this subject). In any case, some category-specific verb disorders are certainly due to a disruption of the semantic representation of actions, and we will focus on this more circumscribed problem in later parts of this chapter.

In particular, we will try to determine: (1) whether the anatomical locus of lesion is different in patients with a category-specific impairment for action names and object names; and (2) whether the neuroanatomical correlates of these category-specific disorders are consistent with the predictions based on the "sensory—motor model of semantic knowledge."

Neuroanatomical correlates of disorders selectively affecting nouns and verbs

Both direct and indirect evidence points to an association between defects for action names and left frontal lesions and between defects for object names and left temporal pathology. The indirect evidence is based on the anatomical locus of lesion in agrammatic patients (where selective verb disorders are usually observed) and in anomia, where disorders mainly concern the production (and sometimes the comprehension) of objects' names. The direct evidence consists of neuroimaging data coming from patients with vascular, neoplastic, and degenerative syndromes (Damasio & Tranel, 1993; Daniele *et al.*, 1994; Bak & Hodges, 1997;

Cappa *et al.*, 1998a; Rapp & Caramazza, 1998; Tranel *et al.*, 2001; Hillis *et al.*, 2002b; Tranel *et al.*, 2003; Saygin *et al.*, 2004), which confirm that a selective impairment of action names is associated with left frontal lesions, and a defect of object names with left temporal pathology. Even if some authors (e.g. Rapp & Caramazza, 1998; Tranel *et al.*, 2001; Hillis *et al.*, 2002b) have interpreted data concerning verbs within the framework of the grammatical category hypothesis (since in their patients selective defect for verbs was apparent only on naming, but not on lexical comprehension tasks), data obtained from other patients (e.g. Damasio & Tranel, 1993; Daniele *et al.*, 1994; Bak & Hodges, 1997; Tranel *et al.*, 2003; Saygin *et al.*, 2004) clearly point to a disorder affecting the semantic representation of actions in patients with left frontal lesions.

Thus, Tranel *et al.* (2003) showed that conceptual knowledge of actions is mainly impaired by lesions encroaching upon the left frontal and parietal cortices, whereas Saygin *et al.* (2004) reported that lesions of the same cortical areas are associated with deficits in nonlinguistic tasts of action comprehension (panto-mime understanding). Analogously, Bak and Hodges (2003) showed a double dissociation between frontal and temporal variants of the fronto-temporal dementia on two conceptual tests based respectively on objects (the "Pyramids and Palm Trees" test) devised by Howard and Patterson (1992) and on actions (the "Kissing and Dancing" test). Patients with left frontal variant were more impaired on the "Kissing and Dancing" test, whereas patients with left temporal atrophy (semantic dementia) were more impaired on the "Pyramids and Palm Trees" test.

Consistency between neuroanatomical data and predictions based on the "sensory–motor model of semantic knowledge"

The above-mentioned data are consistent with the "sensory–motor model of semantic knowledge," which assumes that the brain areas damaged in a given form of category-specific semantic disorder have also been involved in the acquisition of sensory–motor information crucial for the development of that category. According to this model, a selective inability to name or understand action names should usually be due to a lesion of the parts of the left frontal lobe, where action schemata are planned and represented and which become active not only when a motor schema is actually executed, but also when it is simply imagined (Decety *et al.*, 1997) or recognized in other subjects (Gallese *et al.*, 1996; Rizzolatti *et al.*, 1996; Buccino *et al.*, 2001). The "sensory–motor model" receives further support from recent fine-grained investigations of the neural substrate of verb meaning, conducted with neuroimaging procedures by Grossman *et al.* (2002) and with neurophysiological techniques by Pulvermüller *et al.* (2001). With a functional magnetic resonance imaging (fMRI) study, Grossman *et al.* (2002)

observed that a different pattern of activation is associated with verbs of motion (which represent events involving action planning) and verbs of cognition (which contain few associated sensory–motor features), since only the former recruited the prefrontal cortex, whereas the latter activate the left posterolateral temporal cortex. On the other hand, Pulvermüller *et al.* (2001) showed that different parts of the frontal lobe are activated by verbs denoting different kinds of actions. Using high-resolution electroencephalogram (EEG) recordings, these authors investigated the brain activity elicited by verbs referring to actions performed with the face (e.g. "talking") and with the legs (e.g. "walking"). Face-related action verbs produced the strongest in-going currents over the left Sylvian fissure, close to the part of the motor cortex involved in the representation of the face movements, whereas leg-related action verbs produced the strongest in-going currents at the vertex, close to the cortical representation of the lower limbs' movements.

2.2.2 Disorders in identification of living beings and artifacts in brain-damaged patients

Even if several instances of category-specific semantic disorders have been reported in the literature, the most typical and the most frequently reported one consists of a striking dissociation between a severe inability to recognize living beings (animals, flowers, fruits, vegetables, etc.) and a relatively spared capacity to identify artifacts (tools, furniture, clothing, vehicles, etc.). The main characteristics of this syndrome were first reported by Warrington and Shallice (1984) and were afterwards confirmed by other authors (e.g. Basso *et al.*, 1988; Pietrini *et al.*, 1988; Sartori & Job, 1988; Silveri & Gainotti, 1988; Sirigu *et al.*, 1991; Hart & Gordon, 1992; Sartori *et al.*, 1993; Sheridan & Humphreys, 1993; De Renzi & Lucchelli, 1994; Farah *et al.*, 1996; Gainotti & Silveri, 1996; Forde *et al.*, 1997; Samson *et al.*, 1998; Kolinsky *et al.*, 2002; Samson & Pillon, 2003), who have studied the pattern of cognitive impairment and/or the distribution of the anatomical lesions associated with this form of category-specific semantic disorder, which is often observed in patients with herpes simplex encephalitis (HSE). From the cognitive point of view, these patients show a severe inability to identify animals, vegetables (and often food), independently from the verbal or pictorial modality through which information is presented and the patient's response is expressed. This massive impairment of living beings identification is often observed in patients showing no defect of language or of visual–spatial functions and stands in contrast with a relatively spared capacity to identify artifacts and body parts. The opposite dissociation, namely a prevalent impairment of artifacts and body parts, has been much less frequently reported (e.g. Warrington & McCarthy, 1983, 1987; Hillis & Caramazza, 1991; Sacchett & Humphreys, 1992; Silveri *et al.*, 1997; Cappa *et al.*, 1998b) and is, in any case, much less striking than the previously described selective inability to identify living beings. Furthermore, it must be acknowledged that the artifacts category is not necessarily a homogeneous domain since within this category a more fine-grained distinction has been proposed by Warrington and McCarthy (1987) between small manipulable objects, such as tools, and large outdoor objects, such as vehicles. This distinction has proved fruitful, since it has prompted important clinical (e.g. Buxbaum *et al.*, 2000; Buxbaum & Saffran, 2002) and neuroimaging (e.g. Kellenbach *et al.*, 2003) investigations, to which we will return in later sections of this chapter.

Objections addressed to category-specific semantic disorders for living entities

In spite of their dramatic and selective nature, both general and more specific objections have been addressed to category-specific semantic disorders for biological entities reported in the literature. General methodological objections, recently addressed by Laws (2005), have stressed the fact that in most instances the selective nature of the disorder has been assessed in nonrigorously controlled conditions, namely in the absence of an appropriate control group. More specific critiques have concerned the possibility that category-specific semantic disorders for living entities may be an artifact of stimulus selection. Funnell and Sheridan (1992), Stewart *et al.* (1992) and Gaffan and Heywood (1993) have, indeed, hypothesized that category-specific deficits for living entities might simply reflect the fact that members of these categories tend to be of lower frequency and familiarity and of greater visual complexity than nonliving beings. In support of their hypothesis, these authors reported instances of patients who showed an apparent category-specific semantic disorder for biological entities only when these variables were not carefully controlled, but not when living and nonliving categories were matched for frequency, familiarity, and visual complexity. Both the general methodological point stressed by Laws (2005) and the more specific objections raised by Funnell and Sheridan (1992), Stewart *et al.* (1992) and Gaffan and Heywood (1993) are certainly worth stressing. In a later part of this chapter, we will even see that in single case studies the prevalent impairment of some semantic categories can be explained by gender-related familiarity effects. However, neither the general nor the more specific methodological objections can fully explain the most typical instances of category-specific semantic disorders for living beings, since even when frequency, familarity, and visual complexity are taken into account (e.g. Warrington & Shallice, 1984; Hart & Gordon, 1992; Laiacona *et al.*, 1993; Sartori *et al.*, 1993; Sheridan & Humphreys, 1993; Farah *et al.*, 1996; Gainotti & Silveri, 1996, etc.), many patients continue to show disproportionate difficulty in naming or recognizing living things. Furthermore, there are patients who show a disproportionate deficit for the (supposedly easier to process) category of nonliving things and there are instances of patients who showed opposite category-specific deficits when tested with the same battery of living and artifact stimuli (Hillis & Caramazza, 1991; Gainotti & Silveri, 1996; Silveri *et al.*, 1997). It remains, therefore, unquestionable that some kinds of brain lesions (later considered in more detail) give rise to a specific disruption of knowledge of biological entities.

The interpretation of category-specific semantic disorders for living beings and artifacts

Even if general agreement can be found on the existence of category-specific semantic disorders for living and nonliving beings, the interpretation of this distinction remains controversial. To be sure, at least three main theoretical models have been proposed on this subject.

The first and more influential model, called the "sensory–functional theory," was put forward by Warrington and Shallice in their 1984 seminal paper. This model assumes that the living/nonliving distinction may be due to a more basic dichotomy concerning the differential weighting that visuoperceptual and functional attributes have in the identification of members of biological and, respectively, of artifact categories. According to this interpretation, identification of members of living categories mainly relies upon visual properties, whereas identification of artifacts critically depends upon functional attributes, i.e. the subtly different functions for which artifacts were designed. This interpretation was afterwards revised and partly modified on the basis of the distinction between small manipulable objects and large outdoor objects proposed by Warrington and McCarthy (1987) and of the studies that other investigators have conducted following this distinction. All these investigations have, indeed, shown that in the representation of small manipulable objects "function" and "manipulation" are distinct features (Buxbaum *et al.*, 2000; Buxbaum & Saffran, 2002) and that manipulable/action features play a critical role in tool representations (Kellenbach *et al.*, 2003). In spite of these modifications, the model is still usually called the "sensory–functional theory" and is evaluated with reference to the distinction between visual and functional information.

The second theoretical model, more recently proposed by Caramazza and Shelton (1998), is based on the observation that in patients with a category-specific defect for living things there is not necessarily a greater impairment of the visual–perceptual rather than of the functional associative properties of the disrupted category. Starting from this weakness of the "sensory–functional theory" and from the observation that animals and plant life can be independently affected in individual patients [animals were, e.g. selectively impaired in patients KR (Hart & Gordon, 1992) and EW (Caramazza & Shelton, 1998), whereas fruits and vegetables were selectively affected in patients MD (Hart *et al.*, 1985) and

TU (Farah & Wallace, 1992)], Caramazza and Shelton (1998) have rejected the hypothesis assuming that the living/nonliving distinction may be the byproduct of a more basic sensory–functional dichotomy. They have rather proposed that category-specific defects of brain-damaged patients may be due to the disruption of different evolutionary-adapted dedicated neural mechanisms for the domains of "animals" (potential predators), "plant life" (possible source of food and medicine) and "artifacts." This model is usually named the "domain-specific knowledge systems" hypothesis.

The third and last theoretical model, proposed by Gonnerman *et al.* (1997), Garrard *et al.* (1998) and Moss *et al.* (1998), underlines the different levels of interconnections existing between shared (perceptual and functional) attributes of living and nonliving things and assumes that this structural difference may be more important than the differential weighting of perceptual and functional attributes to explain category-specific semantic disorders. To be sure, this model stresses the fact that within the animal category some perceptual properties, such as "having eyes" and "having ears," regularly co-occur with some functional attributes, such as "can see" and "can hear," whereas artifacts have a greater proportion of distinctive properties that are less densely interconnected. This last model is often labeled the "intercorrelations among semantic features" hypothesis.

The main criteria that have been used by various authors to support or reject these competing theoretical models are: the relative impairment of visual and functional knowledge in patients with selective damage to the living or nonliving categories; the pattern of impaired and spared categories that can be found in these patients; and the results of computational studies, which have used a computer simulation to produce category-specific defects for living or nonliving things. I will describe here, as an example of this computational line of research, the implementation of the "sensory–functional" hypothesis, put forward by Farah and McClelland (1991), since I intend to come back to this study in a later section of this chapter. Farah and McClelland (1991) used in their model an assembly of simple neuron-like processing units, forming a peripheral and a semantic layer and linked by means of weighted connections. The peripheral input system was composed by both visual and verbal units, whereas in the semantic layer some units responded mainly to objects with visual properties and other units to objects with functional properties. Living and nonliving things were represented in the model and a lesion was simulated by deleting some proportions of units either in the visual or in the functional semantic pool. The ability of the model to perform a task analogous to a picture naming was then investigated. The model showed: (a) that it is possible to produce a category-specific defect for living things by preferentially damaging sensory inputs and (b) that in this case, not only perceptual, but also functional attributes of biological entities were impaired, because the loss of units mainly contributing to the activation of the system also weakened the activation of the functional features, rendering them inaccessible.

Implications of neuroanatomical data for cognitive interpretations of category-specific disorders for living and nonliving beings

Although less frequently considered, the neuroanatomical correlates of category-specific semantic disorders for living or nonliving things are potentially relevant from the theoretical point of view, since each of the above-mentioned models makes a different set of predictions about extent and localization of the underlying brain pathology.

Thus the sensory–functional hypothesis, stressing the importance of visual–perceptual properties in the semantic representation of biological categories, and the crucial role of functional/action-related attributes in the semantic representation of artifacts, leads to predict that lesions provoking a category-specific semantic impairment for living things should encroach upon brain structures critically involved in processing high-level visual data and integrating them with other kinds of perceptual knowledge, whereas those provoking a selective deficit for artifacts should impinge upon brain areas involved in manipulation and physical use of objects.

Less clear are the predictions made by the "domain-specific knowledge systems" hypothesis. However, Caramazza (1998), Caramazza and Shelton (1998) and Shelton and Caramazza (2001) have made some explicit claims which should have neuroanatomical implications. To be sure, these authors have assumed: (a) that the domains of "animals" and "plant life" should be subserved by dedicated brain structures storing all kinds of perceptual and functional–associative information relevant to identify the category members; and (b) that, because of the "affective/emotional components associated with the flight and feeding responses to animals and plants," the assumed neural circuits for these biological categories should probably involve the limbic system. On the basis of these claims, it should be possible to identify two distinct neural networks, connected with the limbic system and subserving the domains of "animals" and "plant life."

Still different are the predictions made by the "intercorrelations among semantic features" hypothesis, since this model assumes that the severity of brain damage, rather than its precise anatomical location, should play a major role in provoking a category-specific defect for living or nonliving entities. Gonnerman *et al.* (1997) have, indeed, argued that biological entities, having many interconnected features in their semantic structure, should be more resistant than artifacts to a mild diffuse damage of the semantic system. This hypothesis has been confirmed by a computer simulation study, which has shown that with a small degree of damage to the system there was a greater impairment of artifacts, but with increasing damage, there was a dramatic decline of the living categories. On the basis of a different connectionistic model, Moss *et al.* (1998) and Tyler *et al.* (2000) have predicted just the opposite type of interaction between prevalent impairment of biological or artifact categories and stage of disease progression, confirming, in any case, the greater importance of disease severity in the pathophysiology of different kinds of category-specific semantic disorders.

In our attempts to check these alternative predictions, we argued that, since our knowledge of the neuroanatomical correlates of category-specific semantic disorders for living beings and artifacts is almost completely based on single-case studies, a better understanding of this problem could probably be reached by means of detailed reviews of all the available anatomoclinical reports of patients showing these kinds of category-specific semantic disorders. In the next section of this chapter, I shall focus on predictions based on the "sensory–functional" and on the "domains of knowledge" hypothesis, rather than on those based on the "intercorrelations among semantic features" hypothesis, since the latter assumes that the severity of brain damage (and not the anatomical locus of lesions) plays the major role in the pathophysiology of category-specific disorders for living vs. nonliving things. In a later section of this chapter I shall, however, return to results of investigations which have checked the neuroanatomical predictions of the "intercorrelations among semantic features" hypothesis.

Neuroanatomical correlates of disorders specifically affecting living and nonliving things

In our first review of this subject (Gainotti, 2000) we took systematically into account all patients reported in the neuropsychological literature for a disorder selectively affecting living things or artifacts and for whom neuroanatomical data had been reported. Our inclusion criteria were met by 57 patients (47 with a selective defect for living beings and 10 with a prevalent impairment for artifacts). The cognitive and neuroanatomical variables considered in our review were: (a) the locus of cognitive impairment (distinguishing semantic, lexical and visuoperceptual disorders); (b) the etiology of the disease; and (c) the neuroanatomical locus of lesion.

As for the first point, within both category-specific groups, the deficit concerned in most patients (60–70 percent) the semantic level, in a less numerous group (25–30 percent) the output lexicon, and in a small number of subjects (5–10 percent) the visual level.

From the etiological point of view, the large majority of patients with a semantic disorder for living beings (namely 20/38) suffered from a relatively rare disease (i.e. herpes simplex encephalitis), which typically involves the anterior and mesial parts of both temporal lobes. A less important number of patients were affected by other diseases, such as head trauma and semantic dementia, which also tend to encroach upon the anterior parts of the temporal lobes. On the other hand, patients with a purely lexical impairment for living beings were usually affected by a left-sided brain infarct, which in half of them (4/8) selectively damaged the inferomesial aspects of the temporal and occipital lobes. In these patients, plants, fruits, and vegetables were usually more affected than animals. A more detailed analysis of lesion location within the temporal lobes in patients with a semantic impairment for living things showed that lesions were usually bilateral, with a prevalence for the left side, and that they almost invariably encroached upon the anterior, mesial, and inferior parts of the temporal lobes, sparing their lateral and posterior parts.

Very different were etiology and anatomical locus of lesion in patients with a semantic disorder selectively involving artifacts, since all these patients (who also showed a defect in the recognition of body parts) were affected by infarcts in the territory of the left middle cerebral artery, which typically involved the frontoparietal cortices, provoking a severe (usually nonfluent) form of aphasia.

Results obtained in this systematic review of the neuroanatomical correlates of category-specific semantic disorders for living beings and artifacts have been confirmed by results of a second, more recent, review, in which we tried to make a more articulated analysis of the problem (Gainotti, 2005), assessing the influence of lesion location and of gender-related familiarity factors on naming disorders for artifacts, animals, and plant-life categories.

The influence of lesion location and of gender-related familiarity factors on category-specific disorders for artifacts, animals and plant-life categories

The aim of this second review consisted in checking the neuroanatomical implications of the "domains of knowledge" hypothesis (Caramazza, 1998; Caramazza & Shelton 1998; Capitani *et al.*, 2003; Martin & Caramazza, 2003), which suggests that it should be possible to distinguish two different anatomical localizations in patients with category-specific disorders for animals and, respectively, for plant life. Some hints in this direction had been found in our previous review (Gainotti, 2000), in which we had observed some differences between lesions encroaching upon the anterior parts of the temporal lobes and lesions located in the territory of the left posterior cerebral artery, since the latter apparently more specifically affected the plant-life categories. As these putative effects were very mild, we decided to take also into account the influence of gender-related familiarity effects that could be considered as a possible source of confounding, due to the existence of documented interactions between gender and familiarity with different kinds of living and nonliving categories. As a matter of fact, in a normative study conducted by McKenna and Parry (1994), and in further studies conducted in normal subjects by Laws (1999, 2000, 2002, 2004), Capitani, Laiacona, and Barbarotto (1999), Albanese, Capitani, Barbarotto, and Laiacona (2000) and Barbarotto, Laiacona, Macchi, and Capitani (2002), men were usually more familiar with artifacts and women with living things. Furthermore, a more specific gender by category interaction had been found within the biological categories in McKenna and Parry's (1994) normative study, where males fared better with animals and females with fruit and vegetables. This interaction had been partly confirmed in studies conducted by Capitani *et al.* (1999), Albanese *et al.* (2000) and Barbarotto *et al.* (2002), where the female superiority for natural categories concerned only fruit and vegetables, but not animals. I therefore deemed it interesting to take into account the possible influence of these gender-related familiarity effects in patients reported in the neuropsychological literature for a category-specific naming impairment. To be sure, since both gender and anatomical locus of lesion could in part explain a prevalent impairment for animals, plant-life, or artifacts, I took into account both these factors in a systematic review of all patients reported in the neuropsychological literature for a category-specific naming impairment. Due to the nature of this review, which aimed to quantitatively evaluate the effects of lesions location and of gender-related familiarity effects, the anatomical study was less fine-grained in this than in the previous review, and patients were simply classified in three general lesion groups: (a) anterior temporal lesions; (b) temporo-occipital injuries; and (c) other more dorsal lesions.

Results of the review were not consistent with the predictions based on the "domains of knowledge" hypothesis, since they showed that:

1. Lesion location has a strong influence on the distinction between biological and artifacts categories, but not on that between animals and plant-life domains. In patients with a prevalent impairment either for animals or for fruits and vegetables, lesions usually encroach upon the anterior parts of the temporal lobes or (in a less sizable number of patients) on the inferomesial parts of the temporo-occipital cortices, whereas in patients with a prevalent impairment for artifacts they are located elsewhere (usually on more dorsal structures of the brain). This part of the review is consistent with results of the previous survey (Gainotti, 2000) of the brain correlates of category-specific semantic disorders for living beings and artifacts. It is, on the contrary, at variance with the the neuroanatomical implications of the "domains of knowledge" hypothesis (Caramazza, 1998), which assumed that "animals" and "plant-life" categories,

being subserved by distinct neural networks, should present different neuroanatomical correlates in patients with a selective impairment for one of these categories.

2. Gender, on the contrary, does not influence the distinction between living and nonliving things, but has a strong influence, within the biological categories, on the distinction between animals and plant life. In keeping with data obtained in normal subjects, men were, indeed, more impaired with flowers, fruits and vegetables, whereas women were more impaired with animals.

This composite set of data seems to indicate that the distinction between living things and artifacts must be considered as a truly biological phenomenon, resulting from the disruption of brain structures specifically subserving these different categories of knowledge, whereas the distinction between animals and plant life must be considered as a more spurious phenomenon, mainly based on gender-related familiarity factors.

Consistency between neuroanatomical correlates of category-specific semantic disorders for living beings and artifacts and predictions based on the "sensory–motor model of semantic knowledge"

The neuroanatomical data consistently observed in our reviews can be explained if we take into account the main functions of the anteromesial and inferior parts of the temporal lobes, which in our first review (Gainotti, 2000) had been found strictly related to category-specific semantic disorders for biological entities, and of the left frontoparietal areas, which had been usually involved in patients with a semantic disorder for artifacts.

The anteromedial temporolimbic structures and the inferotemporal lobe (ITL) could, indeed, constitute a cortical network, devised to process high-level visual information and to integrate these data with other kinds of perceptual knowledge. Since the seminal work of Ungerleider and Mishkin (1982) and of Mishkin *et al.* (1984), the ITL is, in fact, considered as the main component of the "ventral stream" of the extra-striate visual processing system, which plays a crucial role in object recognition. According to Mishkin *et al.* (1984), the anterior parts of ITL (and in particular area TE) could store the structural description (or the visual templates) of objects, and similar claims have been made by Gross *et al.* (1972) and by Desimone (1991) with respect to area AIT (Brodmann's area 20–21). On the other hand, within the medial temporal lobe (MTL) telencephalic temporo-limbic structures, the parahippocampal region might contain representations of complex conjunctions of visual features (Eichenbaum & Bunsey, 1995; O'Reilly & Rudy, 2001), the perirhinal cortex could play an important role in visual object representation (Bussey & Saksida, 2002; Bussey *et al.*, 2003) and the entorhinal cortex receives convergent, integrated input from all the sensory modalities

(Mesulam *et al.*, 1977; Van Hoesen, 1982) through the perirhinal and the parahippocampal gyri (Suzuki & Amaral, 1994). Finally, the temporal pole is considered by Damasio (1989, 1990) and by Mesulam (1998) as a higher-order convergence zone, i.e. as a transmodal area that binds together the components of a concept distributed through different sensory modalities. Inferior temporal lobe, temporolimbic structures and temporal pole could, therefore, be critically involved in processing, storing and retrieving the representations of those semantic categories whose knowledge is mainly based upon sensory (and above all upon visual) information.

A very different set of functions is usually attributed to the dorsolateral (and in particular to the frontoparietal) areas of the dominant hemisphere. These areas are, in fact, part of the "dorsal stream" of visual processing, involved in spatial and action functions (Goodale *et al.*, 1991) and play a very important role both in action planning and in high-level somatosensory processing. The frontoparietal areas of the dominant hemisphere therefore subserve those somatosensory and motor schemata which (through processes of concrete utilization and of physical contact) could have critically contributed to building the semantic representation of man-made objects and, in particular, of small manipulable objects, such as tools (Warrington & McCarthy, 1987; Buxbaum *et al.*, 2000; Buxbaum & Saffran, 2002; Kellenbach *et al.*, 2003). From this point of view, the joint impairment of the categories of man-made objects and of body parts could be due to the fact that the sensory–motor mechanisms that critically contribute to the construction of the semantic representation of man-made objects are also involved in building the representation of the body parts category.

2.2.3   Category-specific naming disorders in patients with a "visuoverbal disconnection"

The study of the neuroanatomical correlates of category-specific semantic disorders does not constitute the only strategy followed to test the "sensory–motor model of semantic knowledge."

The most important complementary line of research has been represented by the functional neuroimaging investigations which have explored the cortical areas preferentially activated by stimuli belonging to different categories of knowledge. A review of these studies will not be reported here, since detailed surveys of this subject have been made in other chapters of this book. An alternative line of research on which we have recently focused (Gainotti, 2004) is the pattern of impaired and spared naming abilities for different categories of knowledge observed in patients with a visuoverbal disconnection.

A review of this topic was considered worthy of interest to better understand the neuroanatomical organization of categorical knowledge for two main reasons: the first is the observation that action naming (Manning & Campbell, 1992;

Campbell & Manning, 1996; Teixeira-Ferreira *et al.*, 1997) and body parts naming (Forde *et al.*, 1997; Shelton *et al.*, 1998) can be selectively spared in these patients; the second is the observation, made in our previous review (Gainotti, 2000) and mentioned in an earlier section of this chapter, that some patients with a vascular lesion in the territory of the left posterior cerebral artery show a selective naming impairment for fruit and vegetables (e.g. Farah & Wallace, 1992; Goldenberg, 1992). These observations seemed to show that in patients with optic aphasia the access to the lexical output mechanisms could be different for items belonging to different categories of knowledge.

The specific set of predictions advanced in our study was prompted by the classical neurological models of "optic aphasia" and of "visuoverbal disconnection" proposed by Freund (1889) and by Geschwind (1965). According to Freund's (1889) model, a joint lesion of the left visual areas and of the posterior parts of the corpus callosum should prevent visual information, processed by the right hemisphere visual cortices, from reaching the left hemisphere lexical output mechanisms. The inter-hemispheric pathways connecting the right with the left visual cortices pass, in fact, through the splenium (i.e. through the damaged posterior part) of the corpus callosum. Geschwind (1965) observed that, in spite of this lack of connections between right and left hemisphere visual cortices, some visual stimuli are correctly named in these patients and attributed these residual visual naming abilities to the use of alternative inter-hemispheric callosal pathways. According to Geschwind's (1965) model, the vision of an object arouses associations in other sensory modalities and "the arousal of such associations permits the finding of an alternative pathway across uninvolved more anterior portions of the corpus callosum." The rationale of our review was an integration of this model with the "differential weighting hypothesis," since we assumed that the residual naming abilities could be related to the different weight that nonvisual sensory attributes have in the representation of different semantic categories. According to this view, in patients with optic aphasia, visual naming should be spared for conceptual categories, such as action names, body parts (and in part artifacts) whose representations are mainly based upon nonvisual (motor and somatosensory) information. It should, on the contrary, be impaired for living things and in particular for fruits, vegetables, and flowers, whose representations are mainly based upon visual attributes. Results of the review strongly confirmed the predictions concerning body parts and action names, since in all patients where these categories had been taken separately into account, pictures representing actions or body parts were perfectly or preferentially (in comparison with other categories) named. Less clear results were obtained in the comparison between living things and artifacts, since a trend toward a greater impairment of biological stimuli was found, but neither the difference between artifacts and living stimuli, nor the difference (within the latter) between animals and plant life reached the level of statistical significance.

2.3 Main objections addressed to the "sensory–motor model of semantic knowledge"

Data surveyed in previous sections of this chapter and concerning the neuroanatomical correlates of category-specific semantic disorders for actions/ verbs vs. objects/nouns and, respectively, for living beings vs. artifacts are consistent with the "sensory–motor model of semantic knowledge." Also consistent with this model is the pattern of naming impairment for different categories of knowledge observed in patients with a visuoverbal disconnection. Taken together, these data strongly suggest that different semantic categories bear the stamp of the sensory–motor channels through which they were acquired and that lesions provoking a semantic impairment for a given category usually encroach upon brain structures involved in the perceptual–motor functions which have mainly contributed to the development of that category.

It must be acknowledged, however, that important objections have been raised to various aspects of this model. In particular, several critiques have been addressed to Warrington and Shallice's (1984) hypothesis, assuming that the living/nonliving distinction may be the byproduct of a more basic dichotomy concerning the different weighting that visuoperceptual and functional attributes have in the identification of biological entities and artifacts respectively. Caramazza *et al.* (Caramazza, 1998; Caramazza & Shelton, 1998; Shelton & Caramazza, 2001) have, indeed, repeatedly observed that in patients with a category-specific defect for living things the impairment of the visual–perceptual properties is not necessarily greater than that of the functional associative attributes, as should be predicted by the Warrington and Shallice's (1984) hypothesis. On the other hand, Lambon-Ralph *et al.* (1998, 1999, 2003) have noticed that category-specific defects for living things are rarely observed in patients with semantic dementia, in spite of the fact that in these patients the atrophy selectively affects the antero-inferolateral parts of the temporal lobes (including IT) and that these patients provide fewer sensory than functional attributes in their definition of concepts.

Even if these objections are important and well documented, they are not necessarily inconsistent with the "sensory–motor model of semantic knowledge."

Thus the objection raised by Caramazza *et al.* is supported by many empirical data (see Shelton & Caramazza, 2001 and Capitani *et al.*, 2003 for review) but can be mitigated by methodological problems concerning the assessment of perceptual and functional properties of living beings and by results of the previously mentioned computer simulation study conducted by Farah and McClelland (1991). Let us consider first the methodological problems met when we try to operationally define the "functional properties" of living beings, in order to compare the level of impairment for visual and functional attributes of the disrupted categories in patients with a selective impairment for living things. These problems stem from the fact that the term "functional properties" is often used with a different acceptation in the case of living things and of artifacts, as is explicitly recognized by Moss *et al.* (1998). These authors maintain that the key functional properties of living things concern biological actions, such as eating, walking, and growing, whereas the key functional properties of artifacts are the typical actions accomplished with objects by humans. This observation also applies to the choice of questions used to probe the functional knowledge of living and nonliving things by standard batteries, such as that proposed by Laiacona *et al.* (1993). This tendency to use a different acceptation of the term "functional knowledge" when dealing with living and nonliving things is probably due to the extreme difficulty in defining many instances of biological entities that stress the function that these beings have for man. I have personally experienced this difficulty when I have tried to construct a naming-by-definition task and a sentence verification task in which the same (living and nonliving) stimuli were described with reference once to visuoperceptual and once to functional–encyclopedic information (Gainotti & Silveri, 1996). This different acceptation of the term "functional properties" is, however, a source of confusion, as is documented by patients with a category-specific semantic impairment for living things who have shown very different patterns of performance when studied with different kinds of tests devised to explore their knowledge of visual–perceptual and functional knowledge. Thus patient SE, who showed a category-specific defect for living things after recovering from herpes simplex encephalitis (HSE), has shown a prevalent deficit for functional attributes of animals, when studied by Laws *et al.* (1995), but the opposite pattern of results (namely a selective impairment for the visual properties of living things) when studied with a different battery by Moss *et al.* (1997).

Passing now to the computer simulation study of Farah and McClelland (1991), we recall that this study has not only shown that it is possible to produce a category-specific defect for living things by preferentially damaging sensory inputs, but has also demonstrated that both perceptual and functional attributes of biological entities are disrupted by this lesion. Therefore, according to this model of category-specific defects, Warrington and Shallice's (1984) hypothesis does not necessarily predict a greater impairment of the visual–perceptual rather than of the functional associative attributes in the disrupted biological categories.

If we pass now to the objections addressed to Warrington and Shallice's (1984) model by Lambon-Ralph *et al.* (1998, 1999, 2003), we can say that their data could still be compatible with the "sensory–motor" model if we assume: (a) that category-specificity is not an "all-or-nothing", but a graded phenomenon; (b) that the lesion of IT is an important, but not a sufficient, condition for the development of a category-specific disorder for living beings (an equal or even more important role being played by MTL telencephalic temporolimbic structures).

As for the first point, it is interesting to note that almost all patients with semantic dementia (SD) reviewed by Lambon-Ralph *et al.* (2003), namely NV (Basso *et al.*, 1988), DM (Breedin *et al.*, 1994), MF (Barbarotto *et al.*, 1995), SD (Cardebat *et al.*, 1996), TOB (McCarthy & Warrington, 1988) showed a trend toward a greater impairment for living categories and that a similar trend was also observed in the six patients reported in Lambon-Ralph *et al.*'s (2003) study. Lesions observed in SD could, therefore, contribute, but not necessarily fully account for the development of a clear-cut category-specific disorder for living beings.

As for the second point, it must be noted that in patients with semantic dementia the atrophy typically affects the anterior and inferior parts of the temporal lobes, whereas the medial temporal areas are relatively spared (Mummery *et al.*, 2000; Hodges, 2001). Now, in recent years, several authors (e.g. Suzuki & Amaral, 1994; Parker & Gaffan, 1998; Murray & Bussey, 1999; Murray, 2000; Bussey & Saksida, 2002) have stressed the importance of the monkey's MTL temporolimbic structures within the cortical network, devised to process and to integrate high-level visual information with other kinds of perceptual knowledge. Furthermore, Lee *et al.* (2005) have recently challenged the view suggesting that in humans the MTL plays an exclusive role in memory functions, showing that high-level visual activities are also impaired in amnesic patients with MTL damage. From the functional point of view, it is important to note that IT has purely visual processing properties, whereas the MTL structures are considered as multimodal areas, where the rostral parts of the ventral stream of visual processing are integrated with other kinds of non-visual information. It is, therefore, possible that in the cortical network subserving living beings knowledge, MTL temporolimbic structures play a more critical role than IT. This suggestion is supported by clinical data, showing that living things are more impaired than artifacts (Silveri *et al.*, 1991; Daum *et al.*, 1996; Whatmough *et al.*, 2003; Zannino *et al.*, 2002; Marra *et al.*, in press) in Alzheimer's disease (AD), where the atrophy severely affects the MTL (and in particular the hippocampal–entorhinal complex), since the earliest stages of the disease (Braak & Braak, 1991; Jack *et al.*, 1997; Laakso *et al.*, 1998; Galton *et al.*, 2001). A further interesting observation that has been consistently made in studies conducted on AD by Whatmough *et al.* (2003), Zannino *et al.* (2002) and Marra *et al.* (in press) is the stability during the disease progression of the greater impairment for living things. This finding is at variance with the predictions made by models based on the "intercorrelations among semantic features hypothesis," since these models assumed an interaction between stage of disease progression and prevalent impairment of biological or artifact categories. The consistency of the greater impairment of living things across different stages of disease progression suggests that this categorical impairment is due to a neuroanatomical reason (namely to the severe atrophy of MTL structures), rather than to the different resistance to brain damage of categories with different degrees of interconnected semantic features.

2.4   Concluding remarks

We have seen in the last section of this chapter that the general model that we have proposed to account for the anatomoclinical aspects of category-specific semantic disorders is open to criticism and we acknowledge that the "sensory–motor model of semantic knowledge" certainly explains only a part of the variance existing in this area. It is clear, for instance, that idiosyncratic factors (linked to the previous personal experience with different domains of knowledge) play a much more important role in this field than in any other area of cognitive neuropsychology (Funnell *et al.*, 1996; Lambon-Ralph *et al.*, 2002, 2003; Gainotti, 2005). It is, therefore, mandatory that these idiosyncratic factors be systematically controlled (with structured interviews or a checklist considering the premorbid interests of the patient) in new single-case studies of patients with a prevalent impairment for a given category of knowledge.

These notes of caution made, it remains that the complementary study of the neuroanatomical correlates of category-specific semantic disorders and of the patterns of categorical impairment observed in patients with a visuoverbal disconnection strongly supports the "sensory–motor model of semantic knowledge." In particular, I would conclude by stressing two points which underline the importance of neuroanatomical data to clarify the mechanisms subserving category-specific disorders of brain-damaged patients:

• the surprising fact that the majority of patients with a semantic disorder for living beings suffer from a relatively rare disease (i.e. herpes simplex encephalitis), which typically involves the anterior and mesial parts of both temporal lobes (Gainotti, 2000);

• the equally surprising fact that in all patients with a visuoverbal disconnection in whom these categories had been taken separately into account, "actions" and "body parts" were systematically spared in comparison to all other categories (Gainotti, 2004).

These striking anatomoclinical data must, in any case, be taken into account by any theoretical model aiming to explain category-specific semantic disorders.

REFERENCES

Albanese, E., Capitani, E., Barbarotto, R., and Laiacona, M. (2000). Semantic category dissociations, familiarity and gender. *Cortex*, **36**: 733–46.

Allport, D. A. (1985). Distributed memory, modular systems and dysphasia. In S. K. Newman and R. Epstein (eds.), *Current Perspectives in Dysphasia*. Edinburgh: Churchill Livingstone, pp. 32–60.

Anderson, J. R. and Bower, G. H. (1973). *Human Associative Memory*. New York: Winston & Sons.

Bak, T. and Hodges, J. R. (1997). Noun–verb dissociation in three patients with motor neuron disease and aphasia. *Brain and Language*, **60**: 38–40.

Bak, T. and Hodges, J. R. (2003). "Kissing and Dancing" – a test to distinguish the lexical and conceptual contributions to noun/verb and action/object dissociation. Preliminary results in patients with frontotemporal dementia. *Journal of Neurolinguistics*, **16**: 169–81.

Ballard, D. H. (1986). Cortical connections and parallel processing: structure and function. *Behavioral and Brain Sciences*, **9**: 67–120.

Barbarotto, R., Capitani, E., Spinnler, H, and Trivelli, C. (1995). Slowly progressive semantic impairment with category specificity. *Neurocase*, **1**: 107–19.

Barbarotto, R., Laiacona, M., Macchi, V., and Capitani, E. (2002). Picture reality decision, semantic categories and gender. A new set of pictures, with norms and an experimental study. *Neuropsychologia*, **40**: 1637–53.

Basso, A., Capitani, E, and Laiacona, M. (1988). Progressive language impairment without dementia: A case with isolated category specific semantic effect. *Journal of Neurology, Neurosurgery and Psychiatry*, **51**: 1201–7.

Baxter, D. M. and Warrington, E. K. (1985). Category-specific phonological dysgraphia. *Neuropsychologia*, **23**: 653–66.

Bird, H., Howard, D. and Franklin, S. (2000). Why is a verb like an inanimate object? Grammatical category and semantic category deficits. *Brain and Language*, **72**: 246–309.

Braak, H. and Braak, E. (1991). Neuropathological stageing of Alzheimer-related changes. Review. *Acta Neuropathologica (Berlin)*, **82**: 239–59.

Breedin, S. D. and Martin, R. C. (1996). Patterns of verb impairment in aphasia: an analysis of four cases. *Cognitive Neuropsychology*, **13**: 51–91.

Breedin, S. D., Saffran, E, and Coslett, H. (1994). Reversal of the concreteness effect in a patient with semantic dementia. *Cognitive Neuropsychology*, **11**: 617–69.

Buccino, G., Binkofski, F., Fink, G. R., Fadiga, L., Fogassi, L., Gallese, V., *et al.* (2001). Action observation activates premotor and parietal areas in somatotopic manner: An fMRI study. *European Journal of Neuroscience*, **13**: 400–4.

Bussey, T. J. and Saksida, L. M, (2002). The organization of visual object representation: a connectionist model of effects of lesions in perirhinal cortex. *European Journal of Neuroscience*, **15**: 355–64.

Bussey, T. J., Saksida, L. M. and Murray, E. A. (2003). Impairments in visual discrimination after perirhinal cortex lesions: testing "declarative" vs "perceptual–mnemonic" views of perirhinal cortex functions. *European Journal of Neuroscience*, **17**: 649–60.

Buxbaum, L. J. and Saffran, E. M. (2002). Knowledge of object manipulation and object function: Dissociations in apraxic and non-apraxic subjects. *Brain and Cognition*, **82**: 179–99.

Buxbaum, L. J., Veramonti, T, and Schwartz, M. F. (2000). Function and manipulation tool knowledge in apraxia: Knowing "what for" but not "how". *Neurocase*, **6**: 83–97.

Campbell, R. and Manning, L. (1996). Optic aphasia: a case with spared action naming and associated disorders. *Brain and Language*, **53**: 183–221.

Capitani, E., Laiacona, M. and Barbarotto, R. (1999). Gender affects word retrieval of certain categories in semantic fluency tasks. *Cortex*, **35**: 273–8.

Capitani, E., Laiacona, M., Mahon, B. and Caramazza, A. (2003). What are the facts of semantic category-specific deficits? A critical review of the clinical evidence. *Cognitive Neuropsychology*, **20**: 213–61.

Cappa, S., Binetti, G., Pezzini, A., Padovani, A., Rozzini, L, and Trabucchi, M. (1998a). Object and action naming in Alzheimer's disease and frontotemporal dementia. *Neurology*, **50**: 351–5.

Cappa, S., Frugoni, M., Pasquali, P., Perani, D. and Zorat, F. (1998b). Category-specific naming impairment for artefacts: a new case. *Neurocase*, **4**: 391–7.

Caramazza, A. (1998). The interpretation of semantic category-specific deficits: What do they really reveal about the organization of conceptual knowledge in the brain? *Neurocase*, **4**: 265–72.

Caramazza, A. and Hillis, A. (1991). Lexical organization of nouns and verbs in the brain. *Nature*, **349**: 788–90.

Caramazza, A., Hillis, A., Rapp, B. C., and Romani, C. (1990). The multiple semantic hypothesis: multiple confusions? *Cognitive Neuropsychology*, **7**: 161–89.

Caramazza, A. and Shelton, J. R. (1998). Domain-specific knowledge systems in the brain: the animate–inanimate distinction. *Journal of Cognitive Neuroscience*, **10**: 1–34.

Cardebat, D., Demonet, J. F., Celsis, P., and Puel, M. (1996). Living/nonliving dissociation in a case of semantic dementia: A SPECT activation study. *Neuropsychologia*, **34**: 1175–9.

Chambers, D. and Reisberg, D. (1985). Can mental images be ambiguous? *Journal of Experimental Psychology: Human Perception and Performance*, **11**: 317–28.

Churchland, P. S. and Sejnowsky, T. J. (1988). Neural representation and neural computation. L. Nadel (ed.), *Biological Computation*. Cambridge, MA: MIT Press.

Coccia, M., Bartolini, M., Luzzi, S., Provinciali, L., and Lambon-Ralph, M. A. (2004). Semantic memory is an amodal, dynamic system: evidence from the interaction of naming and object use in semantic dementia. *Cognitive Neuropsychology*, **21**: 513–27.

Damasio, A. R. (1989). Time-locked multiregional retroactivation: a systems level proposal for the neural substrates of recall and recognition. *Cognition*, **33**: 25–62.

Damasio, A. R. (1990). Category-related recognition defects as a clue to the neural substrates of knowledge. *Trends in Neurosciences*, **13**: 95–8.

Damasio, A. R. and Tranel, D. (1993). Nouns and verbs are retrieved with different distributed neural systems. *Proceedings of the National Academy of Sciences USA*, **90**: 4957–60.

Daniele, A., Giustolisi, L., Silveri, M. C., Colosimo, C. and Gainotti, G. (1994). Evidence for a possibile neuroanatomical basis for lexical processing of nouns and verbs. *Neuropsychologia*, **332**: 1325–41.

Daum, J., Riesch, G., Sartori, G., and Birbaumer, N. (1996). Semantic memory impairment in Alzheimer's disease. *Journal of Clinical and Experimental Neuropsychology*, **18**: 648–65.

Decety, J., Grezes, J., Costes, N., Perani, D., Jeannerod, M., Procyk, E., *et al.* (1997). Brain activity during observation of actions. Influence of action content and subject's strategy. *Brain*, **120**: 1763–77.

De Renzi, E. and Lucchelli, F. (1994). Are semantic systems separately represented in the brain? The case of living category impairment. *Cortex*, **30**: 3–25.

Desimone, R. (1991). Face-selective cells in the temporal cortex of monkeys. *Journal of Cognitive Neuroscience*, **3**: 1–8.

Eichenbaum, H. and Bunsey, M. (1995). On the binding of associations in memory: Clues from studies on the role of the hippocampal region in paired associate learning. *Current Directions in Psychological Science*, **4**: 19–23.

Farah, M. J. and McClelland, J. L. (1991). A computational model of semantic memory impairment: modality specificity and emergent category-specificity. *Journal of Experimental Psychology: General*, **120**: 339–57.

Farah, M. J., Meyer, M. M., and McMullen, P. A. (1996). The living/non-living dissociation is not an artifact: giving an a priori implausible hypothesis a strong test. *Cognitive Neuropsychology*, **13**: 137–54.

Farah, M. J. and Wallace, M. A. (1992). Semantically-bounded anomia: implications for the neural implementation of naming. *Neuropsychologia*, **30**: 609–21.

Forde, E. M. E., Francis, D., Riddoch, M. J., Rumiati, R. I., and Humphreys, G. W. (1997). On the links between visual knowledge and naming: a single case study of a patient with a category-specific impairment for living things. *Cognitive Neuropsychology*, **14**: 403–58.

Freund, C. S. (1889). Ueber optische Aphasie und Seelenblindheit. *Archiv für Psychiatrie und Nervenkrasse*, **20**: 371–416.

Funnell, E. and De Mornay Davies, P. (1996). JBR: A reassessment of concept familiarity and a category-specific disorder for living things. *Neurocase*, **2**: 461–74.

Funnell, E. and Sheridan, J. (1992). Categories of knowledge: Unfamiliar aspects of living and nonliving things. *Cognitive Neuropsychology*, **9**: 135–54.

Gaffan, D. and Heywood, C. A. (1993). A spurious category-specific visual agnosia for living things in normal humans and non-human primates. *Journal of Cognitive Neuroscience*, **5**: 118–28.

Gainotti, G. (1990). The categorical organization of semantic and lexical knowledge in the brain. *Behavioural Neurology*, **3**: 109–15.

Gainotti, G. (2000). What the locus of brain lesion tells us about the nature of the cognitive defect underlying category-specific disorders: a review. *Cortex*, **36**: 539–59.

Gainotti, G. (2004). A metanalysis of impaired and spared naming for different categories of knowledge in patients with a visuo-verbal disconnection. *Neuropsychologia*, **42**: 299–319.

Gainotti, G. (2005). The influence of gender and lesion location on naming disorders for animals, plants and artefacts. *Neuropsychologia*, **43**: 1633–44.

Gainotti, G. (2006). Disorders of semantic memory. In B. Miller and G. Goldenberg (eds.), *Neuropsychology and Behavior 1*, A volume of the Handbook of Clinical Neurology series, 3rd edn. Amsterdam: Elsevier.

Gainotti, G. and Silveri, M. C. (1996). Cognitive and anatomical locus of lesion in a patient with category specific semantic impairment for living beings. *Cognitive Neuropsychology*, **13**: 357–89.

Gainotti, G., Silveri, M. C., Daniele, A., and Giustolisi, L. (1995). Neuroanatomical correlates of category-specific semantic disorders: a critical survey. *Memory*, **3**: 247–64.

Gallese, V., Fadiga, L., Fogassi, L. and Rizzolatti, G. (1996). Action recognition in the premotor cortex. *Brain*, **119**: 593–609.

Galton, C., Patterson, K., Graham, K., Lambon-Ralph, M. A., Williams, G., Antoun, N., Sahakian, B. J., and Hodges, J. R. (2001). Different patterns of temporal atrophy in Alzheimer's disease and semantic dementia. *Neurology*, **57**: 216–25.

Garrard, P., Patterson, K., Watson, P. C. and Hodges, J. R. (1998). Category-specific semantic loss in dementia of Alzheimer's type. Functional–anatomical correlations from cross-sectional analyses. *Brain*, **121**: 633–46.

Geschwind, N. (1965). Disconnexion syndromes in animals and man. *Brain*, **88**: 237–94.

Geschwind, N. (1967). The varieties of naming errors. *Cortex*, **3**: 97–112.

Goldenberg, G. (1992). Loss of visual imagery and loss of visual knowledge. A case study. *Neuropsychologia*, **12**: 1081–99.

Gonnerman, L. M., Anderson, E. S., Devlin, J. T., Kempler, D., and Seidenberg, M. S. (1997). Double dissociation of semantic categories in Alzheimer's disease. *Brain and Language*, **57**: 254–79.

Goodale, M. A., Milner, A. D., Jakobson, L. S., and Carey, D. P. (1991). A neurological dissociation between perceiving objects and grasping them. *Nature*, **349**: 154–6.

Goodglass, H., Klein, B., Carey, P., and Jones, K. (1966). Specific semantic word categories in aphasia. *Cortex*, **2**: 74–89.

Gross, C. G., Rocha-Miranda, C. E., and Bender, D. B. (1972). Visual properties of neurons in inferotemporal cortex of the macaque. *Journal of Neurophysiology*, **35**: 96–111.

Grossman, M., Koenig, P., DeVita, C., Glosser, G., Aslop, D., Detre, J., and Gee, J. (2002). Neural representation of verb meaning; an fMRI study. *Human Brain Mapping*, **15**: 124–34.

Hart, J., Berndt, R. S., and Caramazza, A. (1985). Category-specific naming deficit following cerebral infarction. *Nature*, **316**: 439–40.

Hart, J. and Gordon, B. (1992). Neural subsystem for object knowledge. *Nature*, **359**: 60–4.

Hillis, A. E. and Caramazza, A. (1991). Category-specific naming and comprehension impairment: a double dissociation. *Brain*, **114**: 2081–94.

Hillis, A. E. and Caramazza, A. (1995). Cognitive and neural mechanisms underlying visual and semantic processing: implications from "optic aphasia". *Journal of Cognitive Neuroscience,* **7**: 457–78.

Hillis, A. E., Tuffiash, E., and Caramazza, A. (2002a). Modality-specific deterioration in naming verbs in nonfluent primary progressive aphasia. *Journal of Cognitive Neuroscience,* **14**: 1099–108.

Hillis, A. E., Tuffiash, E., Wityk, R. J., and Barker, P. B. (2002b). Regions of neural dysfunction associated with impaired naming of actions and objects in acute stroke. *Cognitive Neuropsychology,* **19**: 523–34.

Hodges, J. R. (2001). Frontotemporal dementia (Pick's disease): Clinical features and assessment. *Neurology,* **56**: S6–S10.

Howard, D. and Patterson, K. (1992). *Pyramids and Palm Trees: access from pictures and words.* Bury St. Edmunds (UK), Thames Valley Test Company.

Humphreys, G. W. and Riddoch, M. J. (1988). On the case for multiple semantic systems: a reply to Shallice. *Cognitive Neuropsychology,* **5**: 143–50.

Jack, C. R., Petersen, R. C., Xu, J. C., Waring, S. C., O'Brien, P. C., Tangalos, E. G., *et al.* (1997). Medial temporal atrophy on MRI in normal aging and very mild Alzheimer's disease. *Neurology,* **49**: 786–94.

Jackendoff, R. (1987). On beyond zebra: the relation of linguistic and visual information. *Cognition,* **26**: 89–114.

Jackendoff, R. (1990). *Semantic Structures.* Cambridge, MA: MIT Press.

Kellenbach, M. L., Brett, M., and Patterson, K. (2003). Actions speak louder than functions: The importance of manipulability and action in tool representation. *Journal of Cognitive Neuroscience,* **15**: 30–46.

Kieras, D. (1978). Beyond pictures and words: alternative information-processing models for imagery effects in verbal memory. *Psychological Bulletin,* **85**: 532–54.

Kolers, P. and Brison, S. (1984). Commentary: on pictures, words and their mental representation. *Journal of Verbal Learning and Verbal Behavior,* **23**: 105–13.

Kolinsky, R., Fery, P., Messina, D., Evink, S., and Perez, Morais, J. (2002). The fur of the crocodile and the mooing sheep: The longitudinal study of a patient with a category-specific impairment for biological things. *Cognitive Neuropsychology,* **19**: 301–42.

Laasko, M. P., Soininen, H., Partanen, K., Lehtovirta, H., Hallicainen, M., Hanninen, T., Helkala, E.-L., Vainio, P., and Riekkinen, Sr. P. J. (1998). MRI of the hippocampus in Alzheimer's disease: sensibility, specificity and analysis of incorrectly classified subjects. *Neurobiology of Aging,* **19**: 23–31.

Laiacona, M., Barbarotto, R., and Capitani, E. (1993). Perceptual and associative knowledge in category specific impairment of semantic memory: a study of two cases. *Cortex,* **29**: 727–40.

Lambon-Ralph, M. A., Graham, K. S., Patterson, K., and Hodges, J. R. (1999). Is a picture worth a thousand words? Evidence from concept definitions by patients with semantic dementia. *Brain and Language,* **70**: 309–35.

Lambon-Ralph, M. A., Howard, D., Nightingale, G., and Ellis, A. W. (1998). Are living and nonliving category-specific deficits causally linked to impaired perceptual or associative knowledge? Evidence from a category-specific double dissociation. *Neurocase,* **4**: 311–38.

Lambon-Ralph, M. A., Moriarty, L., and Sage, K. (2002). Anomia is simply a reflection of semantic and phonological impairment: Evidence from a case-series study. *Aphasiology,* **16**: 56–82.

Lambon-Ralph, M. A., Patterson, K., Garrard, P., and Hodges, J. R. (2003). Semantic dementia with category specificity: A comparative case-series study. *Cognitive Neuropsychology,* **20**: 307–26.

Lauro-Grotto, R., Reich, S., and Visadoro, M. (1997). The computational role of conscious processing in a model of semantic memory. In M. Ito, S. Miyashita and E. Rolls (eds.), *Cognition, Computation and Consciousness.* Oxford: Oxford University Press, pp. 249–63.

Laws, K. R. (1999). Gender affects naming latencies for living and nonliving things: implications for familiarity. *Cortex,* **35**: 729–33.

Laws, K. R. (2000). Category-specific naming errors in normal subjects: the influence of evolution and experience. *Brain and Language,* **75**: 123–33.

Laws, K. R. (2002). Category-specific naming and modality-specific imagery. *Brain and Cognition,* **48**: 418–20.

Laws, K. R. (2004). Sex differences in lexical size across semantic categories. *Personality and Individual Differences,* **36**: 23–32.

Laws, K. R. (2005). "Illusions of normality": a methodological critique of category-specific naming. *Cortex,* **41**: 842–51.

Laws, K. R., Evans, J. J., Hodges, J. R., and McCarthy, R. (1995). Naming without knowing and appearance without associations: evidence for constructive processes in semantic memory? *Memory,* **3**: 409–33.

Lee, A. C. H., Bussey, T. J., Murray, E. A., Saksida, L. M., Epstein, R. A., Kapur, R., Hodges, J. R., and Graham, K. S. (2005). Perceptual deficits in amnesia: challenging the medial temporal lobe "mnemonic" view. *Neuropsychologia,* **43**: 1–11.

Manning, L. and Campbell, R. (1992). Optic aphasia with spared action naming: a description of possible loci of impairment. *Neuropsychologia,* **30**: 587–92.

Marin, O. S. M., Saffran, E. M., and Schwartz, M. F. (1976). Dissociations of language in aphasia: implications for normal functions. *Annals of the New York Academy of Sciences,* **280**: 868–84.

Marra, C., Ferraccioli, M., and Gainotti, G. (in press). Gender-related dissociations of categorical fluency in normal subjects and in Alzheimer's disease. *Neuropsychology.*

Marshall, J. (2003). Noun–verb dissociations – evidence from acquisition and developmental and acquired impairments. *Journal of Neurolinguistics,* **16**: 67–84.

Marshall, J., Chiat, S., Robson, J., and Pring, T. (1996a). Calling a salad a federation: an investigation of semantic jargon: Part 2, verbs. *Journal of Neurolinguistics,* **9**: 251–60.

Marshall, J., Pring, T., Chiat, S., and Robson, J. (1996b). Calling a salad a federation: an investigation of semantic jargon. Part 1, nouns. *Journal of Neurolinguistics,* **9**: 237–50.

Martin, A. (1998). Organization of semantic knowledge and the origin of words in the brain. In N. G. Jablonski and L. C. Aiello (eds.), *The Origins and Diversification of Language.* San Francisco: California Academy of Sciences, pp. 69–88.

Martin, A. and Caramazza, A. (2003). Neuropsychological and neuroimaging perspectives on conceptual knowledge: an introduction. *Cognitive Neuropsychology,* **20**: 195–212.

Martin, A. and Chao, L. L. (2001). Semantic memory and the brain: Structure and processes. *Current Opinion in Neurobiology*, **11**: 194–201.

Martin, A., Ungerleider, L. G., and Haxby, J. V. (2000). Category-specificity and the brain: the sensory–motor model of semantic representations of objects. In M. S. Gazzaniga (ed.), *The New Cognitive Neurosciences*. Cambridge, MA: MIT Press, pp. 1023–36.

McCarthy, R. A. and Warrington, E. K. (1985). Category-specificity in an agrammatic patient: the relative impairment of word retrieval and comprehension. *Neuropsychologia*, **23**: 709–27.

McCarthy, R. A. and Warrington, E. K. (1988). Evidence for modality-specific meaning systems in the brain. *Nature*, **334**: 428–30.

McCarthy, R. A. and Warrington, E. K. (1991). *Cognitive Neuropsychology: A Clinical Introduction*. New York: Academic Press.

McKenna, P. and Parry, R. (1994). Category-specificity in the naming of natural and manmade objects: Normative data from adults and children. *Neuropsychological Rehabilitation*, **4**: 225–81.

McKenna, P. and Warrington, E. K. (2000). The neuropsychology of semantic memory. In F. Boller and J. Grafman (eds.), *Handbook of Neuropsychology*, 2nd edn. Vol. 2. Amsterdam: Elsevier, pp. 355–82.

Mesulam, M. M. (1998). From sensation to cognition. *Brain*, **121**: 1013–52.

Mesulam, M. M., Van Hoesen, G. W., Pandya, D. N., and Geschwind, N. (1977). Limbic and sensory connections of the IPL in the rhesus monkey. *Brain Research*, **136**: 393–414.

Miceli, G., Silveri, M. C., Nocentini, U., and Caramazza, A. (1988). Patterns of dissociation in comprehension and production of nouns and verbs. *Aphasiology*, **2**: 351–8.

Miceli, G., Silveri, M. C., Villa, G., and Caramazza, A. (1984). On the basis of the agrammatic's difficulty in producing main verbs. *Cortex*, **20**: 207–20.

Miozzo, A., Soardi, M., and Cappa, S. F. (1994). Pure anomia with spared action naming due to a left temporal lesion. *Neuropsychologia*, **32**: 1101–9.

Mishkin, M., Malamut, B., and Bachevalier, J. (1984). Memories and habits: Two neural systems. In G. Lynch, J. L. McGaugh and N. M. Weinberger. (eds.), *Neurobiology of Learning and Memory*. New York: The Guilford Press, pp. 65–77.

Moran, T. P. (1973). The symbolic nature of visual imagery. Third International Joint Conference on Artificial Intelligence, pp. 472–7.

Moss, H. E., Tyler, L. K., and Jennings, F. (1997). When leopards lose their spots: knowledge of visual properties in category-specific deficits for living things. *Cognitive Neuropsychology*, **14**: 901–50.

Moss, H. E., Tyler, L. K., Durrant-Peatfield, M., and Bunn, E. M. (1998). Two eyes of a see-through: impaired and intact semantic knowledge in a case of selective deficit for living things. *Neurocase*, **4**: 291–310.

Mummery, C. J., Patterson, K., Price, C. J, Ashburner, J., Frackowiak, R. S. J., and Hodges, J. R. (2000). A voxel based morphometry study of semantic dementia: The relation of temporal lobe atrophy to cognitive deficit. *Annals of Neurology*, **47**: 36–45.

Murray, E. A. (2000). Memory for objects in nonhuman primates. In M. S. Gazzaniga (ed.), *The New Cognitive Neurosciences*. London: The MIT Press, pp. 753–63.

Murray, E. A. and Bussey, T. J. (1999). Perceptual—mnemonic functions of perirhinal cortex. *Trends in Cognitive Sciences*, **3**: 142—51.

O'Reilly, R. C. and Rudy, J. W. (2001). Conjunctive representations in learning and memory: principles of cortical and hippocampal function. *Psychological Review*, **108**: 311—45.

Parker, A. and Gaffan, D. (1998). Memory systems in primates: episodic, semantic and perceptual learning. In A. D. Milner (ed.), *Comparative Neuropsychology*. Oxford: Oxford University Press, pp. 109—26.

Patterson, K., Graham, N., and Hodges, J. R. (1994). The impact of semantic memory loss on phonological representations. *Journal of Cognitive Neuroscience*, **6**: 57—69.

Patterson, K. and Hodges, J. R. (2000). Semantic dementia: one window on the structure and organisation of semantic memory. In F. Boller and J. Grafman (eds.), *Handbook of Neuropsychology*. 2nd edn. Vol. 2. Amsterdam: Elsevier, pp. 313—33.

Pietrini, V., Nertempi, P., Vaglia, A., Revello, M. G., Pinna, V., and Ferro-Milone, F. (1988). Recovery from herpes simplex encephalitis: selective impairment of specific semantic categories with neuroradiological correlation. *Journal of Neurology, Neurosurgery and Psychiatry*, **51**: 1284—93.

Pinker, S. (1989). Learnability and cognition. *The Acquisition of Argument Structure*. Cambridge, MA: MIT Press.

Pulvermüller, F., Harle, M., and Hummel, F. (2001). Walking or talking? Behavioral and neurophysiological correlates of action verb processing. *Brain and Language*, **78**: 143—68.

Pylyshyn, Z. W. (1973). What the mind's eye tells to the mind's brain: a critique of mental imagery. *Psychological Bulletin*, **80**: 1—24.

Rapp, B. and Caramazza, A. (1998). A case of selective difficulty in writing verbs. *Neurocase*, **4**: 127—40.

Riddoch, M. J., Humphreys, G. W., Coltheart, M., and Funnell, E. (1988). Semantic systems or system? Neuropsychological evidence re-examined. *Cognitive Neuropsychology*, **5**: 3—25.

Rizzolatti, G., Fadiga, L., Matelli, M., Bettinardi, V., Paulesu, E., and Perani, D., *et al.* (1996). Localization of grasp representations in humans by PET. 1. Observation versus execution. *Experimental Brain Research*, **111**: 246—52.

Rogers, T. T., Lambon-Ralph, M. A., Hodges, J., and Patterson, K. (2004). Natural selection: the impact of semantic impairment on lexical and object decision. *Cognitive Neuropsychology*, **21**: 331—52.

Sacchett, C. and Humphreys, G. W. (1992). Calling a squirrel a squirrel but a canoe a wigwam: a category-specific deficit for artefactual objects and body parts. *Cognitive Neuropsychology*, **9**: 73—86.

Saffran, E. M. and Schwartz, M. F. (1994). Of cabbages and things: semantic memory from a neuropsychological perspective — A tutorial review. *Attention and Performance*, **25**: 507—36.

Samson, D. and Pillon, A. (2003). A case of impaired knowledge for fruit and vegetables. *Cognitive Neuropsychology*, **20**: 373—400.

Samson, D., Pillon, A., and De Wilde, V. (1998). Impaired knowledge of visual and non-visual attributes in a patient with a semantic impairment for living entities: A case of a true category-specific deficit. *Neurocase*, **4**: 273—90.

Sartori, G. and Job, R. (1988). The oyster with four legs: a neuropscholigical study on the interaction of visual and semantic information. *Cognitive Neuropsychology*, **5**: 105–32.

Sartori, G., Job, R., Mozzo, M., Zago, S., and Marchiori, G. (1993). Category-specific form-knowledge deficit in a patient with Herpes Simplex virus encephalitis. *Journal of Clinical and Experimental Neuropsychology*, **15**: 280–99.

Saygin, A. P., Wilson, S. M., Dronkers, N. F., and Bates, E. (2004). Action comprehension in aphasia: linguistic and non-linguistic deficits and their lesion correlates. *Neuropsychologia*, **42**: 1788–804.

Seymour, P. H. K. (1979). *Human Visual Cognition*. London: Collier Macmillan.

Shallice, T. (1988). *From Neuropsychology to Mental Structure*. Cambridge: Cambridge University Press.

Shanon, B. (1988). Semantic representation of meaning: A critique. *Psychological Review*, **104**: 70–93.

Shapiro, K. and Caramazza, A. (2003). The representation of grammatical categories in the brain. *Trends in Cognitive Sciences*, **7**: 201–6.

Shapiro, K., Shelton, J., and Caramazza, A. (2000). Grammatical class in lexical production and morphological processing: evidence from a case of fluent aplasia. *Cognitive Neuropsychology*, **17**: 665–82.

Shelton, J. R. and Caramazza, A. (2001). The organisation of semantic memory. In B. Rapp (ed.), *The Handbook of Cognitive Neuropsychology*. Hove, UK: Psychology Press, pp. 423–43.

Shelton, J. R., Fouch, E., and Caramazza, A. (1998). The selective sparing of body part knowledge: A case study. *Neurocase*, **4**: 339–51.

Sheridan, J. and Humphreys, G. W. (1993). A verbal–semantic category-specific recognition impairment. *Cognitive Neuropsychology*, **10**: 143–84.

Silveri, M. C., Daniele, A., Giustolisi, L., and Gainotti, G. (1991). Dissociation between knowledge of living and non-living things in dementia of the Alzheimer's type. *Neurology*, **41**: 545–6.

Silveri, M. C. and Di Betta, A. M. (1997). Noun–verb dissociations in brain-damaged patients: further evidence. *Neurocase*, **3**: 477–88.

Silveri, M. C. and Gainotti, G. (1988). Interaction between vision and language in category-specific semantic impairment. *Cognitive Neuropsychology*, **5**: 677–709.

Silveri, M. C., Gainotti, G., Perani, D., Cappelletti, J. Y., Carbone, G., and Fazio, F. (1997). Naming deficit for non-living items: neuropsychological and PET study. *Neuropsychologia*, **35**: 359–67.

Sirigu, A., Duhamel, J. R., and Poncet, M. (1991). The role of sensorimotor experience in object recognition. *Brain*, **114**: 2555–73.

Snowden, J. S., Thompson, J. C., and Neary, D. (2004). Knowledge of famous faces and names in semantic dementia. *Brain*, **127**: 860–72.

Stewart, F., Parkin, A. J., and Hunkin, N. M. (1992). Naming impairment following recovery from herpes simplex encephalitis: category-specific? *Quarterly Journal of Experimental Psychology*, **44A**: 261–84.

Suzuki, W. A. and Amaral, D. G. (1994). Topographic organization of the reciprocal connections between the monkey's entorhinal cortex and the perirhinal and parahippocampal cortices. *Journal of Neurosciences*, **13**: 2430–51.

Teixeira-Ferreira, C., Giuliano, B., Ceccaldi, M., and Poncet, M. (1997). Optic aphasia: evidence of the contribution of different neural systems to object and action naming. *Cortex*, **33**: 499–514.

Tranel, D., Adolphs, R., Damasio, H., and Damasio, A. R. (2001). A neural basis for the retrieval of words for actions. *Cognitive Neuropsychology*, **18**: 655–70.

Tranel, D., Kemmerer, D., Damasio, H., Adolphs, R., and Damasio, A. R. (2003). Neural correlates of conceptual knowledge for actions. *Cognitive Neuropsychology*, **20**: 409–32.

Tyler, L. K., Moss, H. E., Durrant-Peatfield, M., and Levy, J. (2000). Conceptual structure and the structure of categories: A distributed account of category-specific deficits. *Brain and Language*, **75**: 195–231.

Ungerleider, L. G. and Mishkin, M. (1982). Two cortical visual systems. In D. J. Ingle, M. A. Goodale and R. J. W. Mansfield (eds.), *Analysis of Visual Behavior*. Cambridge, MA: MIT Press.

Van Hoesen, G. W. (1982). The primate parahippocampal gyrus: New insights regarding its cortical connections. *Trends in Neuroscience*, **5**: 345–50.

Warren, C. and Morton, J. (1982). The effects of priming on picture recognition. *British Journal of Psychology*, **73**: 117–29.

Warrington, E. K. (1975). The selective impairment of semantic memory. *Quarterly Journal of Experimental Psychology*, **27**: 635–57.

Warrington, E. K. (1981). Neuropsychological studies of verbal semantic systems. *Philosophical Transactions of the Royal Society of London*, **B295**: 411–23.

Warrington, E. K. and McCarthy, R. (1983). Category-specific access dysphasia. *Brain*, **106**: 859–78.

Warrington, E. K. and McCarthy, R. (1987). Categories of knowledge: Further fractionations and an attempted integration. *Brain*, **110**: 1465–73.

Warrington, E. K. and McCarthy, R. (1994). Multiple meaning systems in the brain: a case for visual semantics. *Neuropsychologia*, **32**: 1465–73.

Warrington, E. K. and Shallice, T. (1984). Category-specific semantic impairments. *Brain*, **107**: 829–54.

Whatmough, C., Chertkow, H., Murtha, S., Templeman, D., Babins, L., and Kelner, N. (2003). The semantic category effect increases with worsening anomia in Alzheimer's type dementia. *Brain and Language*, **84**: 134–47.

Zannino, G. D., Perri, R., Carlesimo, G. A., Pasqualetti, P., and Caltagirone, C. (2002). Category-specific impairment in patients with Alzheimer's disease as a function of disease severity: A cross-sectional investigation. *Neuropsychologia*, **40**: 2268–79.

Zingeser, L. B. and Berndt, R. S. (1988). Grammatical class and context effect in a case of pure anomia: implications for models of language production. *Cognitive Neuropsychology*, **5**: 473–516.

Zingeser, L. B. and Berndt, R. S. (1990). Retrieval of nouns and verbs in agrammatism and anomia. *Brain and Language*, **39**: 14–32.

Part II

Insights from Electrophysiology

3

Functional modularity of semantic memory revealed by event-related brain potentials

John Kounios

Drexel University

Theorists have faced a lack of consensus about basic properties of mind and brain. Of these basic properties, perhaps the most important is whether mind and brain are best conceived of as consisting of a number of independently functioning processing modules (e.g. Donders, 1868; Posner & Raichle, 1994; Sternberg, 1969, 1998, 2001), or rather as a single entity consisting of a large number of massively interacting parts (e.g. Anderson, 1995; Rumelhart, McClelland, & the PDP Research Group, 1986). Answering this question is extremely important, because the answer necessarily directs the course of both theory construction and experimentation in cognitive psychology and cognitive neuroscience, and the study of semantic memory in particular.

As a contribution toward clarifying this issue, this chapter demonstrates how *event-related potentials* (ERPs) can be used to detect, isolate, and analyze functional neural modules, with special attention to functional modularity in semantic information processing. The method and analyses described in this chapter are also applicable to the closely related technique of magnetoencephalography (MEG; Hämäläinen, Hari, Ilmoniemi, Knuutila, & Lounasmaa, 1993), as well as to ERPs. The approach described here is based on a well-known physical property of electric fields in a volume conductor such as the brain, namely, that electric fields generated by separate sources combine by summation (Kutas & Dale, 1997; Nunez, 1981, 1990). Expanding on earlier work (Kounios, 1996; see also Kounios & Holcomb, 1992; Sternberg, 2001), this chapter shows how factorial experimental design can enable independent manipulation of these separate sources, yielding additive contributions to the aggregate electric field detectable at the scalp. This allows detection of the functional independence of the populations of

The author thanks Theodore Bashore, Phil Holcomb, Frank Norman, and Allen Osman for helpful discussions and suggestions. Special thanks go to Saul Sternberg for many detailed and insightful suggestions and comments on a previous draft of this article. Preparation of this article was supported by PHS Grants MH57501 and DC04818 to J.K. Correspondence may be sent to John Kounios at Department of Psychology, Drexel University, 245 N. 15th Street, MS 626, Philadelphia, PA 19102–1192, or by e-mail to john.kounios@gmail.com.

neurons that generate these fields. These functionally independent neuronal populations are operationally defined as *functional modules*.[1] The view on which this approach is based differs from previous views, in that it describes modularity as a dynamic, emergent property of processing, rather than as a collection of structural constraints. As shown below, this approach clarifies important issues central to research on semantic information processing.

3.1   Modularity versus interactionism

Proponents of modularity (e.g. Posner & Raichle, 1994) often cite the work of Donders (1868) as their intellectual forerunner. Donders assumed that mental processes were organized as a sequence of independent processing stages whose individual durations sum to yield the overall time elapsing between stimulus and response. The assumed independence of these stages formed the basis for his subtraction method in which stages could, by a judicious choice of experimental manipulations, be selectively inserted or deleted from the sequence without influencing the durations of the other stages. Sternberg (1969) extended and refined this conception into the *additive-factor method*, which dispenses with the strong "pure insertion" assumption that underlies the subtraction method. Instead, he proposed the principle that additivity of factor effects on mean reaction time suggests that separate, independent processing stages (or sets of stages) are selectively influenced by the two experimental factors, while an interaction between factor effects indicates that the two factors affect at least one stage in common (see Sternberg, 1998, for a review). Such processing stages may be considered an example of one type of cognitive module, specifically, of processing modules organized in a temporal sequence.

As in Donders' method, brain imaging studies using positron emission tomography (PET) or functional magnetic resonance imaging (fMRI) also frequently employ a type of subtraction that assumes modularity. According to this approach, a brain image acquired in a baseline or control condition is subtracted from an image acquired in one or more experimental conditions. This procedure is assumed to isolate areas of the brain involved in task-relevant processing in the

---

[1] At least two distinct ways of defining *module* can be found in the literature. Many neuroscientists (e.g. Arbib, Erdi, & Szentagothai, 1998; Mountcastle, 1979) use the term to refer to neuroanatomical units (e.g. cortical columns) that combine to form larger and more complex structural entities (e.g. a cortical lobe). In contrast, cognitive psychologists and cognitive neuroscientists typically do not define a module in morphological terms, but rather in terms of its functional independence from other modules. For example, Sternberg (2001) defined a module simply as a distinct part (e.g. a processing stage) that can be modified separately from other parts. This chapter builds on the latter notion and defines a module as a population of neurons that functions independently of other neuronal populations, therefore enabling it to be influenced selectively.

experimental condition that are less active in the control condition. It has been argued that this subtractive approach is a spatial analog of Donders' temporal subtraction method in that it assumes that focal differences in cerebral metabolism or blood volume indicate that specific, localizable neural modules are selectively influenced by experimental manipulations while other modules remain unaffected (Posner & Raichle, 1994).

Neuropsychologists typically study the effects of brain lesions on performance in a variety of cognitive tasks. The fact that such lesions can selectively impair specific cognitive faculties is sometimes understood to mean that brain and mind are of modular construction and that a focal lesion can impair or destroy a single module, leaving others relatively intact (see Farah, 1994, with following commentaries by various authors, for a critical discussion of this view).

In contrast, the massive structural interconnectivity of the brain has been cited as evidence against the existence of strongly independent processing modules. For instance, Mountcastle (1998) wrote:

Cortical nerve cells are organized in highly specific patterns into many systems, which are heavily connected with one another; the number of interconnections between nerve cells in the neocortex reaches an astronomical figure... They are so numerous that it is unlikely that any portion of the brain ever functions in complete isolation from other parts; the signal processing systems of the brain are distributed in nature. (p. xiii)

Consequently, neural network modelers construct parallel distributed processing (PDP) models consisting of hundreds or thousands of primitive, highly inter-connected, neuron-like processors. Such models are thought to be more "neurally plausible" and "brain-like" (e.g. Rumelhart *et al.*, 1986), and have been used in attempts to explain the focal effects of brain lesions on a variety of cognitive functions (e.g. Hinton, Plaut, & Shallice, 1993). In essence, these models are *equipotential* in that they represent knowledge as a pattern of weights on connections between all the units in a network, not over just a particular region of it (Hinton, McClelland, & Rumelhart, 1986).

There are also intermediate positions in this debate. Fodor (1983) has argued that "input systems" subserving perception and language comprehension are reflexive and strongly modular, while downstream "central processes" are neces-sarily nonmodular because they must be able to integrate different types of information from different sources. Such integration presupposes interaction among processes. Fodor further argued that the nonmodularity of central processes makes them difficult or impossible to analyze experimentally, because such analyses presuppose dissection of something that is necessarily unitary.

Another type of intermediate position has been taken by neural network modelers who have incorporated modular principles into hybrid semi-connectionist networks. For example, Jacobs, Jordan, and Barto (1991) proposed an information-processing architecture consisting of a number of independently functioning modules, with each module consisting of a PDP network. Each module learns to compute a different function through competition. This arrangement allows a complex task to be decomposed into independent subtasks that can be individually addressed by the modules. Jacobs *et al.* argued that such an architecture can exhibit superior task generalization, speed of learning, and efficiency in terms of hardware implementation (see also Jacobs, 1997; cf. Kounios, 1993).

Generally speaking, the theoretical and methodological approaches just described either assume some form of modularity or interactionism, or utilize other strong assumptions or models in order to infer some position on this matter. Taking a different approach, this chapter demonstrates how ERPs can be used to reveal the existence of independently functioning processing modules in the brain and, by inference, in the mind. After a brief introduction to relevant aspects of the ERP technique, the foundations and logic of this approach are explained and illustrated with two empirical examples that demonstrate functional modularity in semantic information processing. This is followed by conclusions and suggestions for further developments.

3.2   Event-related brain potentials

If electrodes are attached to a person's scalp, and if the electrical signals measured at these sites are appropriately amplified and filtered, then one can measure that person's ongoing electroencephalogram (EEG), namely, that part of the brain's electrical activity that is measurable at the scalp. If the EEG is recorded while a person participates in a task involving discrete stimulus events, then the segments of EEG following (or preceding) presentations of each instance of that class of stimuli can be averaged, yielding the event-related potential, or ERP. Such signal averaging serves to eliminate the contribution to the ERP of electrical activity not correlated with instances of the critical stimulus event, such as brain activity associated with the control of autonomic or other regulatory functions, or brain activity associated with irrelevant stimuli, whether internal or external, that impinge on the subject. The resulting ERP waveform therefore constitutes a moment-by-moment average record of aggregate brain activity associated with the presentation of members of a class of stimuli. In fact, external stimuli are not the only discrete events that can be used as a basis for averaging EEG signals in order to extract an ERP. For example, one could average segments of EEG preceding behavioral responses (e.g. button presses), thereby yielding a record of brain activity correlated with response preparation and execution (e.g. Coles, 1989; Osman & Moore, 1993). In principle, one could even average segments of EEG preceding or following an internal event, as long as that event has a temporally discrete onset that could be measured precisely. (For a discussion of the technical foundations of the ERP technique, see Picton, Lins, & Scherg, 1995.)

It is important to keep in mind that neural activity measured in this way constitutes only a part of the brain's total electrical activity associated with an event. Some activity of interest is likely to be invisible because it is too faint to be measured through the relatively nonconductive skull. This may be particularly true of certain kinds of subcortical activity. Nevertheless, under appropriate conditions, even brainstem potentials can be measured at the scalp (see Hillyard & Picton, 1987). However, a more interesting (and useful) restriction on the domain of ERP measurement results from a consideration of the origins of these signals.

3.2.1   Prerequisites for ERP generation

Neuronal activity induces extracellular current flow, though the electric field that an individual neuron generates is too weak to be detectable at the scalp. Scalp potentials are therefore understood to reflect the summed extracellular current flow associated with a relatively large number of individual neurons (Martin, 1991; Nunez, 1981; Picton *et al.*, 1995). However, the detection of such summed electrical fields depends on three necessary conditions. First, the activity of these neurons must be nearly synchronous so as to result in temporal summation. Second, sufficient spatial summation of the individual neuronal electrical fields must exist. Such spatial summation occurs when neurons are in close physical proximity. And third, the contributing neurons must be arranged geometrically in parallel (i.e. in a sheet). If this third condition is not met, then the electrical fields of individual neurons will tend to cancel each other out and not yield a measurable scalp potential (for discussions, see Hillyard & Picton, 1987; Kutas & Dale, 1997).

As for the temporal summation requirement, the flow of current that yields a measurable ERP is thought to be primarily associated with postsynaptic potentials rather than much briefer action potentials, the brevity of the latter (e.g. approximately 1–10 ms) likely yielding insufficient synchrony to result in substantial temporal summation (Martin, 1991; Picton *et al.*, 1995). Furthermore, the notion that neurons performing closely related functions are situated in close proximity (i.e. the spatial proximity requirement) is supported by (a) the high degree of structural differentiation of the brain, (b) the focal effects of lesions sometimes, and (c) the fact that the activity of proximal neurons (e.g. those within a cortical column) tends to be more highly correlated than that of distal neurons (e.g. those located within different columns; see Kandel, Schwartz, & Jessell, 1995, ch. 18, 19, 23). And finally, much of the brain does consist of sheets of neurons in parallel formation. This is particularly true of pyramidal cells which proliferate in the cortex and which perform a variety of critical information-processing functions (Crick & Asanuma, 1986).

3.2.2 Conclusions

The fact that ERPs can be measured at the scalp indicates that the conditions of synchrony, spatial proximity, and parallel geometrical configuration that enable the summation of individual neuronal electric fields must hold. The existence of measurable ERPs therefore suggests the existence of localized, functionally related populations of neurons. Furthermore, as discussed below, the fact that features of the ERP correlate with theoretically meaningful experimental manipulations substantiates the notion that the localized populations of neurons that generate these scalp potentials are performing important information-processing functions (for reviews, see Hillyard & Picton, 1987; Kutas & Dale, 1997; Rugg & Coles, 1995).

3.3 Levels of analysis

It is important to note that ERP research can involve several levels of analysis. All of these levels do not necessarily play an active conceptual role in every ERP study. Nevertheless, each level is potentially important and can suggest and constrain theoretical inference. These levels are delineated here, because distinguishing among them clearly is necessary for understanding the logic described below.

3.3.1 Scalp potentials

The first level of analysis concerns the signal-averaged ERPs measured at the scalp. These ERP waveforms exhibit positive and negative deflections which are manifestations of theoretical entities known as *components*, and are named according to their polarity (*P* for positive, *N* for negative), and either their latency in milliseconds (e.g. N400) or poststimulus order (e.g. P3). Various parameters of these components, such as their amplitudes and peak latencies, can provide evidence concerning the complexity and timing of cognitive processes (Rugg & Coles, 1995). In addition, ERPs are almost always measured at multiple sites on the scalp using an array of electrodes. This provides a moment-by-moment *topographic distribution* of scalp potentials that supplements wave morphology.

The amplitudes of these potentials across electrode sites (at a given point in time or averaged over an interval of time) can be plotted as a topographic map (Wong, 1991). Such topographic profiles can be used to distinguish components and can also be used to make inferences concerning the number and location of neural sources (e.g. Mangun, Hillyard, & Luck, 1993; Nobre & McCarthy, 1995a; Wong, 1991).

3.3.2   Intracranial potentials

Scalp potentials afford a selective view of another level of analysis, namely, the electric fields within the brain. These electric fields are attenuated and smeared due to the insulating properties of the skull and scalp (Nunez, 1981), complicating the task of inferring the neural sources of these signals based solely on the measurement of scalp potentials. Intracranial potentials are of great interest because they potentially offer a more detailed view of the electrical activity of the brain and because they are easier to localize. They can sometimes be directly measured in clinical populations using electrodes placed on the cortical surface or implanted within the brain (e.g. McCarthy, Nobre, Bentin, & Spencer, 1995; Nobre & McCarthy, 1995b). However, for ethical and practical reasons, intracranial potentials cannot be measured in healthy brains.

3.3.3   Processors

As mentioned, these electrical fields are generated by the summed postsynaptic activity of populations of temporally synchronous, spatially parallel, neurons in close physical proximity. Such neuronal populations constitute another level of analysis, here termed *neural processors.*[2] These processors are arranged according to a functional architecture, probably at least partially ad hoc in nature, constituting a pattern of interconnection allowing for intercommunication and transmission of information in a purposeful fashion (Schweickert, 1993). As will be shown below, some processors are modular in that they function independently of other processors. Henceforth, processors are abstractly denoted by italicized lowercase letters: *a, b, c,* etc.

3.3.4   Factorial design

Another level of analysis concerns factorial experimental design. A typical ERP study minimally involves at least one experimental factor with two or more levels

---

[2] It is likely that there are neural processors engaged in information processing that do not consist of temporally synchronous, spatially parallel neurons in close physical proximity and which therefore do not yield ERPs detectable at the scalp, for example, subcortical nuclei forming closed fields (see Hillyard & Picton, 1987). Such processors are beyond the scope of this chapter and the method it describes.

(e.g. two types of stimuli) and an electrode-site (i.e. topographic) factor reflecting the use of multiple electrodes (McCarthy & Wood, 1985), or, as required for the method described below, at least two experimental factors with two or more levels each, plus an electrode-site factor.

When at least two types of stimuli are used in an experimental design, it is possible to compare the morphology and topography of the ERP responses in the two experimental conditions. The fact that stimulus factors can differentially influence characteristics of the ERP response indicates that the factors differentially influence the relevant neural processors. Henceforth, experimental factors are denoted by italicized capital letters: *A*, *B*, *C*, etc.

3.4   ERP amplitude

ERP amplitude, the voltage difference between a scalp electrode and a reference electrode, is determined by several factors. As mentioned, the primary determinant is the summed postsynaptic potentials on the dendrites of cortical pyramidal cells aligned in a parallel, sheet-like formation. If there are several regions in the brain fitting this characterization, then the electric fields generated by these sources each contribute (as discussed below) to the scalp potential. There are, however, other important determinants of scalp-recorded potentials, both structural and nonstructural.

3.4.1   Structural factors

As for relevant structural considerations, the depth of the neurons involved is an important determinant. All things being equal, deep processors contribute less to the ERP than do superficial ones. Furthermore, the orientation of the relevant neurons is an important factor. Because of the shape of the electric field generated by a dipolar source, radially oriented cells (e.g. cells on the crest of a gyrus) contribute more to the ERP than do neurons oriented tangentially to the scalp surface (e.g. those on the wall of a sulcus). Other anatomical determinants of the scalp ERP include the thickness and conductivity of the layers of brain tissue, cerebrospinal fluid, skull, scalp, and other tissues interposed between the source of the electric field and an electrode. Such structural features are important considerations when localizing in the brain the sources of the ERP.

3.4.2   Nonstructural factors

There are two major nonstructural influences on the amplitude of the ERP. First, the number of cells contributing to the field potential is an important consideration, as a processor consisting of a relatively small number of neurons is less likely to have a discernible impact on the ERP than a processor consisting of a relatively large number of neurons. Second, the degree of temporal and spatial summation of these neurons is also relevant. For example, increased synchrony of neuronal (postsynaptic) activity will yield greater spatial summation, allowing the relevant neurons to contribute more to the ERP. Such non-structural factors are important to ERP research, because they show that the technique is sensitive to brain activity directly implicated in neural information processing.

3.5   The analysis of ERP topography

ERP scalp topography provides information about task-related functional neuroanatomy, though the relationship between ERP topography and this underlying functional neuroanatomy is not always straightforward (Wong, 1991). There are two uses for such topographic analysis. First, one can use topography as the basis for localizing the neural sources of the ERP (e.g. Gevins, 1996; Pascual-Marqui *et al.*, 1994; Scherg, 1990). Second, a more modest goal of topographic analysis is to determine whether topographic differences obtained in two experimental conditions are the result of differences in the underlying functional neuroanatomy without specifically localizing these differences. While both of these types of analyses are valuable uses of topography, localization is not an immediate goal of the present method. Instead, simply determining that differences between the topographies corresponding to the main effects of two experimental factors are due to differences in the underlying functional neuroanatomy is sufficient for isolating neural modules. The present discussion therefore focuses on the latter type of topographic analysis. One technique for analyzing the topography of ERP amplitudes is to perform an ANOVA using one or more experimental factors and one or more electrode-site factors. For instance, a significant $A \times E$ interaction (where E is an electrode-site factor) might be interpreted as meaning that the different levels of the A factor yield different scalp topographies. However, as McCarthy and Wood (1985) pointed out, for physical reasons, this kind of inference can be incorrect. This is because ANOVA assumes an additive model, whereas an electric field in a volume conductor such as the brain does not diminish as a linear function of the distance of an electrode from the source of the field, but instead, as the inverse square of this distance (Nunez, 1981). This means that a significant $A \times E$ interaction could result solely from a difference between the levels of Factor A in ERP amplitude, even if the different levels of A have the same topographic contour over the scalp.

By way of analogy, two objects could have identical shapes but differ only in size. In this case, the two objects are physically different. However, if the size difference were eliminated, then, given that the objects have the same shape, they would be identical. Similarly, by eliminating amplitude (i.e. "size") differences, one can more easily ascertain whether there are any purely topographic (i.e. "shape") differences.

In order to avoid interactions that spuriously suggest topographic differences between two experimental conditions, McCarthy and Wood (1985) recommended that significant $A \times E$ interactions be followed up by re-analysis after normalizing the amplitudes in each condition in order to eliminate the main effect of Factor A. In other words, after the mean amplitudes for each level of Factor A have been equated (leaving untouched the distribution of amplitudes across the scalp within each level of A), a significant $A \times E$ interaction would therefore indicate that the different levels of A exhibit significantly different topographic distributions of amplitudes.

Since the method described here requires at least two experimental factors, an important goal of a topographic analysis is to determine whether the main effect of Factor A has a topography different from that of Factor B. In an experimental design consisting of two experimental factors with two levels each, the relevant interaction is therefore $[A - B] \times E$, where $[A - B]$ is the difference between the main effects of A and B. In other words, if the main effect of A (i.e. $A_1 - A_2$ for each electrode site) minus (for each electrode site) the main effect of B (i.e. $B_1 - B_2$ for each electrode site) has any topographic distribution other than a uniform (i.e. flat) one, then the main effects of A and B have different topographies, and therefore elicit qualitatively different patterns of brain activation. This, of course, presupposes that the amplitudes have been normalized such that the magnitudes of the main effects of A and B are the same (leaving intact the topographic distributions of these main effects). There are various ways to accomplish this. For the analyses described below, $(A - B) \times E$ interactions are reported as significant only if they reach statistical significance after the amplitudes of the main effects of A and B have been normalized by being vector scaled according to the procedure described by McCarthy and Wood (1985).

3.6   The additive-amplitude method

The *additive-amplitude method* for detecting and analyzing functional neural modules is based on three important principles: (a) linear superposition of electric fields, (b) spatial distinctiveness of neurocognitive systems, and (c) selective influence on neural processors.

3.6.1 Linear superposition

The physical principle of *linear superposition* states that electric fields generated by separate sources in a volume conductor such as the brain combine by summation (Kutas & Dale, 1997; Nunez, 1981, 1990). Consequently, the voltage (V) measured at a specific electrode on the scalp (e_1) is the weighted sum of contributions from various electrical sources ($s_1, s_2, \ldots s_n$),

$$V_{e1} = W_{e1s1}S_1 + W_{e1s2}S_2 + \ldots + W_{e1sn}S_n$$

where w_{es} represents a weight specific to each combination of electrode location and electrical source in the brain.

On a small scale, linear superposition of electric fields generated by the individual neurons constituting a processor results in a larger electric field in the brain that is, under certain circumstances, detectable at the scalp. On a larger scale, linear superposition enables the summing of electric fields generated by separate populations of neurons (i.e. separate neural processors) resulting in an aggregate electric field detectable at the scalp.

3.6.2 Spatial distinctiveness

The principle of *spatial distinctiveness* holds that "different cognitive systems will tend to be more spatially distinct within the brain than will a single cognitive system" (Holcomb, Kounios, Anderson, & West, 1999, p. 723). This implies that different cognitive mechanisms will yield different ERP scalp topographies (see below). More precisely, ERP topography results from the fact that the electrical brain sources that contribute to the ERP have different strengths, and that the contribution of each source to the voltage measured at an electrode is determined by a weight associated with the source and the electrode,

$$V_{e1} = W_{e1s1}S_1 + W_{e2s2}s_2 + \ldots + W_{e1sn}S_n$$

$$V_{e2} = W_{e2s1}S_1 + W_{e2s2}S_2 + \ldots + W_{e2sn}S_n$$

$$V_{e3} = W_{e3s1}S_1 + W_{e3s2}S_2 + \ldots + W_{e3sn}S_n$$

and so forth (where the weights are determined by structural and nonstructural factors, such as those described above). Obviously, if the relative strengths of the sources change, then the distribution of voltages across electrode sites will change. This can happen if an experimental manipulation causes a change in the relative strengths of the same sources, or if an experimental manipulation alters the set of brain sources that provide significant contributions to the ERP, thereby changing s and its associated W.

3.6.3 Selective influence

The principle of *selective influence* can, in this context, be considered an experimental strategy derived from a testable hypothesis about functional neuro-anatomy. This principle asserts that some neural processors can be selectively influenced by appropriate experimental manipulations, because these processors function independently of each other. In other words, if a particular experimental manipulation influences only Processor *a*, then Processor *a* can be selectively influenced. Another way to frame this notion is that, in a given situation, the operation of Processor *a* may be *invariant* with respect to the operation of all other task-relevant processors and, conversely, that the operation of all other task-relevant processors is invariant with respect to the operation of Processor *a*. This principle is related to the notion of separate modifiability and invariance of cognitive processes (Sternberg, 2001) as employed in the additive-factor method for analyzing reaction-time data from factorial experiments (Sternberg, 1998). However, the additive-factor method is based on a general model in which cognitive processes are organized in a temporal sequence of independent stages whose individual durations combine by summation to yield total reaction time. In contrast, the additive-amplitude method makes no assumption about a combination rule – it is well known from physics that simultaneous electric fields in a volume conductor combine by summation. Consequently, the additive-amplitude method does not require strong assumptions about neural information-processing architecture.

3.7 Overview of the method

The basic principle underlying the additive-amplitude method can be summarized (and oversimplified) as follows: If two or more processors function independently of each other during a given time-window (i.e. *epoch*) in a factorial experiment, that is, if the operation of each of these processors is invariant with respect to the other (and all other task-relevant processors), then the electric fields generated by these neuronal populations will yield additive contributions to the amplitude of the scalp ERP during this same time-window. Because the term "additivity" indicates that the effects of one factor are *invariant* with respect to the effects of another factor (Sternberg, 1998), there is additivity even at an electrode site at which one factor has a significant effect while a second factor has no discernible effect due, for instance, to the distance of the electrode from the source of the electric field influenced by the second factor or the geometrical orientation of this source with respect to one or more electrodes. If these processors do not function independently of each other (e.g. because of intercommunication enabling mutual influence between processors or because their corresponding neuronal populations overlap), then they will yield interacting contributions to ERP amplitude within that time-window. This logic is, in principle, straightforward, though in practice it is more complicated. The various empirical possibilities and their corresponding theoretical interpretations are presented below. In particular, an important scenario in which two experimental factors have additive effects at some electrode sites, but not at every electrode site, is discussed. This is followed by two examples from recent experiments that illustrate the use of the method.

3.7.1   Case 1: Amplitude additivity at every electrode site

The first case minimally involves an $A \times B \times E$ factorial experiment in which A and B are experimental factors (e.g. stimulus variables) and E is an electrode-site factor. If additivity between the effects of the A and B factors is obtained, that is, if the main effect of Factor A on ERP amplitude is invariant with respect to the levels of Factor B (and vice versa) within a given epoch, then the independence of (inferred) Processors a and b is tentatively suggested (where Processors a and b are selectively influenced by Factors A and B, respectively). For the purpose of explication, we restrict the discussion to a simple case in which there is a one-to-one mapping between factors and processors (Factor A influences Processor a, Factor B influences Processor b, etc.). In fact, it may frequently be the case that the activity of multiple processors located in different regions of the brain can form a single distributed network such that these processors effectively constitute a single functional unit (i.e. a *processor complex*) and therefore respond in concert to the manipulation of a particular factor. Fortunately, principles of the additive-amplitude method described within the context of the simple scenario utilized for the purpose of exposition apply equally well to these more complex situations. Specifically, any processor isolated using the additive-amplitude method in a particular experiment may actually be a processor complex to be further analyzed by including additional factors into the experimental design. Including additional factors makes it possible to selectively influence and decompose the component neuronal populations comprising the complex.

Next, suppose that the topographic distribution of the Factor A effect on ERP amplitude is different from the topographic distribution of the Factor B effect (i.e. a significant $[A - B] \times E$ interaction, see below). In this case, additivity of the effects of A and B in conjunction with different topographies for the main effects of these two factors yields two important conclusions: (a) that two nonidentical neural processors (or sets of processors — see below), a and b, are involved, and (b) that these processors function independently of each other. Again, this conclusion results from two premises: (1) amplitude additivity indicates independent contributions to ERP amplitude, and (2) different scalp topographies corresponding to the main effects of Factors A and B indicate that nonidentical neuronal populations are generating these effects (Wong, 1991). This logic makes an additional minor assumption. As noted above, a difference in ERP topography between two experimental conditions can occur when the experimental manipulation involved serves to change which processors are involved, or serves to change only the relative strengths of the electric fields generated by the processors involved. The latter can occur when the synchrony of the postsynaptic potentials associated with the processors changes without necessarily influencing which neurons are participating in these processors. According to this latter scenario, a difference in topography can result from changing the relative (phase-locked) synchrony of neuronal populations associated with each processor without changing the neuronal populations themselves. In this highly specific case, a change in topography does not reflect a qualitative difference in the underlying functional neuroanatomy.

In contrast, additive effects of A and B combined with topographies that are not discernibly different suggest three possibilities. First, the issues of statistical power and spatial resolution of the ERP scalp topography must be examined, as an insufficiency of either could make it difficult to resolve topographic differences and detect a real underlying $(A - B) \times E$ interaction. A second, alternate, interpretation is that additivity of the main effects of Factors A and B combined with the absence of an $(A - B) \times E$ interaction could suggest that a single processor may be responsible for the obtained additivity. For instance, such a pattern could result if the processor in question linearly sums outputs from two other selectively influenced (and undetected) processors. This might occur if the detected processor sums inputs correlated with the summed postsynaptic potentials of the neurons in the two undetected processors, a highly specific and perhaps unlikely scenario. A third possibility is that additivity of A and B combined with the absence of an $(A - B) \times E$ interaction could result from two independently functioning processors, a and b, that, in a sense, occupy the "same" physical location in the brain, hence yielding the same topographic distribution. This could occur, for example, if the two processors consist of nonoverlapping sets of spatially interleaved cortical columns. This interpretation has a well-known precedent, namely, the existence in striate cortex of alternating ocular dominance columns preferentially responding to the right or left eye.

In any event, though additivity of the effects of A and B combined with different topographies suggests the presence of independent a and b modules (or sets of modules), this should be followed up by tests for an $A \times B$ interaction separately at each electrode site. If additivity does not hold at all electrode sites, that is, if there is an $A \times B$ interaction at a minimum of one electrode site, then the situation reverts to the last scenario (Case 3), in which there is at least one additional processor, c.

3.7.2   Case 2: Factors interact at all electrode sites

Another common pattern of results occurs when there is a significant $A \times B$ interaction, suggesting that Processors a and b are non-independent (e.g. because of mutual influence or because their corresponding neuronal populations overlap). The inference that these nonindependent processors are also nonidentical would be substantiated by the existence of different topographies for the main effects of Factor A and Factor B. If, on the other hand, the main effects of Factors A and B have the same topography (assuming ample statistical power and an optimal electrode configuration), then either two (or more) interacting processors are occupying approximately the same physical space in the brain, or only one processor is responsible for the observed interaction. In either case, there is no direct evidence of independent modules.

As in the previous scenario, tests should be done to determine whether there is an $A \times B$ interaction at all electrode sites. If additivity is present at a minimum of one electrode site, then, as explained next, there is evidence of modularity.

3.7.3   Case 3: Factors interact at some sites

Suppose that Factors A and B have different scalp topographies, and follow-up tests are done to determine whether there is a significant $A \times B$ interaction at each electrode site. If the $A \times B$ interaction is significant at every electrode site, then the interpretation given above holds: there is no evidence of modularity. However, a more interesting and complicated scenario occurs when there are significant $A \times B$ interactions at some sites, while additivity is evident at other sites.

If additivity is evident at a minimum of one electrode site, then the basic interpretation of additivity given above holds: it is caused by the independent functioning of two neural processors. However, additivity of two electric fields should theoretically be present everywhere (i.e. at every electrode site) because of the principle of linear superposition in a volume conductor. The failure to find additivity everywhere, when present anywhere, is therefore inferred to be due to the presence of at least one additional processor (i.e. separate from the modular neural Processors a and b) that generates an electric field that regionally obscures the detection of the additivity of the electric fields generated by Processors a and b. This third processor, c (or set of Processors $c, d, e, \ldots$, etc.), could obscure this additivity at only a subset of the total set of electrode sites because its geometrical orientation and location may limit the spatial scope of its detectability over the scalp. More specifically, the dipolar source constituting Processor c might be oriented so that its contribution to the aggregate electric field is detectable over only a circumscribed area of the scalp. These considerations lead to the principle that additivity at any electrode site indicates that there is an underlying additivity that would be detectable at every electrode site if the contribution of one or more "obscuring" processors could be removed.

This principle carries with it an important implication that must always be kept in mind during any analysis of ERP topography. Specifically, the presence of an obscuring Processor c (or multiple obscuring Processors c, d, e, etc.) could, under certain circumstances, obscure underlying additivity of a and b at *every* electrode site, or at least at every electrode site exhibiting significant main effects of Factors A and B. This implies that an $A \times B$ interaction present at each electrode site could be masking an underlying independence between a and b, and that such independence may or may not be uncovered by more detailed analyses or further experimentation. How could Processor c obscure additivity between Processors a and b (or obscure additive effects produced by a single processor) at any or all electrode sites? For c to obscure $a + b$ independence, the minimal requirement is that the activity of c be influenced by both Factors A and B and that their effect on c be interactive. For instance, an additive relationship between the effects of Factors A and B can be disrupted when an additional contribution is made to the measured amplitude in just one cell of an $A(2) \times B(2)$ factorial design. In contrast, if Processor c is influenced only by Factor A or only by Factor B, then observed $A + B$ additivity is preserved at all electrode sites. Another way to think about this is that if Processor c were influenced only by Factor A and not by Factor B, then Processors a and c could be grouped together as a single functional unit (or *processor complex*) that functions independently of b. Similarly, if Processor c were only influenced by Factor B, then Processors c and b could be thought of as a single processor complex that functions independently of Processor a.

Nevertheless, it should be kept in mind that such a pattern does not necessarily imply communication or mutual influence between the obscuring Processor c and either a or b. Processor c could also be a module. For instance, c could theoretically lie on a separate parallel stream of information processing such that a, b, and c are simultaneously and independently responding to information transmitted to them by processors that were active in an earlier epoch. According to this scenario, if Processor c is directly and interactively influenced by the same experimental factors (A and B) that selectively influence Processors a and b, then effects on Processor c arising from a conjunction of levels of Factors A and B can obscure $A + B$ factor additivity at some (or all) electrode sites. In this case, Processor c is a module because its function is independent of a and b. This also means that Processor c would not be influencing Processors a or b, because this would disrupt the observed functional independence of a from b and b from a that would be manifested as $A + B$ additivity at some electrode sites. (This is because B could then influence a indirectly through c, and A could then influence b indirectly through c.) Alternately, Processor c could respond to the conjunction of levels of

Factors A and B because of direct or indirect influence of Processors a and b on c. In this case, Processor c would not be a module.[2]

Does additivity at a subset of the electrodes necessarily implicate the participation of one or more obscuring processors responding to both Factors A and B? There is one scenario under which topographically circumscribed additivity could be a result of two interactive processors. Specifically, if two interactive neural processors yield statistical interactions of opposite sign and if the neurons constituting these processors are oriented radially with respect to the scalp, then the respective statistical interaction effects corresponding to these processors may perfectly cancel each other out at a subset of electrodes. Such an alternate explanation for additivity can be assessed by examining the scalp topography of the $A \times B$ interaction effect. If the plotted interaction effect shows a region of additivity (i.e. zero interaction) sandwiched between a region of positive interaction and a region of negative interaction, then canceling interaction effects may be producing the region of additivity.

Another interesting scenario (strictly speaking belonging to Case 2) occurs when a close approximation to additivity does not occur at any individual electrode sites, but the largest $A \times B$ interaction effect (i.e. at any electrode site) showing the joint influence of Factors A and B (i.e. $[(A_1B_1 - A_2B_1) - (A_1B_2 - A_2B_2)]$) is of very small magnitude relative to the size of the main effects of Factors A and B, but is statistically significant. Under these circumstances, the most useful characterization of the neural information-processing architecture is either "leaky" modularity, in which Processors a and b exhibit only a small degree of interactivity, or an alternate situation in which a third (interactive) Processor c has only a faint electrophysiological signature on the scalp (e.g. due to its depth, nonoptimal geometrical configuration, etc.). According to the leaky modularity notion, the topographic distribution of the $A \times B$ interaction effect should be similar to the topographic distributions of the main effects, because Processors a and b generate both the main effects and the interaction effect. In contrast, if this weak interaction effect has a scalp topography that is qualitatively different from those of the main effects, then there is at least one interactive Processor c present which yields an electrophysiological signature which is faint not because of leaky modularity, but rather for other reasons, such as the depth of the interactive source.

3.8   Modularity as revealed by the additive-amplitude method

What is the nature of the modularity potentially revealed by the additive-amplitude method? Fodor (1983) listed a number of characteristics of modularity, consonant with his theoretical scheme (see also Coltheart, 1999). Arguably, the most important of these characteristics are that a putative module must be: (a) *reflexive*, in that its operation should be automatically triggered by appropriate stimuli and be difficult to alter or inhibit once begun; (b) *domain specific*, in that it should process only a particular type of information and not process other types of information; and (c) *encapsulated* from the influence of other processes. The additive-amplitude method does not directly address the issues of reflexivity and domain specificity, although appropriate ERP experimentation taking advantage of principles of the method may shed light on these properties. Instead, the additive-amplitude method reveals the existence of independently functioning, separately modifiable, neural processors, and allows inferences to be made about the nature of these processors. However, such modules need not function independently of each other across tasks, or even across different epochs within a particular task. In fact, there is no a priori reason why a specific neural processor might not be engaged more than once over the time-course of processing (or for an extended period of time defined as a single epoch), enjoying functional independence during certain time-windows, but not during others. Consequently, the modules in question are defined less stringently than Fodor's modules. They are context-specific in that they are defined only in terms of encapsulation from other processes active in a particular task during a particular epoch. Fortunately, employing a less specific definition of modularity does not weaken the theoretical implications of results obtained with the additive-amplitude method. For instance, as will be evident from the empirical examples presented below, modules defined according to these less stringent criteria need not be confined to upstream "input systems," as hypothesized by Fodor; instead, such modularity can be present during late epochs of processing that should, according to Fodor, be dominated by integrative, domain general, equipotential, "central" processes.

3.9   Statistical considerations

3.9.1   Additivity and acceptance of the null hypothesis

As described, the additive-amplitude method is essentially a tool for detecting and analyzing neural modules. However, the determination that encapsulated modules are present is dependent on the necessary (but insufficient) failure of an $A \times B$ interaction term to achieve statistical significance at one or more electrode sites. Acceptance of the null hypothesis is, obviously, a delicate matter, as impractical levels of statistical power may be necessary in order to detect a minute, but real, interaction (see recent discussions by Frick, 1995a; Hagen, 1997; commentaries by Edgell, 1995; Falk, 1998; Granaas, 1998; Malgady, 1998; McGrath, 1998; Thompson, 1998; Tryon, 1998; and replies by Frick, 1995b; Hagen, 1998). (This issue is also a concern in applying Sternberg's additive-factor method.)

However, in the case of the additive-amplitude method, the interpretation of such situations is more complicated. A significant $A \times B$ interaction present at each electrode site used in an experiment does not necessarily mean that an additive relation between A and B would not have been detected at one or more sites if other scalp sites had been sampled (i.e. by placing the electrodes at other locations). This will become much less of an issue as more ERP laboratories acquire the capability of recording electrical brain activity from dense electrode arrays, thereby improving the spatial sampling of electrical brain activity. Nevertheless, as explained above, even if an $A \times B$ interaction were detected at every possible location on the scalp, this does not necessarily indicate the absence of encapsulated modules, because interactive obscuring processors could, in principle, hinder the detection of additivity everywhere on the scalp. So, for the present purposes, the detection of additivity is much more useful than the failure to detect it.

These considerations suggest the application of strict criteria for accepting the null hypothesis, certainly stricter than the failure of an interaction term to achieve statistical significance. However, under some circumstances, one might be inclined to mitigate such rigor, so as to avoid "throwing the baby out with the bathwater," because a very small, but statistically significant, interaction could suggest that if one electrode had been placed perhaps 1 or 2 cm away from its actual location (i.e. to a new location at which the electric field generated by an obscuring processor cannot be detected), then additivity could have been observed. Nevertheless, it is probably unproductive to speculate about what results would have been obtained if an experiment had been executed differently. It is more productive to simply rearrange or increase the number of electrodes in order to improve spatial sampling. Consequently, there is no profit in adopting relaxed criteria for declaring additivity. Such a conclusion should be based only on a very close approximation to additivity obtained at a minimum of one electrode site.

3.9.2 Multiple comparisons

A related issue concerns the relatively large number of statistical tests that may be involved in applying the additive-amplitude method. Conventional statistical practice requires the use of special procedures (e.g. Bonferroni, Scheffe, etc.) when multiple comparisons are performed, in order to safeguard against statistically significant effects that are random and spurious. However, in the case of the additive-amplitude method, it is specifically the absence of such interactions that is of potential theoretical importance. Hence, adjustments of alpha to compensate for a large number of comparisons would increase the risk of incorrectly failing to reject the null hypothesis (of additivity). Consequently, no such adjustments were made in the analyses presented below. Instead, in order to minimize both Type 1 and Type 2 error, modularity was inferred only when the obtained results closely approximated additivity, and not just when an interaction term failed to achieve statistical significance.

The relative theoretical ambiguity of significant and omnipresent interactions coupled with the greater inferential power of additive results illustrate the important point that standard notions of hypothesis testing are not precisely applicable to additive-amplitude analyses. In conventional statistical analyses, rejection of the null hypothesis is typically given a strong interpretation, while failure to reject the null hypothesis is typically treated as ambiguous because there may actually have been an effect that was too small to detect with the available statistical power. However, according to the additive-amplitude method, a statistically significant $A \times B$ interaction at every electrode site is treated as a comparatively "weak" result that does not, by itself, support strong inference, because such an interaction may, or may not, be masking true $a + b$ independence (i.e. modularity). Again, only a very close approximation to additivity at a minimum of one electrode site can permit a strong theoretical inference (except for the "leaky modularity" scenario described above). One possible criticism of this approach is that the absence of procedures to compensate for the execution of multiple comparisons could make it probable that randomly obtained additivity is obtained at one electrode site. This should not be a serious concern, because the stricter the criterion for accepting the null hypothesis and declaring additivity (e.g. an arbitrarily small interaction effect), the less likely it will be that such results are obtained by chance. Of course, in the extreme case, if perfect additivity is the criterion, then obtaining additivity is, for all practical purposes, impossible (see the discussion of this point by Hagen, 1997).

It should also be kept in mind that such ERP data are usually infested with noise from many more sources than are likely to influence, for instance, reaction-time data. For example, electrodes will inevitably not be placed on precisely the same locations on the heads of different participants. Furthermore, there are considerable individual differences in both head shape and size, as well as in brain morphology and functional neuroanatomy. Additionally, if a particular time-window is used for measuring average ERP amplitude, then both within- and between-subject variability in the latency of one or more target ERP components could mean that this time-window is not optimal (for each trial or each participant) for measuring the amplitudes of those components. These are just a few of the sources of noise that should conspire against obtaining additive amplitudes. Given these statistical considerations, the failure of an interaction term to achieve statistical significance should not be surprising. Conversely, these same considerations render a close approximation to additivity all the more salient.

The following examples consist of additive-amplitude analyses of ERP data from two semantic memory experiments. These examples illustrate important patterns of results yielded by the method. The first reveals additivity at a subset of the electrode sites, indicating the presence of at least two modules plus a processor responding to both factors in the 2×2 design. The second reveals additivity at all the electrode sites, which provides evidence for only two modules. More importantly, these examples demonstrate functional modularity of semantic processing.

3.10   Example 1: Concreteness, context, and modularity in sentence comprehension

The first example is based on data from a study of concreteness effects on sentence comprehension (Holcomb, Kounios, Anderson, & West, 1999, corresponding conditions of Experiments 1 and 2, combined) that was originally intended to test competing predictions of the dual-coding theory of Paivio (1986) and the context-availability model of comprehension (e.g. Kieras, 1978; Schwanenflugel & Shoben, 1983; for a comparison and discussion, see Holcomb *et al.*, 1999; Kounios & Holcomb, 1994). More specifically, these theories seek to explain the pervasive finding that concrete verbal materials (e.g. the word *eagle*) are generally processed more quickly and accurately than abstract verbal materials (e.g. the word *liberty*). Dual-coding theory posits separate imaginal and verbal representation and processing systems, and explains the processing advantage for concrete materials as resulting from their being represented and processed in both systems, while abstract materials are represented and processed only in the verbal system. In contrast, the context-availability model argues against multiple systems or types of representations, and explains concreteness effects as resulting from greater internal supportive context (i.e. more or stronger links to related concepts) associated with concrete words. Consistent with this notion, Schwanenflugel and Shoben (1983) have shown that the (reaction-time) processing advantage for concrete words disappears when both concrete and abstract words are embedded in an external supportive context intended to compensate for the relative lack of internal context associated with abstract words. They therefore concluded that the concreteness factor is reducible to a manipulation of context. However, these findings have been reinterpreted to signify that concreteness and context are, in fact, theoretically separate factors that both influence the duration of a common stage of processing (Holcomb *et al.*, 1999; Kounios & Holcomb, 1994).

Furthermore, Holcomb *et al.* showed that the main effects of word concreteness and contextual fit of the final word of a sentence into the preceding sentence frame (i.e. context) have different topographic ERP distributions, indicating that concreteness and context have different functional neuroanatomical substrates, thereby supporting some variant of dual-coding theory.

An additive-amplitude analysis of data from the Holcomb *et al.* study is presented next. The goal is to provide a more stringent test of the notion that the concreteness and context factors manipulate fundamentally different neural and cognitive processes. In particular, the analyses presented below were undertaken with the aim of determining whether concreteness and context might be processed by independently functioning neural modules, with the integration of these two types of information occurring in one or more additional processors that respond interactively to both factors.

Only those aspects of the data relevant to the analysis and interpretation of ERP amplitude additivity are described here. Similarly, the experimental design, selection of stimuli, and specific procedures are only summarized. For a detailed description, see Holcomb *et al.* (1999).

Forty right-handed native English-speaking participants viewed sentences, one word at a time, on a computer monitor. Each word was displayed for 200 ms with an 800 ms stimulus–onset asynchrony. The final word of each sentence (which included the sentence-ending period) rendered the sentence either congruous (i.e. meaningful) or anomalous (i.e. without a straightforward meaning). Half of these final words were concrete (e.g. *rose*) and half were abstract (e.g. *fun*). Similarly, half of the sentence stems leading up to the final word were concrete (e.g. *Armed robbery implies that the thief used a* _____), and half were abstract (e.g. *Lisa argued that this had not been the case in one single* _____). It is the ERPs to the final words of the anomalous sentences that are the focus of the present example, in particular, the anomalous-sentence conditions forming a 2 (abstract versus concrete sentence-stem) × 2 (abstract versus concrete final-word) design.

Subjects' EEGs were measured with 13 electrodes distributed across the scalp (referenced to the left mastoid). These consisted of midline frontal (Fz), central (Cz), and parietal (Pz) electrodes, plus left and right frontal (F7/8), left and right anterior-temporal (ATL/R), left and right temporal (TL/R), left and homologous-right Wernicke's area (WL/R), and left and right occipital (O1/2) electrodes.

The grand-average final-word ERPs for the four types of anomalous sentences were computed. For the purposes of the present analyses, average ERP amplitudes were calculated for each of these conditions for two separate epochs: 300–500 and 500–800 ms. These epochs correspond roughly to the latencies of the N400 and LPC (Late Positive Complex) waves observed in previous studies employing visually presented linguistic materials (e.g. Kounios & Holcomb, 1992, 1994; for reviews, see Kounios, 1996; Kutas & van Petten, 1994; Osterhout & Holcomb, 1995). These two epochs are focused on here because they are relatively late during the time-course of processing and might therefore be expected to reflect integrative control processes (e.g. Fodor, 1983). In particular, the N400 component has been specifically hypothesized to reflect a semantic integration mechanism (e.g. Kounios, 1996; Osterhout & Holcomb, 1995).

For each time-window, these average ERP amplitudes were subjected to separate repeated-measures analysis of variance (ANOVAs) using data from the lateral and from the midline electrode sites using the Geisser–Greenhouse correction where appropriate (Geisser & Greenhouse, 1959). The significance of interactions involving an electrode-site factor (e.g. Word-Concreteness × Hemisphere) was checked by an identical analysis using normalized ERP amplitudes (see below); analyses of the normalized amplitudes are reported here where appropriate. Main effects and interactions involving only topographic factors (i.e. Hemisphere and Anterior–Posterior electrode-site) were ignored, as were three- and four-way interactions involving the Stem, Word, and one or both topographic factors. Different topographies for the stem-concreteness and final-word concreteness main effects were detected by examining the (Word–Stem) × Electrode-Site interactions. A significance criterion of 0.05 was used.

In addition to the overall ANOVAs described above, tests were done to determine the significance at each electrode site of the 2×2 interaction of the stimulus factors. This test was done for each electrode site irrespective of the results of the overall ANOVA, because the significance of interactions in the overall ANOVA is influenced (in unpredictable ways) by the number and placement of electrode sites used in the analysis. Furthermore, as discussed, performing a large number of such follow-up tests does not risk inappropriate inference, because any spuriously significant interactions that result from using this criterion would not indicate additivity, but instead would suggest a relatively ambiguous pattern of results. Only a close approximation to additivity present at a minimum of one electrode site can, by itself, permit a strong theoretical inference.

3.10.1 Results

300–500 ms

Global analyses were performed in order to detect overall main effects, interactions, and topography. These global analyses demonstrated main effects of the Stem and Word factors, and scalp topographies that differed along the anterior–posterior dimension for these main effects. There was, however, no evidence of an interaction between the stimulus factors. Specifically, an ANOVA on the lateral-electrode amplitudes for the 300–500 ms (i.e. N400) time-window yielded significant main effects of sentence Stem ($F[1,39] = 29.77$, $p < 0.0001$) and Word ($F[1,39] = 60.73$, $p < 0.0001$) concreteness, and a significant Word × Anterior–Posterior ($F[4,156] = 33.61$, $p < 0.0001$) interaction. An ANOVA on the midline-electrode amplitudes yielded significant main effects of Stem ($F[1,39] = 48.10$, $p < 0.0001$) and Word ($F[1,39] = 30.29$, $p < 0.0001$), and a significant Word × Anterior–Posterior interaction ($F[2,78] = 12.25$, $p < 0.001$). The (Word–Stem) × Hemisphere × Anterior–Posterior test for distinguishing between the topographies of the Stem and Word effects yielded a significant (Word–Stem) × Anterior–Posterior interaction ($F[4,156] = 13.63$, $p < 0.0001$). The analogous test for the midline electrodes yielded a significant (Word–Stem) × Anterior–Posterior interaction ($F[2,78] = 5.60$, $p = 0.005$). The most important results from the 300–500 ms epoch are depicted graphically in Figure 3.1 and can be summarized as follows. Figure 3.1 shows the ERP amplitudes (y-axis, in microvolts) of the Word (i.e. Concrete-Word minus Abstract-Word)

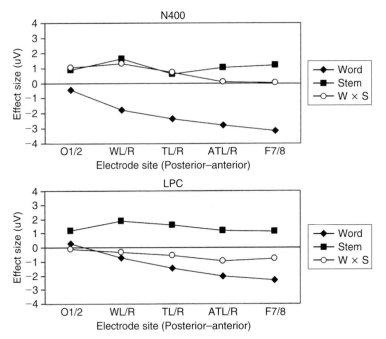

Figure 3.1.   Plot of Word and Stem main effects and Word × Stem interaction effect (in microvolts, on y-axis) as a function of electrode site (posterior to anterior sites shown from left to right on the x-axis). The top panel shows results for the 300–500 ms time-window; the bottom panel shows corresponding results for the 500–800 ms time-window. See text for explanation.

and Stem (i.e. Concrete-Stem minus Abstract-Stem) main effects and the Word × Stem interaction effect (i.e. [(Concrete-Stem/Concrete-Word minus Concrete-Stem/Abstract-Word) minus (Abstract-Stem/Concrete-Word minus Abstract-Stem/Abstract-Word)]) at lateral electrode sites going from the back of the head to the front (i.e. left to right on the x-axis). For simplicity of presentation, and because there were no relevant hemispheric effects, the x-axis collapses across homologous left- and right-hemisphere electrode sites. The corresponding results for the midline electrodes follow the pattern shown for the lateral electrodes and are not shown in Figure 3.1. This graphical summary of effect-size topographies shows that the Word effect is largest at anterior sites and gradually diminishes (i.e. towards zero) posteriorly. In contrast, the Stem effect has a relatively flat topography across the scalp, with a maximum at the Wernicke sites. ANOVA shows that the Word and Stem effects had significantly different topographies (see below), suggesting nonidentical neuroanatomical substrates. The topography of the Word × Stem interaction effect showed another pattern, namely, it was largest at the Wernicke sites and virtually non-existent at anterior sites. The interaction effects are only 0.09 and 0.02 microvolts at the anterior–temporal and lateral–frontal electrodes, respectively. In contrast, the interaction effects at the posterior electrodes are much larger, for example, 1.56 microvolts at the parietal-midline electrode. Furthermore, the main effects are even larger, for example, greater than 3 microvolts at some sites.

These observations are substantiated by the individual-electrode analyses, which, for the sake of brevity, are summarized as follows. For the lateral sites, there was a significant main effect of Stem at each electrode, and a significant main effect of Word at all but the occipital sites (which yielded a marginally significant Word effect). The Wernicke sites yielded a significant Stem × Word interaction; this interaction was marginally significant at the occipital sites and nonsignificant at the temporal ($F[1,39] = 2.00$, $p > 0.16$), anterior–temporal ($F[1,39] = 0.00$, $p > 0.98$), and lateral–frontal sites ($F[1,39] = 0.01$, $p > 0.91$). For the midline electrodes, there were significant main effects of Stem and Word at each site, with the Stem X Word interaction being non-significant at the central ($F[1,39] = 2.44$, $p > 0.12$) and frontal ($F[1,39] = 0.25$, $p > 0.62$) sites.

To summarize, there are two important points to keep in mind. First, according to the additive-amplitude method, the additivity (i.e. a virtually nonexistent interaction effect) at frontal sites indicates that processors influenced by the Stem and Word factors are independent of each other, but that there is at least one additional processor with a posterior scalp focus that obscures this additivity at posterior electrodes. Second, the fact that the two stimulus factors exhibit different topographic distributions suggests the involvement of nonidentical functional neuroanatomies corresponding to the two main effects.

500–800 ms

Analyses of data from the 500–800 ms epoch again demonstrate significant main effects of the two stimulus factors that differ in topography along the anterior–posterior dimension. Specifically, an overall ANOVA on the lateral-electrode amplitudes yielded main effects of Stem ($F[1,39] = 29.14$, $p < 0.0001$) and Word ($F[1,39] = 27.80$, $p < 0.0001$). The midline analysis also yielded main effects of Stem ($F[1,39] = 51.14$, $p < 0.0001$) and Word ($F[1,39] = 13.98$, $p < 0.001$). The (Word–Stem) × Hemisphere × Anterior–Posterior test yielded significant (Word–Stem) × Anterior–Posterior interactions for the lateral ($F[4,156] = 13.63$, $p < 0.0001$) and midline ($F[2,78] = 5.36$, $p < 0.0005$) electrodes indicating different topographies for the two stimulus factors. The bottom panel of Figure 3.1 graphically depicts the magnitudes of the Word, Stem, and interaction effects for the 500–800 ms interval in exactly the same way as for the 300–500 ms epoch. Note once again the tendency toward a frontal focus for the Word effect compared to the flatter topography of the Stem effect. Examination of the interaction effect yields no evidence of the frontal additivity of the Stem and Word factors seen in the 300–500 ms epoch. There was a significant Stem × Word interaction at the anterior–temporal sites ($F[1,39] = 5.51$, $p < 0.03$). The other electrodes sites do not show a significant interaction between these factors, though the inference of additivity is persuasive only at the occipital sites (Stem × Word interaction for occipital sites: $F[1,39] = 0.03$, $p > 0.86$; interaction effect: -10.10 microvolts). The occipital sites showed a significant effect of Stem ($F[1,39] = 16.37$, $p < 0.001$), though they did not show a significant effect of Word ($F[1,39] = 1.24$, $p > 0.27$). Nevertheless, this does not complicate the interpretation of additivity, because the Stem effect was apparently invariant with respect to the levels of the Word factor at the occipital sites, even though the electrophysiological manifestation of the Word effect was not detectable at that location. In contrast, the midline sites showed no evidence of additivity.

ANOVAs for the lateral sites yielded a significant main effect of Stem at each site, and a significant main effect of Word at each site, except for the occipital ones. The Stem × Word interaction was significant only at the anterior–temporal sites ($F[1,39] = 5.51$, $p < 0.03$). The individual-electrode analyses for the midline electrodes yielded a significant main effect of Stem at each midline site. The Word effect was significant at the central and frontal sites, but was nonsignificant at the parietal site.

3.10.2 Discussion

The results from Example 1 show evidence of ERP amplitude additivity at a subset of the electrodes during both of the epochs examined. This additivity was particularly striking during the 300–500 ms epoch employed in the analysis of activity during the time-window of the N400 component. According to the additive-amplitude method, this indicates the involvement of at least three neural processors, at least two of which were modular and responded to one of the stimulus factors. The third was influenced by both the Stem and Word factors. These results are consistent with a model in which information about the final word and information about the preceding context are represented separately and independently, while a third processor is responsible for the attempt to integrate these two types of information. This interpretation is particularly interesting because it suggests that the attempt at integration does not automatically override, overwrite, or absorb the separate representations of the word and context information. This is logical, as any attempt at integration subsequent to an initial unsuccessful attempt (as might be the case for such anomalous sentences) must avail itself of the separate pieces of information to be integrated. Overwriting these original representations during the initial attempt would render this impossible, thereby precluding error correction. These results also provide evidence against the context availability model of comprehension, because they show that concreteness is not reducible to context; these two types of information are processed by separate modules and integrated in a nonequipotential fashion.

3.11   Example 2: Repetition, relatedness, and semantic satiation

Example 2 is a re-analysis of data drawn from a study of semantic verification (Kounios, Holcomb, & Kotz, 2000, Experiments 2a and 2b, combined) designed to examine neural correlates of the *semantic satiation effect*, whereby massed repetitions of a word can lead to a subjective and temporary loss of the meaning of the word and can interfere with associated semantic processing (e.g. Balota & Black, 1997; L. C. Smith, 1984; L. C. Smith & Klein, 1990). One goal of this study was to determine whether the semantic satiation effect is truly semantic in origin, or whether it is a byproduct of sensory satiation or adaptation. Consequently, the number of prime repetitions and the semantic relatedness of the prime and critical item were factorially manipulated with the goal of determining whether repetition and relatedness interact.

This study involved auditory presentation of sequences of 17 nouns (embedded in a continuous stream) with a stimulus–onset asynchrony of 750 ms. Five percent of the words referred to a part of the body (e.g. hand, ear, etc.). The subject's task was to press a button immediately upon hearing such a word. This task was adopted in order to induce subjects to attend to the meaning of the words, but was not itself of primary interest. The other items in each sequence consisted of a single critical noun following either 1 or 15 presentations (i.e. "low" versus "high" levels of the prime *Repetition* factor) of another (context) noun which was either semantically related or unrelated to the critical noun (i.e. the *Relatedness* factor). The focus here is on the ERP responses to these critical related and unrelated nouns which followed either 1 or 15 presentations of the context noun. The number and placement of electrode sites were identical to those used in the study discussed in Example 1, as were other details of the EEG recording. Thirty-six right-handed, native English speakers participated.

3.11.1 Results

The ERPs for related and unrelated critical words following low and high prime repetition are shown in Figure 3.2. This figure displays the same electrode sites shown in Figure 3.1 (for a detailed discussion, see Kounios *et al.*, 2000). The present additive-amplitude analyses focus on quantified ERP amplitudes for two epochs: 400–600 (N400) and 600–800 (Late Positive Complex) ms. The ERPs from Example 2 were parsed into time-windows that were slightly

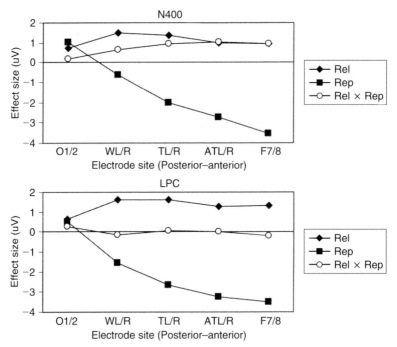

Figure 3.2.   Plot of Repetition and Relatedness main effects and Repetition X Relatedness interaction effect (in microvolts, on *y*-axis) as a function of electrode site (posterior to anterior sites shown from left to right on the *x*-axis). The top panel shows results for the 400–600 ms time-window; the bottom panel shows corresponding results for the 600–800 ms time-window. See text for explanation.

different from those used in Example 1 (i.e. 400–600 and 600–800 ms, rather than 300–500 and 500–800 ms) because auditory linguistic stimuli such as those used in Example 2 yield ERPs with a somewhat different morphology and time-course relative to those resulting from comparable visual linguistic stimuli.

400–600 ms

As was done for Example 1, global analyses were performed in order to detect overall main effects, interactions, and topography. A repeated-measures ANOVA on the ERP amplitudes from the lateral electrodes for the 400–600 ms epoch yielded significant main effects of Repetition ($F[1,35] = 20.90$, $p = 0.0001$) and Relatedness ($F[1,35] = 32.03$, $p < 0.0001$), plus the following interactions: Repetition $\times$ Relatedness ($F[1,35] = 6.81$, $p = 0.01$), Repetition $\times$ Hemisphere ($F[1,35] = 10.67$, $p < 0.0025$), Repetition $\times$ Anterior–Posterior ($F[4,140] = 35.56$, $p < 0.0001$), Relatedness $\times$ Anterior–Posterior ($F[4,140] = 5.37$, $p < 0.02$), and Repetition $\times$ Hemisphere $\times$ Anterior–Posterior ($F[4,140] = 5.24$, $p < 0.005$). The corresponding ANOVA for the midline electrodes yielded a significant main effect of Relatedness ($F[1,35] = 42.99$, $p < 0.0001$), and the following significant interactions: Repetition $\times$ Relatedness ($F[1,35] = 7.08$, $p < 0.02$), Repetition $\times$ Anterior–Posterior ($F[2,70] = 75.63$, $p < 0.001$), and Relatedness $\times$ Anterior–Posterior ($F[2,70] = 3.70$, $p < 0.05$). A (Repetition – Relatedness) $\times$ Hemisphere $\times$ Anterior–Posterior analysis for the lateral sites demonstrated that the main effects of Repetition and Relatedness had different scalp topographies. This analysis yielded a significant interaction of the (Repetition–Relatedness) difference with the Anterior–Posterior electrode-site factor ($F[4,140] = 18.40$, $p < 0.001$), indicating a different front–back distribution for the two factors. An ANOVA for the midline electrode sites yielded a comparable interaction ($F[2,78] = 70.63$, $p < 0.001$). Figure 3.2 (top panel) depicts the Repetition, Relatedness, and interaction effects across lateral sites (collapsed across hemispheres). The most important aspects of this figure can be summarized as follows. There was convincing evidence of additivity of the Repetition and Relatedness effects only at the occipital sites (interaction effect at occipital sites: 0.18 microvolts). The other lateral sites all indicate a Repetition $\times$ Relatedness interaction. The Repetition effect has a more anterior focus than the Relatedness effect.

To summarize the statistical analyses of the lateral sites, there was a significant main effect of Relatedness at each level of the Anterior–Posterior electrode-site factor, as well as a significant main effect of Repetition at each site except the Wernicke sites. In addition, there was a significant Repetition $\times$ Relatedness interaction at each site except for the occipital sites (and the lateral frontal sites which had a marginally significant interaction, $p < 0.10$). At the midline sites, there was a significant main effect of Relatedness at each site, and a significant main effect of Position at the frontal and central sites, and a marginally significant effect of Position at the parietal site ($p < 0.10$). The Position × Relatedness interaction did not approach significance at any of the midline sites.

600–800 ms

Again, global analyses were performed in order to detect overall main effects, interactions, and topography. An ANOVA on the amplitudes at the lateral electrodes from the 600–800 ms epoch yielded significant main effects of Repetition ($F[1,35] = 29.96$, $p < 0.0001$) and Relatedness ($F[1,35] = 61.84$, $p < 0.0001$). The following interactions were also significant: Repetition × Hemisphere ($F[1,35] = 5.32$, $p < 0.03$), Repetition × Anterior−Posterior ($F[4,140] = 22.31$, $p < 0.0001$), Relatedness × Anterior−Posterior ($F[4,140] = 4.63$, $p < 0.03$), and Repetition × Hemisphere × Anterior−Posterior ($F[4,140] = 4.21$, $p = 0.01$). The corresponding midline analysis yielded significant main effects of Position ($F[1,35] = 28.25$, $p < 0.001$) and Relatedness ($F[1,35] = 52.90$, $p < 0.001$), with the following significant interactions: Position × Anterior−Posterior ($F[2,70] = 90.32$, $p < 0.001$) and Relatedness × Anterior−Posterior ($F[2,70] = 5.49$, $p < 0.02$). Neither the Position × Relatedness ($F[1,35] = 0.02$, $p = 0.89$) nor the Position × Relatedness × Anterior−Posterior interactions approached significance ($F[2,70] = 0.05$, $p = 0.88$). A (Repetition−Relatedness) ×Hemisphere × Anterior−Posterior analysis (lateral sites) yielded significant interactions of the (Repetition−Relatedness) difference with the Anterior−Posterior electrode-site factor ($F[4,140] = 10.96$, $p < 0.001$) and with the Hemisphere factor ($F[1,35] = 4.95$, $p = 0.03$), indicating different front−back topographic distributions for the two factors. The corresponding midline-site analysis also yielded a significant interaction with the Anterior−Posterior factor ($F[2,78] = 65.96$, $p < 0.001$).

Figure 3.2 (bottom panel) shows the topographies and magnitudes of the Repetition, Relatedness, and interaction effects. The most striking finding is that additivity is closely approximated at all the sites. The average main effects (across electrode sites) of Repetition and Relatedness were 2.44 and 1.62 microvolts, respectively. In contrast, the average Repetition × Relatedness interaction effect was only 0.03 microvolts. In addition, it is apparent that the Repetition effect had a more anterior focus than the Relatedness effect.

3.11.2 Discussion

Example 2 shows evidence of amplitude additivity at both a subset of the sites (i.e. the occipital sites from 400 to 600 ms) and at all sites (from 600 to 800 ms).

According to the additive-amplitude method, the results from the 400–600 ms epoch suggest the operation of at least three processors (or three sets of processor complexes), two of which were modular and were influenced by only one factor each, while the third processor was influenced by both experimental factors. In the 600–800 ms epoch, the evidence suggests omnipresent additivity. In combination with the different scalp topographies of the Repetition and Relatedness effects, such additivity indicates at least two neural modules.

The results from Example 2 bear an interesting relationship to the results from Example 1. In both examples, there was evidence of at least two independently functioning modules, each responding to one of the experimental factors. Furthermore, both examples showed evidence of at least one additional processor that was influenced by both stimulus factors. This latter processor (or processor complex) hypothetically represents an integration mechanism that somehow utilizes or attempts to combine different types of information. Speculatively, the two stimulus factors employed in Example 2 may have selectively influenced automatic and attentional priming mechanisms (Neely, 1977; Posner & Snyder, 1975). For instance, it is likely that subjects realized that as a run of repeated items progresses, it becomes increasingly probable that the next stimulus will be different. The Repetition effect may represent a mechanism sensitive to such strategic concerns. In contrast, the knowledge that the identity of the next stimulus is likely to be different from that of the last stimulus is uninformative about the semantic relationship between successive items: the next item may be different from the current one, but this does not predict whether that different item will be closely related to the current one. This lack of predictability suggests that the Relatedness effect reflects an automatic semantic priming mechanism. It is plausible that these two types of information are somehow integrated during word recognition, in this case by the interactive processor operating during the 400–600 ms epoch. This interactive processor is not discernibly active during the 600–800 ms epoch, possibly because word recognition is likely complete by 600 ms. The persistence of activity in the modules sensitive to relatedness and prime repetition may, as was hypothesized in Example 1, reflect a property of retaining primitive information that would be available to subsequent integrative processes, in this case, processes that may involve the next word in the sequence. This contrasts with Example 1, which presented results from the final words of sequences that formed sentences; the end of each sentence may have elicited a closure operation that purged the primitive pre-integration information (i.e. the *sentence-ending positivity*, see Osterhout & Holcomb, 1995; cf. Verleger, 1988). Interestingly, the topographies of these two effects are broadly consistent with this scenario. The Repetition effect had a frontal focus, suggesting a frontal source. The frontal lobes have been implicated in expectancy and the operation of strategic processes (Knight & Grabowecky, 1995). In contrast, the Relatedness effect appears to have a relatively flat topography, suggesting either deep (e.g. inferior temporal) or distributed sources. Foci of the Relatedness effect appear at the Wernicke and temporal electrodes, areas which are thought to be important to semantic information processing (e.g. McCarthy, Nobre, Bentin, & Spencer, 1995; Nobre & McCarthy, 1995b).

3.12   General discussion

The present chapter has focused on the classic issue of equipotentialism versus localizationism of brain function and its implications for the cognitive and neural substrates of semantic memory. In particular, it has been shown how a new method of analyzing electrophysiological data, the additive-amplitude method, combines the physical property of linear superposition of electrical fields with factorial experimental design to reveal the existence of encapsulated neurocognitive modules without relying on strong assumptions. Not only has the existence of these functional modules been demonstrated online, in intact brains, but these modules have also been demonstrated to function during a relatively late phase of the time-course of semantic information processing, a phase that even proponents of modularity such as Fodor (1983) have argued should be characterized by integrative "central" processes. Such results are incompatible with the pan-interactive, equipotential approach to conceptualizing neural and cognitive function embodied in many parallel-distributed processing models. Instead, these findings indicate a modular information-processing architecture possibly akin to the general framework proposed by Jacobs (1997; Jacobs *et al.*, 1991).

3.12.1   Integration

What implications do the present results have for the integrative processes that Fodor (1983) argued must exist? While few would call into question the need for processes that integrate different types of information (see McClelland, 1996, for a survey), Fodor's characterization of such processes may have been overspecified. Integration does not necessitate equipotentiality. For example, during the 300−500 ms (N400) epoch of Experiment 1, there was evidence for at least three processors, two frontally distributed ones which were modular and responded to only one experimental factor each (i.e. final-word or sentence-stem concreteness), and a third posteriorly distributed one which responded to both experimental factors. Because it responded to both experimental factors, this third processor may have subserved the role of attempting to integrate information about the final word with the preceding context, and is therefore a candidate for being a Fodorian central process. Apparently, this interaction-yielding posteriorly distributed processor coexists with the frontally distributed modules, indicating that it is not neurally equipotential and does not subsume the modules. As suggested above, such an arrangement allows for the possibility of repeated attempts at integration of the separate pieces of information, thereby enabling error correction of the integrative mechanisms. Hypothesized repeated attempts at integration may be manifested as reactivation of a processor (or processor complex), perhaps the one responsible for generating the N400. Detection of such a repeated component is possible, though it requires minimizing the between-trial variability that leads to temporal jitter that tends to blur ERP waves.

As previously discussed, such an additivity-obscuring processor can be responsible for a spatially regional interaction between two experimental factors in at least two different ways, namely, through influence from other concurrent processors which feed information into it, or through influence from earlier processors. According to the latter of these two scenarios, the interaction-yielding processor could itself be a module and not be directly influenced by concurrent processors.

3.12.2 Disclaimers

In addition to discussing what has been demonstrated with the additive-amplitude method, it is also important to note what these results do not show.

First, though the present evidence of modularity is incompatible with a pure (i.e. fully interconnected) parallel-distributed processing account of semantic processing, neither can the evidence be construed as support for the extreme form of neuropsychological inference (criticized by Farah, 1994) in which focal brain damage can obliterate a single module, leaving all the others functioning normally. In fact, the ERP results described above provide no evidence for the view that the brain incorporates fully encapsulated modules, a prerequisite for a strongly modular neuropsychology. For instance, the present results are not incompatible with a model in which a single neural processor could, in a specific task, function as an independent module during certain epochs, yet could function interactively with other processors during other epochs, either performing the same informa-tion processing function or a different one. Such context specificity is inconsistent with a strongly modular neuropsychology.

Second, it should be kept in mind that modules isolated with the additive-amplitude method are demonstrated to exist during a particular epoch. The issue of whether sequentially organized modules (e.g. discrete processing stages) exist in a specific task is orthogonal to the issue of whether such independent processors coexist during a given (relatively small) window of time. For instance, a discrete-stage architecture could be compatible either with different sets of simultaneous modules active during each stage, or with a group of massively interactive processors active during each stage, as long as task-related computations are performed sequentially with discrete transitions between successive stages (see Rumelhart, Smolensky, McClelland, & Hinton, 1986; Sternberg, 1998). Demonstration of such sequential organization of modules can be aided by behaviorally based methodologies (e.g. Kounios, 1996; Meyer *et al.*, 1988; R. W. Smith & Kounios, 1996; R. W. Smith, Kounios, & Osterhout, 1997; Sternberg, 1998).

And last, it should be kept in mind that ERPs, like all psychophysiological and brain-imaging techniques, are inherently correlational. By themselves, these techniques can only tell us that a particular brain region is active and that activity in this region is correlated with task performance. However, these techniques do not conclusively demonstrate that any particular brain region is actually performing a critical role in task-relevant information processing. One might therefore argue that while the additive-amplitude method may tell us that two or more neuronal populations are functioning independently of each other during a task, it cannot, by itself, conclusively prove that these independent neuronal populations are task relevant.

Fortunately, for at least two reasons, this problem is irrelevant to the general demonstration of neural modularity with the additive-amplitude method. First, while the additive-amplitude method in its present form does not absolutely guarantee that detected modules are relevant to performance in a given task, it nevertheless demonstrates the existence of functional neural modularity. The discovery of independently functioning neuronal populations, even if activity in these populations is really only correlated with activity in other, task-relevant, neuronal populations, still weighs against equipotential views of brain function in which all areas of the neocortex potentially influence each other. So the (unlikely) scenario in which epiphenomenal modules coexist with task-critical neural processors still implies that brain and mind have a modular structure.

Second, further experimentation should be able to establish that particular brain regions are playing a real functional role in task performance in three ways: (a) systematic comparison of activity across experiments should provide evidence that a specific brain region is playing a functional role; (b) lesion and transcranial magnetic stimulation studies can demonstrate the task-relevance of a brain structure by interfering with its function; and (c) localizing the neuronal populations responsible for ERP generation (see below) to specific areas of the brain facilitates using knowledge gained from other techniques as converging evidence.

3.13   Future directions

The additive-amplitude method yields new insights into semantic information-processing architecture. Additional insights can be gained with further development of this approach. First, the additive-amplitude method has the potential to more fully reveal the time-course of modular and non-modular processors. If additive-amplitude analyses are conducted using a series of small (e.g. 50–100 ms) epochs spanning the time-course of processing, then this should yield valuable evidence by pinpointing temporal regions of additivity at each electrode site, thereby helping to trace the time-course of modular and interactive processors.

Second, it would ultimately be highly desirable to know, by judicious manipulation of experimental factors, whether specific processors can be selectively inserted or deleted from the processing architecture without otherwise altering this architecture, as Donders' method of subtraction attempts for modules in the time-domain. Accomplishing this, however, requires spatially localizing these modules. If processors can be spatially localized in the brain, then their neuroanatomical locations can serve to uniquely identify each processor revealed by the method, making it possible to determine whether a specific processor is being inserted into or deleted from the overall processing architecture during a given epoch without otherwise altering this processing architecture. Furthermore, once processors are localized, it will then be possible to determine whether or not a specific processor is functioning across long epochs. These goals are now practical because the field of ERP source localization has undergone dramatic advances in recent years (e.g. see Gevins, 1996; Pascual-Marqui et al., 1994; Scherg, 1990), though the effective application of such techniques requires greater spatial sampling of electrical brain activity than could be accomplished with the number of electrodes available for the present experiments. However, with the increasingly common capability to use dense electrode arrays, possibly in conjunction with co-registered structural magnetic resonance imaging (MRI) (Kounios et al., 2001), such source localization techniques should greatly extend the power of the additive-amplitude method.

And finally, it should be noted that because the additive-amplitude method focuses on a fundamental property of mind and brain, it is applicable to a broad range of areas within psychology and neuroscience. In fact, this approach can be applied to any area that can be studied using the ERP (and MEG) techniques, including sensation, perception, attention, memory, language, thinking, action, and emotion, thereby raising general questions about functional modularity and the architecture of neural and cognitive information processing. For example, are interactive/integrative processors ever modular? If so, what differences are there between integrative and non-integrative modules? Is functional modularity organized or orchestrated by some type of central executive? Does functional modularity develop during childhood or is it hardwired from birth? Does modularity break down in old age, or does processing become overly modularized and thereby ossified? Does modularity emerge with practice during skill acquisition? Does modularization involve a cost in terms of the flexibility of processing? Is there a relationship between extent of modularization and personality, psychopathology, or various types of brain damage? Undoubtedly, pursuit of the answers to these questions will raise other issues not yet envisaged.

REFERENCES

Anderson, J. A. (1995). *An Introduction to Neural Networks.* Cambridge, MA: MIT Press.

Arbib, M. A., Erdi, P., and Szentagothai, J. (1998). *Neural Organization: Structure, function, and dynamics.* Cambridge, MA: MIT Press.

Balota, D. A. and Black, S. (1997). Semantic satiation in healthy young and older adults. *Memory & Cognition,* **25**: 190–202.

Coles, M. G. H. (1989). Modern mind–brain reading: psychophysiology, physiology, and cognition. *Psychophysiology,* **26**: 251–69.

Coltheart, M. (1999). Modularity and cognition. *Trends in Cognitive Sciences,* **3**: 115–20.

Crick, F. and Asanuma, C. (1986). Certain aspects of the anatomy and physiology of the cerebral cortex. In J. L. McClelland, D. E. Rumelhart, and the PDP Research Group (eds.), *Parallel Distributed Processing: Explorations in the microstructure of cognition. Volume 2: Psychological and biological models.* Cambridge, MA: MIT Press, pp. 333–71.

Donders, F. C. (1868). Over de snelheid van psychische processen. *Onderzoekingen gedaan in het Physiologisch Laboratorium der Utrechtsche Hoogeschool,* **2**: 92–100. Translated by W. G. Koster (1969) as *On the speed of mental processes.* In: *Attention and performance* **II**. Acta *Psychologica,* **30**: 312–41.

Edgell, S. E. (1995). Commentary on "Accepting the null hypothesis". *Memory & Cognition,* **23**: 525.

Falk, R. (1998). In criticism of the null hypothesis statistical test. *American Psychologist,* **53**: 798–9.

Farah, M. J. (1994). Neuropsychological inference with an interactive brain: a critique of the "locality assumption," *Behavioral & Brain Sciences,* **17**: 43–61.

Fodor, J. A. (1983). *The modularity of mind: An essay on faculty psychology.* Cambridge, MA: MIT Press.

Frick, R. W. (1995a). Accepting the null hypothesis. *Memory & Cognition,* **23**: 132–8.

Frick, R. W. (1995b). A reply to Edgell. *Memory & Cognition,* **23**: 526.

Geisser, S. and Greenhouse, S. (1959). On methods in the analysis of profile data. *Psychometrika,* **24**: 95–112.

Gevins, A. (1996). High resolution evoked potentials of cognition. *Brain Topography*, **8**: 189–99.

Granaas, M. M. (1998). Model fitting: a better approach. *American Psychologist*, **53**: 800–1.

Hagen, R. (1997). In praise of the null hypothesis statistical test. *American Psychologist*, **52**: 15–24.

Hagen, R. (1998). A further look at wrong reasons to abandon statistical testing. *American Psychologist*, **53**: 801–3.

Hämäläinen, M., Hari, R., Ilmoniemi, R., Knuutila, J., and Lounasmaa, O. V. (1993). Magnetoencephalography: theory, instrumentation, and applications to non-invasive studies of the working human brain. *Reviews of Modern Physics*, **65**: 413–97.

Hillyard, S. A. and Picton, T. W. (1987). Electrophysiology of cognition. In F. Plum (ed.), *Handbook of Physiology: Section 1. Neurophysiology*. Bethesda, MD: American Physiological Society.

Hinton, G. E., McClelland, J. L., and Rumelhart, D. E. (1986). Distributed representations. In D. E. Rumelhart, J. L. McClelland, and the PDP Research Group (eds.), *Parallel Distributed Processing: Explorations in the microstructure of cognition. Volume 1: Foundations*. Cambridge, MA: MIT Press, pp. 77–109.

Hinton, G. E., Plaut, D. C., and Shallice, T. (1993). Simulating brain damage. *Scientific American*, October, 76–82.

Holcomb, P. J., Kounios, J., Anderson, J. E., and West, W. C. (1999). Dual coding, context availability, and concreteness effects in sentence comprehension: an electrophysiological investigation. *Journal of Experimental Psychology: Learning, Memory, and Cognition*, **25**: 721–42.

Jacobs, R. A. (1997). Nature, nurture, and the development of functional specializations: a computational approach. *Psychonomic Bulletin & Review*, **4**: 299–309.

Jacobs, R. A., Jordan, M. I., and Barto, A. G. (1991). Task decomposition through competition in a modular connectionist architecture: the what and where vision tasks. *Cognitive Science*, **15**: 219–50.

Kandel, E. R., Schwartz, J. H., and Jessell, T. M. (1995). *Essentials of neural science and behavior*. New York: McGraw-Hill. Appleton & Lange.

Kieras, D. (1978). Beyond pictures and words: alternative information processing models for imagery effects in verbal memory. *Psychological Bulletin*, **85**: 532–54.

Knight, R. T. and Grabowecky, M. (1995). Escape from linear time: prefrontal cortex and conscious experience. In M. Gazzaniga (ed.), *The Cognitive Neurosciences*. Cambridge, MA: MIT Press, pp. 1357–71.

Kounios, J. (1993). Process complexity in semantic memory. *Journal of Experimental Psychology: Learning, Memory, and Cognition*, **19**: 338–51.

Kounios, J. (1996). On the continuity of thought and the representation of knowledge: electrophysiological and behavioral time-course measures reveal levels of structure in semantic memory. *Psychonomic Bulletin & Review*, **3**: 265–86.

Kounios, J. and Holcomb, P. J. (1992). Structure and process in semantic memory: evidence from event-related potentials and reaction times. *Journal of Experimental Psychology: General*, **121**: 459–79.

Kounios, J. and Holcomb, P. J. (1994). Concreteness effects in semantic processing: ERP evidence supporting dual-coding theory. *Journal of Experimental Psychology: Learning, Memory, and Cognition*, **20**: 804–23.

Kounios, J., Holcomb, P. J., and Kotz, S. (2000). Is the semantic satiation effect really semantic? Evidence from event-related brain potentials. *Memory & Cognition*, **28**: 1366–77.

Kounios, J., Smith, R. W., Yang, W., Bachman, P., and D'Esposito, M. (2001). Cognitive association formation in human memory revealed by spatiotemporal brain imaging. *Neuron*, **29**: 297–306.

Kutas, M. and Dale, A. (1997). Electrical and magnetic readings of mental functions. In M. D. Rugg (ed.), *Cognitive Neuroscience*. Cambridge, MA: MIT Press, pp. 197–242.

Kutas, M. and van Petten, C. (1994). Psycholinguistics electrified. In M. Gernsbacher (ed.), *Handbook of Psycholinguistics*. San Diego, CA: Academic Press, pp. 83–143.

Malgady, R. G. (1998). In praise of value judgments in null hypothesis testing . . . and of "accepting" the null hypothesis. *American Psychologist*, **53**: 797–8.

Mangun, G. R., Hillyard, S. A., and Luck, S. (1993). Electrocortical substrates of visual selective attention. In D. E. Meyer and S. Kornblum (eds.), *Attention & Performance XIV*. Cambridge, MA: MIT Press, pp. 219–44.

Martin, J. H. (1991). The collective electrical behavior of cortical neurons: the electroencephalogram and the mechanisms of epilepsy. In E. R. Kandel, J. H. Schwartz, and T. M. Jessell (eds.), *Principles of Neural Science*. East Norwalk, CT: Appleton & Lange, pp. 777–91.

McCarthy, G., Nobre, A., Bentin, S., and Spencer, D. (1995). Language-related field potentials in the anterior-medial temporal lobe: I. Intracranial distribution and neural generators. *Journal of Neuroscience*, **15**: 1080–9.

McCarthy, G. and Wood, C. C. (1985). Scalp distributions of event-related potentials: an ambiguity associated with analysis of variance models. *Electroencephalography and Clinical Neurophysiology*, **62**: 203–8.

McClelland, J. L. (1996). Integration of information: reflections on the theme of attention and performance XVI. In T. Inui and J. L. McClelland (eds.), *Attention and Performance XVI: Information integration in perception and communication*. Cambridge, MA: MIT Press, pp. 633–56.

McGrath, R. E. (1998). Significance testing: Is there something better? *American Psychologist*, **53**: 796–7.

Meyer, D. E., Irwin, D. E., Osman, A. M., and Kounios, J. (1988). The dynamics of cognition and action: mental processes inferred from speed-accuracy decomposition. *Psychological Review*, **95**: 183–237.

Mountcastle, V. B. (1979). An organizing principle for cerebral function: the unit module and the distributed system. In F. O. Schmitt and F. G. Worden (eds.), *The neurosciences: A fourth study program*. Cambridge, MA: MIT Press, pp. 21–42.

Mountcastle, V. B. (1998). *Perceptual neuroscience: The cerebral cortex*. Cambridge, MA: Harvard University Press.

Neely, J. H. (1977). Semantic priming and retrieval from lexical memory: roles of inhibitionless spreading activation and limited-capacity attention. *Journal of Experimental Psychology: General*, **106**: 226–54.

Nobre, A. C. and McCarthy, G. (1995a). Language-related ERPs: scalp distributions and modulation by word type and semantic priming. *Journal of Cognitive Neuroscience*, **6**: 233−55.

Nobre, A. C. and McCarthy, G. (1995b). Language-related field potentials in the anterior-medial temporal lobe: II. Effects of word type and semantic priming. *Journal of Neuroscience*, **15**: 1090−8.

Nunez, P. (1981). *Electric Fields of the Brain*. Oxford: Oxford University Press.

Nunez, P. (1990). Physical principles and neurophysiological mechanisms underlying event-related potentials. In J. W. Rohrbaugh, R. Parasuraman, and R. Johnson, Jr. (eds.), *Event-Related Brain Potentials: Basic issues and applications*. New York: Oxford University Press, pp. 19−36.

Osman, A. M. and Moore, C. M. (1993). The locus of dual-task interference: psychological refractory effects on movement-related brain potentials. *Journal of Experimental Psychology: Human Perception and Performance*, **19**: 1292−312.

Osterhout, L. and Holcomb, P. J. (1995). Event-related potentials and language comprehension. In M. Rugg and M. G. H. Coles (eds.), *Electrophysiology of Mind*. Oxford, UK: Oxford University Press, pp. 171−215.

Paivio, A. (1986). *Mental Representations: A dual coding approach*. Oxford: Oxford University Press.

Pascual-Marqui, R. D., Michel, C. M., and Lehmann, D. (1994). Low resolution electromagnetic tomography: a new method for localizing activity in the brain. *International Journal of Psychophysiology*, **18**: 49−65.

Picton, T. W., Lins, O. G., and Scherg, M. (1995). The recording and analysis of event-related potentials. In R. Johnson and J. C. Baron (eds.), *Handbook of Physiology, Volume 10*. Amsterdam: Elsevier, pp. 3−73.

Posner, M. I. and Raichle, M. E. (1994). *Images of Mind*. New York: Scientific American Library.

Posner, M. I. and Snyder, C. R. R. (1975). Facilitation and inhibition in the processing of signals. In P. M. A. Rabbitt and S. Dornic (eds.), *Attention and Performance V*. New York: Academic Press, pp. 669−82.

Rugg, M. and Coles, M. G. H. (eds.) (1995). *Electrophysiology of Mind*. Oxford: Oxford University Press.

Rumelhart, D. E., McClelland, J. L., and the PDP Research Group (1987). *Parallel Distributed Processing: Explorations in the microstructure of cognition. Volume 1: Foundations*. Cambridge, MA: MIT Press.

Rumelhart, D. E., Smolensky, P., McClelland, J. L., and Hinton, G. E. (1987). Schemata and sequential thought processes, In J. L. McClelland, D. E. Rumelhart, and the PDP Research Group (eds.), *Parallel Distributed Processing: Explorations in the microstructure of cognition. Volume 2: Psychological and biological models*. Cambridge, MA: MIT Press, pp. 7−57.

Scherg, M. (1990). Fundamentals of dipole source potential analysis. In F. Grandori, M. Hoke, and G.L. Romani (eds.), *Advances in Audiology, Volume 6: Auditory evoked magnetic fields and electric potentials*. Basel: Karger, pp. 40−69.

Schwanenflugel, P. and Shoben, E. (1983). Differential context effects in the comprehension of abstract and concrete verbal materials. *Journal of Experimental Psychology: Learning, Memory, and Cognition*, **9**: 82−102.

Schweickert, R. (1993). Information, time, and the structure of mental events: a twenty-five-year review. In D. E. Meyer and S. Kornblum (eds.), *Attention & Performance XIV*. Cambridge, MA: MIT Press, pp. 535–66.

Smith, L. C. (1984). Semantic satiation affects category membership decision time but not lexical priming. *Memory & Cognition*, **12**: 483–8.

Smith, L. C. and Klein, R. (1990). Evidence for semantic satiation: repeating a category slows subsequent semantic processing. *Journal of Experimental Psychology: Learning, Memory, and Cognition*, **16**: 852–61.

Smith, R. W. and Kounios, J. (1996). Sudden insight: all-or-none processing revealed by speed-accuracy decomposition. *Journal of Experimental Psychology: Learning, Memory, and Cognition*, **22**: 1443–62.

Smith, R. W., Kounios, J., and Osterhout, L. (1997). On the applicability and robustness of speed-accuracy decomposition, a technique for investigating partial information. *Psychological Methods*, **2**: 95–120.

Sternberg, S. (1969). The discovery of processing stages: Extensions of Donders' method. In W. G. Koster (ed.), *Attention and performance II. Acta Psychologica*, **30**: 276–315.

Sternberg, S. (1998). Discovering mental processing stages: the method of additive factors. In D. Scarborough and S. Sternberg (eds.), *An Invitation to Cognitive Science, Volume 4: Methods, Models, and Conceptual Issues*. Cambridge, MA: MIT Press, pp. 365–454.

Sternberg, S. (2001). Separate modifiability, mental modules, and the use of pure and composite measures to reveal them. *Acta Psychologica*, **106**: 147–246.

Thompson, B. (1998). In praise of brilliance: where that praise really belongs. *American Psychologist*, **53**: 799–800.

Tryon, W. W. (1998). The inscrutable null hypothesis. *American Psychologist*, **53**: 796.

Verleger, R. (1988). Event-related potentials and cognition: a critique of the context updating hypothesis and an alternate interpretation of the P3. *Brain and Behavioral Sciences*, **11**: 343–56.

Wong, P. K. H. (1991). *Introduction to Brain Topography*. New York and London: Plenum Press.

4

Bilingual semantic memory revisited – ERP and fMRI evidence

Sonja A. Kotz and Kerrie E. Elston-Güttler

Max-Planck-Institute of Human Cognitive and Brain Sciences

Half a century ago, the linguist Uriel Weinreich (Weinreich, 1953) first characterized the way a bilingual's two languages relate to one another. Based on the way a bilingual actually acquired his or her two languages, he described so-called co-ordinative, sub-ordinative, and compound bilingualism (A, E, and F, respectively, in Figure 4.1). If we use a working definition of bilingualism in this chapter to pertain to anyone who can speak two or more languages, then a great deal of bilinguals are likely to be sub-ordinative, i.e. a native speaker of the first language (L1) and a late, or typical "school learner" of a second language (L2). However, the world is full of cultures and cross-cultural families in which individuals grow up with two or more languages. Right from the very start, such individuals can consequently be defined as compound bilinguals. Fifty years later, psycholinguistic experimental methodologies are well established, and measures such as event-related brain potentials (ERPs) and functional magnetic resonance imaging (fMRI) are increasingly used in the investigation of bilingual language processing. These methods now allow us to model the actual representations and neural basis of bilingual semantic memory based on Weinreich's initial typologies, expanding the typologies to refer to mental representations and not merely the way the L1 and L2 were acquired.

Most of the behavioral data that pertain to the models below were collected in the 1980s until now, using the methodologies of repetition and semantic priming (for semantic priming studies, see discussion below; for repetition priming, see Kirsner *et al.*, 1980, 1984; Scarborough *et al.*, 1984) and the picture—word interference paradigm (see Kroll & De Groot, 1997 for a review). Overall, these studies aimed to determine whether (1) there is a common conceptual system mapping onto the L1 and L2 (as in models C, E, F, G, and H); (2) there are (also) processing linkages at the word form level between translation equivalents (as in B, D, E, G, H); (3) L1—L2 linkages are symmetrical across the L1 and the L2 (as in B, D, F, and G); or (4) whether they are asymmetrical, i.e. that L1 words are linked more strongly to concepts

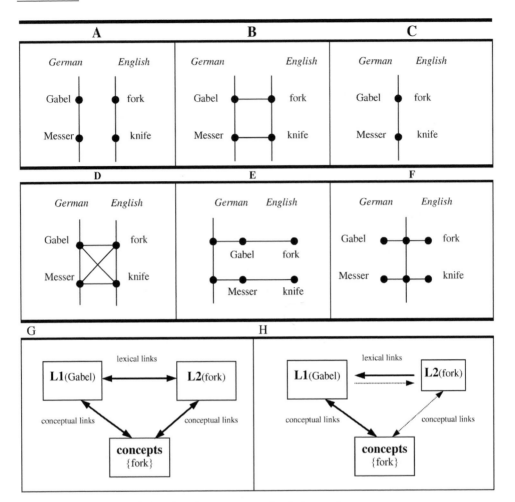

Figure 4.1.   Summary of Theories of L1–L2 Interaction in Processing

A   Co-ordinative bilingualism assumes two separate meaning stores and language-specific "concepts".

B   A combined co-ordinative + sub-ordinative hypothesis (De Groot & Nas, 1991) that assumes separate meaning stores but strong inter-lingual lexical-level translation connections.

C   A hypothesis that assumes word units and meaning of both languages in one integrated system without language-specific meaning or even information on the language to which a word belongs in the network.

D   A modification of co-ordinative bilingualism that assumes separate meaning stores but strong inter-lingual lexical-level *associative* connections as well as lexical-level translation connections.

E   Sub-ordinative bilingualism assumes that the only access to "concepts" from the L2 is via L1 lexical forms and that there are strong inter-lingual lexical-level translation connections. Also called the *Word Association Model* (cf. Potter *et al.*, 1984).

than L2 words are (as in G), or that the only access to concepts is via L1 words
(as in E).

4.1   A shared semantic memory?

Considering cross-language semantic priming tasks, the evidence primarily
supports the idea that there is a shared conceptual system between the L1 and
L2, but also L1–L2 word-to-word connections between translation equivalents.
Cross-language priming tasks operate on the premise that if the prime is *fork*,
a related target such as *Gabel* (the German translation of *fork*) should be judged
to be a word in a lexical decision task more quickly than if the target is preceded
by an unrelated prime such as *Kuh* (*cow*). If such translation priming is obtained
(see Altarriba, 1992; Chen & Ng, 1989; Gollan *et al.*, 1997; Fox, 1996; Jin, 1990;
Schwanenflugel & Rey, 1986; Williams, 1994), this is seen as an argument for
shared conceptual information across languages such as that represented in
Model F. Furthermore, other types of cross-language semantic priming support
variations of concept mediation models: if cross-language semantically related
words (cf. Frenck & Pynte, 1987; Williams, 1994) are primed, Model B is
supported, and if cross-language associates (i.e. *fork–Messer* (*knife*)) are primed
(cf. Grainger & Beauvillain, 1988; Frenck & Pynte, 1987), then model D is possible.
However, once primes are masked to prevent predictive strategies that can arise
from awareness of prime–target relationships (post-access coherence checking,
cf. De Groot, 1984), associates across languages do not prime one another
(De Groot & Nas, 1991; Keatley & De Gelder, 1992; Williams, 1994). Williams
(1994) took this fact to argue that there are limits to the *type* of information
stored at the shared conceptual level rather than evidence of separate semantic
stores for words in the L1 and L2 as depicted in Models A, B, and D.

Caption for Figure 4.1. (*cont.*)   F   Compound bilingualism assumes that there are two specific language-
tagged lexical forms that map onto a shared concept. Also called the *Concept Mediation
Model* (cf. Potter *et al.*, 1984).

G   A combined compound + sub-ordinative hypothesis (De Groot & Nas, 1991)
that assumes a common meaning store as in Model F but strong inter-lingual lexical-level
connections as in Model E.

H   A modification of the combined compound + sub-ordinative hypothesis called
the *Revised Hierarchical Model* that assumes a shared meaning store but stronger
concept-lexical connections in the L1, and stronger inter-lingual, lexical-level translation
connections from the L2 to the L1 than from the L1 to the L2 (Kroll & Stewart, 1994).
The smaller L2 lexicon depicts the fact that it may not be as developed as the L1 lexicon.

Indeed investigations on *types of semantic information* and whether their corresponding concepts are likely to be shared across languages (De Groot, 1992b, 1993, 1995; De Groot & Nas, 1991; De Groot *et al.*, 1994; Van Hell & De Groot, 1998a, 1998b) suggest that a model such as G is needed to account in particular for the processing of cognates (*gut–good*), whose shared semantic and word form information increase cross-language priming effects and suggest dual routes at the semantic and word-form levels. However, De Groot and Nas (1991) also argued for separate conceptual stores in the L1 and L2 as in Model B for noncognates, whose priming effects did not appear to be conceptually mediated. Not only are there differences in processing between cognates and noncognates (cf. De Groot & Nas, 1991; Van Hell & De Groot, 1998a), but taken with studies on word-class effects (De Groot & Keijzer, 2000; De Groot, 1993, 1995; Lotto & De Groot, 1998; Van Hell & De Groot, 1998b), it appears that noncognates, abstract words, and verbs are more likely to be represented in two separate L1 and L2 semantic memory systems (Model B), while concrete words, cognates, and nouns are more likely to be conceptually mediated and represented in compound fashion as in Model G.

However, as it is more parsimonious to assume the same fundamental memory system that applies to all different kinds of words, De Groot suggested the "Distributed Feature Model" (1992a and 1992b; see also Van Hell & De Groot, 1998a) in which it is assumed that a range of overlapping semantic features, and not whole concepts, are shared across languages. Of course on this view, concrete words, nouns, and cognates share more features than do abstract words, verbs, and noncognates. With the assumption of semantic features, this model is similar to so-called two-level theories of semantic memory (Bierwisch & Schreuder, 1992; see also Pavlenko, 1999) in which nonlinguistic concepts are distinct from sets of language-specific features, or semantic forms, that only partially overlap across languages. Another similar two-level model aimed specifically to account for the processing for words with more than one translation (similar to polysemous words in the L1) is the Sense Model by Finkbeiner *et al.* (2004). Here, words such as *black* in English (L2) and *kuroi* in Japanese (L1) have a shared set of features and can be considered translation equivalents, though each language has its own language-specific senses (in the case of *black–kuroi*, the overlapping features reflect 1/8 of the Japanese L1 feature set, but all of the English L2 set). So in Figure 4.1, the dots may really refer to a set of overlapping features across languages, not to actual shared concepts. An alternative to a view involving semantic features is to assume so-called lexical concepts (cf. Levelt *et al.*, 1999; Roelofs, 2000) that can differ across languages and that are distinct from universal nonlinguistic concepts. On this view, *lexical* concepts are slightly different for translation equivalents such as *shade* and *Schatten*, though nonlinguistic concepts are accessible independent of the language (for evidence that different lexicalization patterns affects processing, see Ameel *et al.*, 2005; Elston-Güttler & Williams, accepted). On this latter view, the dots in Figure 4.1 refer to lexical concepts. If we consider the behavioral data to date, we can conclude that at least lexical concepts or semantic features are shared across languages (essentially ruling out Models A, B, and D), and that both lexical-level linkages as well as word—concept linkages are needed to explain stronger priming effects for cognates (as in Models G and H). However, what is still debated is the possible asymmetry between word representations in the L1 and L2 and their linkages to a shared semantic store (i.e. Model G versus Model H).

4.2   Evidence for L1–L2 asymmetry in processing

The asymmetrical model H called the "Revised Hierarchical Model" (RHM; Kroll & Stewart, 1994) predicts several phenomena. First, the model predicts longer latencies for L1-to-L2 (forward) translation than for L2-to-L1 (backward) translation, an effect consistently borne out in the data (Kroll & Sholl, 1992; Kroll & Curley, 1988; Kroll & Stewart, 1989, 1990). Furthermore, the effect appears stronger for less proficient learners than for highly proficient learners (McElree *et al.*, 2000; Cheung & Chen, 1998). Second, the model predicts similarly asymmetric sensitivity to semantic variables of the translation process in category interference or Stroop tasks (studies reviewed in Kroll & Stewart, 1994). Third, the RHM predicts that cross-language semantic priming will be greater from the L1 to the L2 than from the L2 to the L1 in lexical decision tasks (LDT). Following the summary by Kroll & Sholl (1992), seven studies showed greater magnitudes of L1-to-L2 than L2-to-L1 semantic priming (Meyer & Ruddy, 1974; Kirsner *et al.*, 1984; Schwanenflugel & Rey, 1986; Frenck & Pynte, 1987; Chen & Ng, 1989; Keatley *et al.*, 1994; Altarriba, 1990), but several similar studies have demonstrated comparable L1 and L2 semantic priming (Jin, 1990; Frenck-Mestre & Prince, 1997; Meyer & Ruddy, 1974). However, the latter studies have been criticized (cf. Williams, 1994) on the grounds that subjects either processed target words by checking the prime—target relationship or translating the L2 target into L1 (e.g. Altarriba, 1990). Bilingual studies carried out since then that have explicitly induced automatic semantic priming with very short stimulus—onset asynchronies (SOAs) and/or a low relatedness proportion have indeed reported asymmetrical semantic priming effects comparing L1 and L2 (Altarriba, 1990, 1992; De Groot & Nas, 1991 (noncognates); Gerard & Scarborough, 1989; Beauvillain & Grainger, 1987; Keatley *et al.*, 1994; Larsen *et al.*, 1994; Scarborough *et al.*, 1984, Experiment 2).

Even disregarding the issue of masked versus unmasked priming, the asymmetry proposal is still not without its critics (Altarriba & Mathis, 1997;

De Groot *et al.*, 1994; De Groot and Poot, 1997; La Heij *et al.*, 1990, 1996; see Kroll & De Groot, 1997 for a discussion). Most of the critiques come from tasks that involve word translating in Stroop-like situations where there is indeed evidence of as much conceptual mediation in translating from the L2 to L1 as there is from the L1 to the L2 (La Heij *et al.*, 1996). Lee (1994) discussed in detail some problems of generality with La Heij *et al.*'s (1996) interpretation of their data, while Kroll and De Groot (1997) discuss more general problems with precisely defining subject proficiency. They suggest that the inability to do so may have affected many of the studies that appear to support the asymmetry hypothesis. Another problematic aspect of the RHM is the assumption of simple lexical-level links and concepts, without truly defining the specifics involved at either level. Word production data (Levelt *et al.*, 1999) suggest that the idea of a lexical level is too simple: likely, there are phonological, orthographic, and so-called lemma-level representations. The lemma level is thought to exist based primarily on speech error data and on data from the tip-of-the-tongue state (for arguments for the existence of the lemma level, see, e.g. Levelt *et al.*, 1999, but see Caramazza, 1997; Caramazza & Miozzo, 1997 for an alternative view). The lemma level is proposed to concern morphosyntactic and possibly some semantic specifications and acts as an interface to syntax and as an abstract, intermediate level of representation linked to conceptual information and word form (or the lexeme level, cf. Levelt *et al.*, 1999). So even if the basic proposal of asymmetry is accurate, several researchers (cf. Roelofs, 2000; Lee, 1994; see also a discussion in Elston-Güttler, Paulmann & Kotz, 2005) suggest that due to this lack of specification in the RHM, the actual locus of the L1–L2 translation links is not clear: are they at the word form (orthography and phonology) level or at the lemma level? With the use of ERPs in which different components point toward different loci of translational connections between languages, some of the ambiguity of the RHM can be settled.

4.3   Proficiency effects

If there are two routes as suggested by the RHM and concepts are at least partially shared in terms of features or lexical concepts, then how does semantic memory differ for bilinguals of varying ability levels or so-called L2 proficiency? Proficiency, also sometimes referred to as fluency, has been variously defined in terms of years of experience, residence in another country, language attitudes, and language testing; for example, high-proficiency learners are more likely than low-proficiency learners to have more immersion experience abroad, to perform better in tests, and feel confident about their speaking skills in particular. Researchers have yet to agree on the exact definition, but most agree in terms of characterizing bilinguals into low- and high-proficiency groups when the two groups statistically differ in several factors (see Kotz & Elston-Güttler, 2004 for a discussion). Several studies using the picture naming/category interference paradigm (cf. Chen & Leung, 1989; Kroll & Curley, 1988) suggest that less proficient learners are likely to form lexical, not conceptual, links (as in Models B, D, or E), while proficient speakers form conceptual links between their two L1 and L2 lexicons (as in Model F). Researchers have also interpreted proficiency effects in terms of a so-called developmental version of the RHM (Dufour & Kroll, 1995; McElree *et al.*, 2000) in which proficiency is a function of the strength of L2-concept connections, i.e. highly proficient bilinguals have relatively strong L2-concept connections, while less proficient bilinguals have weak L2-concept connections and rely more extensively on the lexical-level word connections (see also Kotz & Elston-Güttler, 2004 for supporting ERP evidence). For example, McElree *et al.* (2000) reported that balanced (highly proficient) bilinguals were equally competent in translating into the L1 and L2, but unbalanced bilinguals retrieved conceptual information in verbal translating more slowly and less accurately in the L2 than in the L1. This phenomenon suggests that the dominant language provided access to conceptual information "whenever mappings of the nondominant language cannot sustain direct retrieval of conceptual information" (McElree *et al.*, 2000, p. 229).

4.4   ERPs and bilingual semantic memory

Especially considering the subtle processing differences observed between different bilingual proficiency groups, the use of behavioral methodologies and response times (RTs) alone (Snodgrass, 1993) might not suffice to monitor the different processing stages during L2 word recognition. An online measure such as ERPs provides a more precise evaluation of such processes. In contrast to RTs, which are measured at a discrete point in time, ERPs measure ongoing electrical brain activity and multidimensional data points such as latency, amplitude, polarity, and scalp distribution of a component (a series of peaks and valleys in the EEG) under investigation. In theory, given the high temporal resolution, ERPs can measure a process on line, as it unfolds.

The method of ERPs has already been used to investigate L2 semantic processing (Ardal *et al.*, 1990; Hahne & Friederici, 2001; Kutas & Kluender, 1991) and has even addressed the issue of maturational effects on L2 processing (Weber-Fox & Neville, 1996). The above studies have examined semantic and/or syntactic processing in the so-called violation paradigm, where electrophysiological responses to semantic/syntactic anomalies are measured. Generally, L2 semantic processing appears to be qualitatively the same as L1 semantic processing, but slowed down slightly. For natives, semantic anomalies are realized in the N400 ERP component (Kutas & Hillyard, 1980), a central parietal negativity with a peak at about 400 ms (anomalies more negative than controls). In the violation paradigm, the N400 effect has been observed in L2 learners, though slightly delayed (Ardal *et al.*, 1990; Kotz & Elston-Güttler, 2004; Kutas & Kluender, 1991; Weber-Fox & Neville, 1996), or with slightly reduced amplitude (Kutas & Kluender, 1991). In a direct comparison of different groups whose age of acquisition (AoA) of the L2 varied, Weber-Fox and Neville (1996) found that the N400 is only delayed in learners who began acquiring the L2 later in life (AoA of between 11 and 13 or > 16 years). Generally, semantic processing appears not be as sensitive to maturational effects (Weber-Fox & Neville, 1996) and to general differences between L1 and L2 processing as is syntactic processing (Hahne & Friederici, 2001).

Though the above studies provide detailed online analysis of processing words and sentences as they unfold, only one type of semantic process — anomaly detection — is measured in the violation paradigm, and it is questionable how much this actually tells us about bilingual semantic memory. Semantic priming performed in the L2 and measured by ERPs, on the other hand, actually tests the nature of and relative strength of connections within the bilingual lexicon (both L2 word–concept and L1 word–L2 word) and therefore serves as a better task to measure proficiency or AoA differences regarding the processing of semantics specifically. Semantic priming is reflected in a larger N400 for unrelated targets (*pond–boy*) during word and sentence processing (see Anderson & Holcomb, 1995; Van Petten & Kutas, 1990) and a reduced N400 for related words (*girl–boy*). Though post-lexical integration may be underlying this effect (e.g. Holcomb, 1993), results from ERP LDT studies suggest that the N400 may also measure automatic processes (i.e. spread of activation; Neely, 1991), so the N400 has been argued to reflect both post-lexical integration and automatic spread of activation (e.g. Besson *et al.*, 1992; Deacon *et al.*, 2000; Holcomb, 1988; Kiefer, 2002, but see for counterevidence Brown & Hagoort, 1993; Chwilla *et al.*, 1995, 2000).

Recent semantic priming studies using ERPs (Kotz, 2001; Kotz & Elston-Güttler, 2004) have generally supported the RHM, but have argued that effects are strongly modulated not only by language proficiency, but also by AoA (i.e. whether learners are "early" and acquired the L2 from early childhood on, or "late" and began the L2 after about ten years of age). Kotz (1996, 1998, 2001) used associatively related word pairs (*girl–boy*) and categorically related word pairs (*junior–boy*) to test whether semantic priming in the N400 component would be observed for these word types the same way for natives (Kotz, 1996, 1998) and parallel bilinguals (Kotz, 2001). Kotz (2001) found that for natives, an N400 priming effect was found for both associative and categorically related pairs, and *early learners* (AoA was 4.5 years) showed comparable, though slightly later, effects for both types as well. In a further study, Kotz and Elston-Güttler (2004) used the same material on two *late learner* groups that were comparable in AoA (about 12 years) but differed in terms of L2 language proficiency. The *low-* and *high-proficiency* groups were defined by various factors on an extensive language questionnaire including number of months of language immersion, vocabulary test scores, and self-ratings in reading, writing, listening, and speaking. Kotz and Elston-Güttler (2004) found that for the high-proficiency, late learner group, an N400 priming effect was observed for associative words, but the effect was very long-lasting with a broad scalp distribution as compared to the early learners and natives from Kotz (2001). For categorical pairs, the high-proficiency group did not show any significant N400 priming effects. Furthermore, the low-proficiency, late learner group did not show any significant N400 priming for either associative or categorical pairs. The data were interpreted to indicate that categorical processing is sensitive to a so-called critical period, or AoA, while associative processing is sensitive to proficiency level. In terms of bilingual semantic memory, the links from L2 words to semantic representations appear to be especially weak for late learners, extending the development argument (cf. Dufour & Kroll, 1995; McElree *et al.*, 2000) to apply to both AoA and proficiency.

4.5   Bilingual semantic access in sentences: RTs and ERPs

There have also been several studies addressing bilingual semantic memory that have appealed to sentence-level processing without necessarily using the violation paradigm. Such studies have used semantic priming as single words and with primes at the end of full sentences. The data suggest that bilinguals have similar access mechanisms in the L1 and L2, but that sentence-level context information is managed differently in the L2 if learners have a late AoA or a low proficiency level. For example, Elston-Güttler and Friederici (2005) used homonyms such as *sentence* or *trip* in English to test the way that native English speakers and German−English bilinguals (English L2) use sentence context cues in determining the correct homonym meaning. Sentences such as "The judge announced the *sentence*" were followed by contextually appropriate (*prison*) or inappropriate (*grammar*) targets after an SOA of 200 and 500 ms, respectively. At the 200 ms SOA, both native and L2 late learners of high proficiency (AoA was 12) showed a more negative waveform for both target types than when the same targets followed an unrelated sentence-final word as in "The judge announced the *guest*." This was evidence that for both L2 learners and natives, both possible meanings at an early SOA can be accessed, an effect previously reported for natives in behavioral studies (cf. Conrad, 1974; Lucas, 1987; Onifer & Swinney, 1981; Seidenberg *et al.*, 1982; Swinney, 1979). However, at the longer SOA of 500 ms, only the natives showed a context effect with a modulation of the N400 component for contextually appropriate targets only. Late learners, on the other hand, showed N400 priming modulations for both target types, suggesting that although both meanings were initially accessed automatically, they were active longer, despite a context that could cause deactivation of the contextually appropriate meanings. However, RTs measured later in time showed deactivation of the inappropriate meanings by the L2 learners. This suggests that the initial semantic access mechanisms in sentence processing are very automatic, even in an L2, but later processes involving the application of context information are not dysfunctional, but merely slower, for late L2 learners.

Another study testing bilingual sentence processing involves a direct comparison of single word and sentence processing as measured by RTs and ERPs and the locus of the translational links assumed in the RHM (Elston-Güttler, Paulmann & Kotz, 2005). In a lexical decision semantic priming task measuring RTs and ERPs, the two translations (e.g. *pine, jaw*) of German L1 homonyms (*Kiefer*) served as primes and targets. Both high- and low-proficiency German learners of English (late AoA of 11 years) performed the task, which was all in English. There was a single word version (*pine—jaw* related and *oak—jaw* unrelated) and a sentence version of the same task, i.e. "The beautiful table was made of *pine (oak)*" followed by the target *jaw*. In both single-word and sentence version, only low-proficiency participants showed a modulation of the N200 (but interestingly, not in the N400) for targets in pairs such as *pine—jaw*, while high-proficiency learners showed effects in the single-word version only. In both single-word and sentence versions, English natives showed no significant N200 modulations. A reversed priming effect in the N200 was argued to indicate L1 interference at the level of orthography. These data suggest that the locus of interference, which is the translation link between the L1 and the L2, was not reflected by the N400, but rather by the N200: this may mean that the locus of the lexical-level translation links in the RHM is indeed at the level of word form, not at the lemma level. Though the N200 has been interpreted as a reflection of phonological mismatch in auditorily presented tasks (e.g. Connolly *et al.*, 1992; Connolly & Philips, 1994; Van den Brink *et al.*, 2001), the N200 has also been proposed to reflect orthographic processing in visually presented tasks (Bentin *et al.*, 1999; Compton *et al.*, 1991). Furthermore, the data suggest another proficiency effect: while interference was found at the word and sentence level for less proficient participants, the higher proficient group was able to use sentence information to prevent strong L1 translation interference, suggesting that the relative strength of L2—L1 lexical connections may decrease with higher proficiency.

The contrast of single-word versus sentence processing using ERPs has also shed light on a very crucial issue in bilingual semantic access referred to as *language or cognitive control*, i.e. how well a bilingual can inhibit or deactivate the irrelevant language while processing in the other. This issue has been primarily investigated using the case of interlingual homographs, or false friends, where a single-word form such as *chef* presents a bilingual with two completely different L1 and L2 meanings (*chef* refers to "cook" in English and "boss" in German). Some earlier behavioral studies argue for language selectivity (e.g. Soares & Grosjean, 1984; Scarborough *et al.*, 1984; Gerard & Scarborough, 1989), a position that assumes that only one language is activated at a time. However, various phenomena observed in more recent studies support a non-selective bilingual word recognition system, i.e. a system that allows for parallel activation of both languages where influence of one language while processing in the other is likely (Chen & Ho, 1986 in Stroop interference; Smith & Kirsner, 1982 in bilingual picture—word distractor tasks; Beauvillain & Grainger, 1987; Grainger & Dijkstra, 1992; De Bruijn *et al.*, 2001; De Moor, 1998; Van Heste, 1999 in primed lexical decision tasks (LDT); Dijkstra *et al.*, 1999; De Groot *et al.*, 2000 in non-primed LDTs).

In a study using both RTs and ERPs, De Bruijn *et al.* (2001) showed with Dutch—English bilinguals that significant RT priming and N400 priming was obtained for targets that were semantically related to the English reading of a preceding Dutch—English homograph. Crucially, the effect was obtained regard-less of whether the pair was preceded by an English-only or Dutch-only word (i.e. there was priming of *heaven* in both the triplets *house—angel—heaven* and *zaak—angel—heaven* in which *angel* means "sting" in Dutch and *zaak* means "case" or "shop"). These data suggest parallel semantic access in the L1 and L2, even when a particular L1 or L2 context has been set. However, the language switching in the experiment itself may have caused the bilingual word recognition system to set threshold levels that allow for both languages to be active (for the Bilingual Interactive Activation (BIA+) model, which explains nonselective data; see Dijkstra and Van Heuven, 2002). To rule this out, Paulmann *et al.* (2006) conducted an RT/ERP experiment in which German—English interlingual homographs such as *chef* were presented to German late learners of English in an entirely English experiment. Here, the language context was set at a more global level, i.e. a film presented in either German or English before the experiment. Results showed significant overall RT and N400 priming of, e.g. *chef—boss* regardless of whether the English or German film was presented first. These data make a strong case for nonselective access, even in very strong all-L2 contexts that are not characterized by language switching. However, Elston-Güttler *et al.* (2005) showed that once primes appear at the end of English sentence con-texts, the film manipulation affects L1 activations during L2 processing. In an all-English experiment including full sentences, there was only RT and N400 priming of L1 interlingual homograph meanings after the German (L1) film presentation and, moreover, only during the first half of the experiment when L1 activations were still strong enough to affect processing. The results of these studies can be accounted for in the BIA+ model (Dijkstra & Van Heuven, 2002), which assumes that bilingual lexical access is fundamentally nonselective, but can be affected by task and sentence context. In language control, the introduction of sentence contexts appears to make the system much more sensitive to task changes.

Even though behavioral data may be similar between native and L2 learners, the underlying mechanisms reflected by ERPs are much more likely to differ between L2 learners and natives (cf. Elston-Güttler & Friederici, 2005) or between learners of different proficiency levels and AoA (cf. Kotz & Elston-Güttler, 2004). Furthermore, the introduction of sentence-level processes can tell us a great deal about bilingual semantic access: (1) access is similar in natives and non-natives, but context management differs; (2) sentences help highly proficient learners deactivate L2−L1 translational links during L2 processing (cf. Elston-Güttler, Paulmann & Kotz, 2005); and (3) sentences help the bilingual recognition system zoom into the correct language and respond to global language context more effectively (cf. Elston-Güttler, Gunter & Kotz, 2005). In the next section, the discussion of functional magnetic resonance imaging (fMRI) data will augment our understanding of the aspects of semantic memory representation and access that have been established so far with behavioral and electrophysiological data.

4.6 The neural basis of bilingual semantic memory: neuroimaging evidence

Next to ERPs, both positron emission tomography (PET) and functional magnetic resonance imaging (fMRI) have been used to test bilingual semantic memory. Stimulated by early evidence on differential impairment and recovery in bilingual aphasics, these methods have been used in the healthy bilingual brain to explore: (1) whether bilingual semantic memory is represented separately or as a common conceptual store; and (2) how AoA and/or proficiency affect such representation. Recently, factors such as task demands (e.g. Gollan & Kroll, 2001), semantic feature complexity (e.g. Faust & Chiarello, 1998; Kotz *et al.*, 2002; Ullman, 2001) as well as domain general resources (e.g. Green, 2005) have been critically noted as influential in the way brain activation may reflect bilingual semantic memory organization. That is, whether semantic memory is tested with a semantic categorization task or a lexical decision task, whether associative or categorical features are investigated, or whether cognitive strategies involved depend on attentional or working memory resources may modulate which brain areas are in concert when testing bilingual semantic memory. Note, though, that most of these factors also play a role in monolingual semantic memory investigations. Last, similar questions have been asked in terms of phonological, morphological, and syntactic knowledge, areas beyond semantic memory and therefore outside the scope of this chapter.

Clinical and neurosurgical research of language and language disturbance has resulted in a number of studies exploring the question of whether the languages of a bilingual are neuroanatomically distinct or not. The debate centers around two principal types of impairment and recovery (but see Paradis, 1977 for at least six distinct recovery patterns in bilinguals). Parallel impairment and recovery implies that two or more languages share a neural representation and/or processing system, while differential impairment and recovery gives prima facie evidence for distinct neural representation and processing. Primarily, evidence from crossed aphasia (Albert & Obler, 1978; Karanth & Rangamani, 1988) has implicated the right hemisphere in bilingual language processing. Furthermore, select case reports (e.g. Abutalebi *et al.*, 2001; Gomez-Tortosa *et al.*, 1995; Paradis, 2001; Vaid & Hull, 2002) support distinct language representation of the L1 and L2. From a functional neuroanatomical point of view, it is, however, critical to consider that a cortical lesion does not necessarily correlate with a specific function, as the function could be supported by a distributed network in which the lesioned site is one of many players (see Green, 2005). In other words, if, for example, a bilingual suffers from a stroke that results in a selective semantic deficit for L1 or L2, this does not imply that the particular stroke site is the representation site for semantic memory in L1 or L2. Thus, any one of the described recovery patterns (Paradis, 1977) could result from the manner in which a dynamic network underlying language function in L1/L2 is affected by a respective stroke. Seminal neurosurgical work by Ojemann and colleagues (1978, 1983, 1990) showed that the languages of a bilingual undergoing neurosurgery might be neurologically separable in the language-dominant hemisphere. Stimulation mapping of cortical areas during naming of an object in two languages revealed interferences with naming in both languages, but also clear dissociations between languages. For example, Lucas *et al.* (2004) showed that L2 sites for object naming were located in the posterior temporal and parietal regions, whereas the L1 and shared sites were found throughout the mapped regions. These data, while constrained by the nature of clinical profiles, demonstrate that L1 and L2 language production involves distinct, but overlapping, brain areas.

As discussed in the previous section on ERPs, the neural organization of semantic memory is strongly influenced by the level of L2 proficiency. Even though there is strong evidence that AoA is more critical for syntactic processes (e.g. Wartenburger *et al.*, 2003), proficiency cannot be viewed completely independent of AoA as often those with higher proficiency have also acquired the L2 earlier in life (e.g. Johnson & Newport, 1989; Kotz, 1996, 2001; Kotz & Elston-Güttler, 2004). However, the general consensus is that AoA may not be a particularly crucial factor in semantic processes. Rather, AoA may influence the extent of activation and/or the processing effort required to perform semantic tasks in the L2 (Marian *et al.*, 2003; Wartenburger *et al.*, 2003).

The level of attained L2 proficiency has been tested in several neuroimaging studies involving multiple language pairs (Mandarin/English; French/English; English/French; Italian/English; Spanish/Catalan) and tasks (stem completion, passive listening, word generation, and word repetition). While language performance rather than semantic knowledge was in the foreground in these studies (Chee *et al.*, 1999, 2001; Klein *et al.*, 1994, 1995; Perani *et al.*, 1996, 1998), the data indirectly support the conclusion that semantic knowledge is largely shared in L1 and L2, and this to a larger extent for those with high L2 proficiency than those with less advanced L2 skills.

4.7   fMRI proficiency and AoA effects

Only a few bilingual neuroimaging studies have directly tested the so-called convergence hypothesis for semantic memory, i.e. the theory that L2 processing becomes more and more L1-like with increased L2 proficiency. Illes and colleagues (1999) used fMRI to test this hypothesis in fluent late bilinguals (English/Spanish and Spanish/English) using both a visual semantic judgment (concrete/abstract) and a visual nonsemantic judgment (upper-/lower-case letter) in English and Spanish. Based on monolingual evidence, the authors focused particularly on the activation of the left inferior prefrontal cortex, a brain area that has been implicated in semantic selection (e.g. Wagner *et al.*, 1997; Thompson-Schill *et al.*, 1997). The results show that fluent bilinguals were above 90 percent correct in L1 and L2 semantic judgment and at ceiling in both languages for the nonsemantic task. A contrast between semantic and nonsemantic judgment revealed consistent activation — independent of L1 or L2 — in the left inferior frontal gyrus (LIFG) and to a weaker extent, in the right inferior frontal gyrus (see also Chee *et al.*, 2001). These results confirm data on French bilingual word generation (Klein *et al.*, 1995) and clearly show that: (1) fluent late bilinguals recruit the same brain region during semantic judgment in L1 and L2; and (2) that activation of the left LIFG is comparable between monolingual and highly proficient bilinguals during semantic judgment. Work by Chee and colleagues (2001) confirms that language proficiency plays a crucial role during semantic processing. Contrasting semantic judgment of words and characters in English—Mandarin bilinguals with varying levels of proficiency, they showed that higher proficiency correlated with reduced response times and error rates as well as a smaller degree of activation in left prefrontal and parietal brain areas. Low-proficiency participants, in contrast, engaged the left and right frontal cortex in addition to the other brain areas. Xue *et al.* (2004) tested low proficient 10- to 12-year-old bilingual children (Chinese/English) in a semantic decision task at the word level (visual modality). In both L1 and L2, the children showed activation of the left inferior frontal cortex, but additional activation of the left inferior parietal and cingulate cortex in L2, which the authors interpret as a correlate of attentional demands in L2. Combining eye-tracking and fMRI, Marian *et al.* (2003) proposed that in general, the same brain structures are active in L1 (Russian) and late learners of L2 (English), but differences within these structures can occur as a function of level of processing and across languages. In particular, L1–L2 differences were found during phonological processing (word level) in the bilateral inferior frontal gyrus, with L2 phonological processing extending across a larger area in the IFG than in L1. Such differences were not found in the superior temporal gyrus (STG). Lexical–semantic processing resulted in a similar pattern of activation in the IFG, but not in the STG. The authors concluded that L2 STG activation confirms the role of this brain area during phonological processing (see also Kim *et al.*, 1997 for similar results on L1 and L2 production).

A few studies have also investigated sentence-level semantic processing in different proficiency or AoA groups. Chee *et al.* (1999) compared sentence comprehension against fixation or pseudo-word strings in fluent bilinguals (L2 AoA before the age of six years with a subgroup of participants with an L2 AoA of 12 years or later). The data reveal comparable activation patterns (prefrontal, temporal, superior parietal, and anterior supplementary motor area) in Mandarin Chinese and English independent of AoA. Wartenburger *et al.* (2003) investigated both AoA and level of proficiency in Italian–German bilinguals using both grammatical and semantic visual judgment. AoA affected the brain activation during grammatical judgment with L2 syntactic processing resulting in different activation patterns than L1 syntactic processing. During semantic judgment, early AoA participants showed no activation differences between L1 and L2, but late learners with high proficiency showed higher activation in the bilateral IFG (BA 47) and insula in L2, and late learners with low proficiency showed left IFG (BA 44/6) and right IFG (BA 47) as well as right insula activation. Rueschemeyer *et al.* (2005) investigated late but proficient Russian–German bilinguals in a semantic violation paradigm (violation of semantic expectancy) and found comparable activation of the left anterior IFG between native and non-native speakers of German.

Summarizing the evidence presented here, several aspects are apparent. There is a paucity of neuroimaging research on bilingual semantic memory and the underlying processing mechanisms at both the word and sentence level.

The current evidence supports the notion that there is a rather similar network underlying language processing in L1 and L2 in terms of semantic processes in particular. Furthermore, it is obvious that when processing semantic information in L2, areas of the language network may be employed differentially or to a larger extent than in the L1. These modulations may be due to proficiency rather than AoA (see Perani *et al.*, 1998, 2003; Wartenburger *et al.*, 2003). However, as critically noted by Green (2005), aspects such as task demands and the resources processing information in the L2 may also play a significant role. What almost all studies show in common is that activation of left, and in some cases, also right inferior frontal areas are more strongly activated in L2 semantic tasks. Furthermore, there seems to be a relative trade-off between frontal areas and the superior temporal activation. What remains to be clarified is whether the diverse enhanced activation patterns in the left frontal areas are due to more effortful semantic selection or due to less proficient phonological decoding in the L2. The fact that only few studies report STG activation may suggest that frontal areas compensate for less sufficient phonological processing in the L2 (see also Rueschemeyer *et al.*, 2005).

4.8   Conclusion

In conclusion, behavioral, ERP, and fMRI data suggest rather strongly that the L1 and L2 share at least some of the same semantic representations and process-ing mechanisms. However, the extent to which these processes are the same over time and the extent to which the relevant brain areas are recruited for L2 semantic processing depends quite profoundly on proficiency level and somewhat on AoA. With the precise time-course information obtained from evoked potentials, ERP studies provide particularly useful insight into time-course differences between the L1 and L2, i.e. we know from several studies that the N400 is indeed present for L2 learners, but can be observed, especially in late learners with low proficiency, with a later onset and/or an extended modulation (Kotz & Elston-Güttler, 2004; Weber-Fox & Neville, 1996). In addition, sentence context information affects the N400 obtained in semantic priming similarly, but is delayed, in L2 learners when compared to natives (Elston-Güttler & Friederici, 2005). These types of effects suggest that while the fundamental processing mechanisms are similar across L1 and L2, certain processes such as using sen-tence context information to resolve ambiguity simply take longer in the L2. Studies using fMRI, in contrast, lack the specific time-course information but offer instead much more precise localization of the neural basis of bilingual semantic processing. Again, L1 and L2 processing share similar brain structures, but the extent of activation along with recruitment of additional areas not observed in L1 semantic processing might differ from patterns reported for semantic processing in the L1. Just as the combined measurement of RTs and ERPs in one task is very useful in determining whether the underlying processes in semantic priming are the same as the behavioral outcome, a promising endeavor is to conduct ERP and fMRI experiments with the same stimuli to explore both the precise time-course and localization of bilingual semantic processing. This, along with the careful control of both the factors of AoA and proficiency, will help disentangle exactly which L1 and L2 processes and representations are always shared, and which are shared due to early L2 acquisition or a high proficiency level.

REFERENCES

Abutalebi, J., Cappa, S. F., and Perani, D. (2001). The bilingual brain as revealed by functional neuroimaging. *Bilingualism: Language and Cognition*, **4**: 179–90.

Albert, M. L. and Obler, L. K. (1978). *The Bilingual Brain*. New York: Academic Press.

Altarriba, J. (1990). *Constraints in interlingual facilitation effects in priming in Spanish-English bilinguals*. Ph.D. Dissertation, Vanderbilt University.

Altarriba, J. (1992). The representation of translation equivalents in bilingual memory. In R. J. Harris (ed.), *Cognitive Processing in Bilinguals*. Amsterdam: North-Holland, pp. 157–74.

Altarriba, J. and Mathis, K. M. (1997). Conceptual and lexical development in second language acquisition. *Journal of Memory and Language*, **36**, 4: 550–68.

Ameel, E., Storms, G., Malt, B. C., and Sloman, S. A. (2005). How bilinguals solve the naming problem. *Journal of Memory and Language*, **52**: 60–80.

Anderson, J. E. and Holcomb, J. P. (1995). Auditory and visual semantic priming using different stimulus onset asynchronies: an event-related brain potential study. *Psychophysiology*, **32**: 177–90.

Ardal, S., Donald, M. W., Meuter, R., Muldrew, S., and Luce, M. (1990). Brain responses to semantic incongruity in bilinguals. *Brain and Language*, **39**: 187–205.

Beauvillain, C. and Grainger, J. (1987). Accessing inter-lexical homographs: some limitations of language-selective access. *Journal of Memory and Language*, **26**: 658–72.

Bentin, S., Mouchetant-Rostaing, Y., Giard, M. H., Echallier, J. F., and Pernier, J. (1999). ERP manifestations of processing printed words at different psycholinguistic levels: time course and scalp distribution. *Journal of Cognitive Neuroscience*, **11**: 235–60.

Besson, M., Kutas, M., and Van Petten, C. (1992). An event-related potential (ERP) analysis of semantic congruity and repetition effects in sentences. *Journal of Cognitive Neuroscience*, **4**: 132–49.

Bierwisch, M. and Schreuder, R. (1992). From concepts to lexical items. *Cognition*, **42**: 23–60.

Brown, C. M. and Hagoort, P. (1993). The processing nature of the N400: evidence from masked priming. *Journal of Cognitive Neuroscience*, **5**: 34–44.

Caramazza, A. (1997). How many levels of processing are there in lexical access? *Cognitive Neuropsychology*, **14**: 177–208.

Caramazza, A. and Miozzo, M. (1997). The relation between syntactic and phonological knowledge in lexical access: evidence from the "tip-of-the-tongue" phenomenon. *Cognition*, **64**: 309–43.

Chee, M., Tan, E., and Thiel, T. (1999). Mandarin and English single word processing studied with functional magnetic resonance imaging. *Journal of Neuroscience*, **19**: 3050–56.

Chee, M., Hon, N., Lee, H. L., and Soon, C. S. (2001). Relative language proficiency modulates BOLD signal change when bilinguals perform semantic judgments. *NeuroImage*, **13**: 1155–63.

Chen, H. C. and Ho, C. (1986). Development of Stroop interference in Chinese–English bilinguals. *Journal of Experimental Psychology: Learning, Memory, and Cognition*, **12**: 397–401.

Chen, H. C. and Leung, Y. S. (1989). Patterns of lexical processing in a non-native language. *Journal of Experimental Psychology: Learning, Memory, and Cognition*, **15**: 316–25.

Chen, H. C. and Ng, M. L. (1989). Semantic facilitation and translation priming effects in Chinese–English bilinguals. *Memory and Cognition*, **17**: 454–62.

Cheung, H. and Chen, H. C. (1998). Lexical and conceptual processing in Chinese–English bilinguals: further evidence for asymmetry. *Memory and Cognition*, **26**: 1002–13.

Chwilla, D. J., Brown, P., and Hagoort, P. (1995). The N400 as a function of the level of processing. *Psychophysiology*, **32**: 274–85.

Chwilla, D. J., Kolk, H. J., and Mulder, G. (2000). Mediated priming in the lexical decision task: evidence from event-related potentials and reaction times. *Journal of Memory and Language*, **42**: 314–41.

Compton, P. E., Grossbacher, P., Posner, M. I., and Tucker, D. M. (1991). A cognitive–anatomical approach to attention in lexical access. *Journal of Cognitive Neuroscience*, **3**: 304–12.

Connolly, J. F. and Phillips, N. A. (1994). Event-related potential components reflect phonological and semantic processing of the terminal word of spoken sentences. *Journal of Cognitive Neuroscience*, **6**: 256–66.

Connolly, J. F., Phillips, N. A., Stewart, S. H., and Brake, W. G. (1992). Event-related potential sensitivity to acoustic and semantic properties of terminal words in sentences. *Brain and Language*, **43**: 1–18.

Conrad, C. (1974). Context effects in sentence comprehension: a study of the subjective lexicon. *Memory and Cognition*, **2**: 130–38.

Deacon, D., Hewitt, S., Yang, Chien-Ming, and Nagata, M. (2000). Event-related potentials indices of semantic priming using masked and unmasked words: evidence that the N400 does not reflect a post-lexical process. *Cognitive Brain Research*, **9**: 137–46.

De Bruijn, E., Dijkstra, T., Chwilla, D., and Schriefers, H. (2001). Language context effects on interlingual homograph recognition: Evidence from event-related potentials and response times in semantic priming. *Bilingualism: Language & Cognition*, **4**: 155–68.

De Groot, A. M. B. (1984). Primed lexical decision: combined effects of the proportion of related prime–target pairs and the stimulus–onset asynchrony of prime and target. *Quarterly Journal of Experimental Psychology, Section A – Human Experimental Psychology*, **36A**: 253–80.

De Groot, A. M. B. (1992a). Determinants of word translation. *Journal of Experimental Psychology: Learning, Memory, and Cognition*, **18**: 1001–18.

De Groot, A. M. B. (1992b). Bilingual lexical representation: a closer look at conceptual representations. In R. Frost and L. Katz (eds.), *Orthography, Phonology, Morphology, and Meaning.* Amsterdam: Elsevier, pp. 389–412.

De Groot, A. M. B. (1993). Word-type effects in bilingual processing tasks: Support for a mixed-representation system. In R. Schreuder and B. Weltens (eds.), *The Bilingual Lexicon*, Amsterdam and Philadelphia, PA: John Benjamins, pp. 27–51.

De Groot, A. M. B. (1995). Determinants of bilingual lexicosemantic organization. *Computer Assisted Language Learning*, **8**: 151–80.

De Groot, A. M. B. and Keijzer, R. (2000). What is hard to learn is easy to forget: the roles of word concreteness, cognate status, and word frequency in foreign-language vocabulary learning and forgetting. *Language Learning*, **50**: 1–56.

De Groot, A. M. B. and Nas, G. L. J. (1991). Lexical representation of cognates and noncognates in compound bilinguals. *Journal of Memory and Language*, **30**: 90–123.

De Groot, A. M. D. and Poot, R. (1997). Word translation at three levels of proficiency in a second language: the ubiquitous involvement of conceptual memory. *Language Learning*, **47**: 215–64.

De Groot, A. M. B., Dannenburg, L., and Van Hell, J. G. (1994). Forward and backward translation by bilinguals. *Journal of Memory and Language*, **33**: 600–29.

De Groot, A. M. B., Delmaar, P., and Lupker, S. J. (2000). The processing of interlexical homographs in translation recognition and lexical decision: support for non-selective access to bilingual memory. *The Quarterly Journal of Experimental Psychology, Section A – Human Experimental Psychology*, **53A**: 397–428.

De Moor, W. (1998). Visual word recognition in bilinguals. Unpublished Master's Thesis, University of Ghent.

Dijkstra, T. and Van Heuven, W. J. B. (2002). The architecture of the bilingual word recognition system: from identification to decision. *Bilingualism: Language & Cognition*, **5**: 175–97.

Dijkstra, T., Grainger, J., and Van Heuven, W. J. B. (1999). Recognition of cognates and interlingual homographs: the neglected role of phonology. *Journal of Memory and Language*, **41**: 496–518.

Dufour, R. and Kroll, J. F. (1995). Matching words to concepts in two languages: a test of the concept mediation model of bilingual representation. *Memory and Cognition*, **23**: 166–80.

Elston-Güttler, K. E. and Friederici, A. D. (2005). Native and L2 processing of homonyms in sentential context. *Journal of Memory and Language*, **52**: 256–83.

Elston-Güttler, K. E., Gunter, T. C., and Kotz, S. A. (2005). Zooming into L2: Global language context and adjustment affect processing of interlingual homographs in sentences. *Cognitive Brain Research*, **25**: 57–70.

Elston-Güttler, K. E., Paulmann, S., and Kotz, S. A. (2005). Who's in control?: Proficiency and L1 influence on L2 processing. *Journal of Cognitive Neuroscience*, **17**: 1593–610.

Faust, M. and Chiarello, C. (1998). Sentence context and lexical ambiguity resolution by the two hemispheres. *Neuropsychologia*, **36**: 827–35.

Finkbeiner, M., Forster, K., Nicol, J., and Nakamura, K. (2004). The role of polysemy in masked semantic and translation priming. *Journal of Memory and Language*, **51**: 1–22.

Fox, E. (1996). Cross-language priming from ignored words: evidence for a common representational system in bilinguals. *Journal of Memory and Language*, **35**: 353–70.

Frenck, C. and Pynte, J. (1987). Semantic representation and surface forms: a look at cross-language priming in bilinguals. *Journal of Psycholinguistic Research*, **16**: 383–96.

Frenck-Mestre, C. and Prince, P. (1997). Second language autonomy. *Journal of Memory and Language*, **37**: 481–501.

Gerard, L. D. and Scarborough, D. L. (1989). Language-specific access of homographs by bilinguals. *Journal of Experimental Psychology: Learning, Memory, and Cognition*, **15**: 305–15.

Gollan, T. H., Forster, K. I., and Frost, R. (1997). Translation priming with different scripts: masked priming with cognates and noncognates in Hebrew–English bilinguals. *Journal of Experimental Psychology: Learning, Memory, and Cognition*, **23**: 1122–39.

Gollan, T. H. and Kroll, J. F. (2001). Lexical access in bilinguals. In B. Rapp (ed.), *A Handbook of Cognitive Neuropsychology: What deficits reveal about the human mind*. New York: Psychology Press, pp. 321–45.

Gomez-Tortosa, E., Martin, E. M., Gaviria, M., Charbel, F., and Ausman, J. I. (1995). Selective deficit of one language in a bilingual patient following surgery in the left perisylvian area. *Brain and Language*, **48**: 320–5.

Grainger, J. and Beauvillain, C. (1988). Associative priming in bilinguals: some limits of interlingual facilitation effects. *Canadian Journal of Psychology*, **42**: 261–73.

Grainger, J. and Dijsktra, T. (1992). On the representation and use of language information in bilinguals. In R. J. Harris (ed.), *Cognitive Processing in Bilinguals*. Amsterdam: North-Holland, pp. 207–20.

Green, D. W. (2005). The neurocognition of recovery patterns in bilingual aphasics. In J. F. Kroll and A. M. B. de Groot (eds.), *Handbook of Bilingualism: Psycholinguistic perspectives*. New York: Oxford University Press, pp. 516–30.

Hahne, A. and Friederici, A. D. (2001). Processing a second language: late learners' comprehension mechanisms as revealed by event-related brain potentials. *Bilingualism: Language and Cognition*, **4**: 123–41.

Holcomb, P. J. (1988). Automatic and attentional processing: an event-related brain potential analysis of semantic priming. *Brain and Language*, **35**: 66–85.

Holcomb, P. J. (1993). Semantic priming and stimulus degradation: implications for the role of the N400 in in language processing. *Psychophysiology*, **30**: 47–61.

Illes, J., Francis, W. S., Desmond, J. E., Gabrieli, J. D., Glover, G. H., Poldrack, R., Lee, C. J., and Wagner, A. D. (1999). Convergent cortical representation of semantic processing in bilinguals. *Brain and Language*, **70**: 347–63.

Jin, Y. S. (1990). Effects of concreteness on cross-language priming in lexical decisions. *Perceptual and Motor Skills*, **70**: 1139–54.

Johnson, J. S. and Newport, E. L. (1989). Critical period effects in second language learning: the influence of maturational state on the acquisition of English as a second language. *Cognitive Psychology*, **21**: 60–99.

Karanth, P. and Rangamani, G. N. (1988). Crossed aphasia in multilinguals. *Brain and Language*, **34**: 169–80.

Keatley, C. W. and De Gelder, B. (1992). The bilingual primed lexical decision task: cross-language priming disappears with speeded responses. *European Journal of Cognitive Psychology*, **4**: 273–92.

Keatley, C. W., Spinks, J., and De Gelder, B. (1994). Asymmetrical cross-language priming effects. *Memory and Cognition*, **22**: 70–84.

Kiefer, M. (2002). The N400 is modulated by unconsciously perceived masked words: further evidence for an automatic spreading activation account of N400 priming effects. *Cognitive Brain Research*, **13**: 27–39.

Kim, K. H. S., Relkin, N. R., Lee, K. M., and Hirsch, J. (1997). Distinct cortical areas associated with native and second languages, *Nature*, **388**: 171–4.

Kirsner, K., Brown, H., Abrol, S., Chadha, N. K., and Sharma, N. K. (1980). Bilingualism and lexical representation. *Quarterly Journal of Experimental Psychology, Section A – Human Experimental Psychology*, **32A**: 585–94.

Kirsner, K., Smith, M. C., Lockhart, R. S., King, M. L., and Jain, M. (1984). The bilingual lexicon: language-specific units in an integrated network. *Journal of Verbal Learning and Verbal Behavior*, **23**: 519–39.

Klein, D., Zatorre, R., Milner, B., Meyer, E., and Evans, A. (1994). Left putaminal activation when speaking a second language: evidence from PET. *Neuroreport*, **5**: 2295–7.

Klein, D., Milner, B., Zatorre, R., Meyer, E., and Evans, A. (1995). The neural substrates underlying word generation: a bilingual functional-imaging study. *Proceedings of the National Academy of Science*, **92**: 2899–903.

Kotz, S. A. (1998). Comparing the auditory and visual sequential priming paradigm: an event-related potential study. *Journal of Cognitive Neuroscience Supplement*, 54.

Kotz, S. A. (1996). Bilingual Memory revisited: An electrophysiological investigation of lexical and semantic representations in fluent bilinguals. Unpublished Ph.D. Dissertation. Tufts University.

Kotz, S. A. (2001). Neurolinguistic evidence for bilingual language representation: a comparison of reaction times and event-related brain potentials. *Bilingualism: Language and Cognition*, **4**: 143–54.

Kotz, S. A. and Elston-Güttler, K. E. (2004). The role of proficiency on processing categorical and associative information in the L2 as revealed by reaction times and event-related brain potentials. *Journal of Neurolinguistics*, **17**: 215–35.

Kotz, S. A., Cappa, S. F., von Cramon, D. Y., and Friederici, A. D. (2002). Modulation of the lexical–semantic network by auditory semantic priming: an event-related functional MRI study. *Neuroimage*, **17**: 1761–72.

Kroll, J. F. and Curly, J. (1988). Lexical memory in novice bilinguals: the role of concepts in retrieving second language words. In M. M. Gruneberg, P. Morris, and R. Sykes (eds.), *Practical Aspects of Memory: Current research and issues.* London: John Wiley & Sons, pp. 389–95.

Kroll, J. F. and De Groot, A. M. B. (1997). Lexical and conceptual memory in the bilingual: Mapping form to meaning in two languages. In A. M. B. De Groot and J. Kroll (eds.), *Tutorials in Bilingualism: Psycholinguistic perspectives.* Mahwah, NJ: Lawrence Erlbaum, pp. 169–99.

Kroll, J. F. and Sholl, A. (1992). Lexical and conceptual memory in fluent and nonfluent bilinguals. In R. J. Harris (ed.), *Cognitive Processing in Bilinguals.* Amsterdam: North-Holland, pp. 191–206.

Kroll, J. F. and Stewart, E. (1989). Translating from one language to another: the role of words and concepts in making the connection. Paper presented at the meeting of the Dutch Psychonomic Society, Noordwijkerhout, The Netherlands.

Kroll, J. F. and Stewart, E. (1990). Concept mediation in bilingual translation. Paper presented at the 31st annual meeting of the Psychonomic Society, New Orleans, November.

Kroll, J. F. and Stewart, E. (1994). Category interference in translation and picture naming: evidence for asymmetric connections between bilingual memory representations. *Journal of Memory and Language,* **33**: 149–74.

Kutas, M. and Hillyard, S. A. (1980). Reading senseless sentences: brain potentials reflect semantic incongruity. *Science,* **207**: 203–5.

Kutas, M. and Kluender, R. (1991). What is who violating? A reconsideration of linguistic violations in light of event-related brain potentials. In H. J. Heinze, T. F. Munte, and G. R. Mangun (eds.), *Cognitive Electrophysiology: Basic and clinical applications.* Boston, MA: Birkauser, pp. 183–210.

La Heij, W., De Bruyn, E., Elens, E., Hartsuiker, R., Helaha, D., and Van Schelven, L. (1990). Orthographic facilitation and categorical interference in a word-translation variant of the Stroop task. *Canadian Journal of Psychology,* **44**: 76–83.

La Heij, W., Hooglander, A., Kerling, R., and Vendervelden, E. (1996). Nonverbal context effects in forward and backward translation: evidence for concept mediation. *Journal of Memory and Language,* **35**: 648–65.

Larsen, J. D., Fritsch, T., and Gravia, S. (1994). A semantic priming test of bilingual language storage and compound versus coordinate bilingual distinction with Latvian–English bilinguals. *Perceptual and Motor Skills,* **79**: 459–66.

Lee, M. W. (1994). Functional architecture of the bilingual lexicon. *Working Papers in English and Applied Linguistics,* **1**: 1–14.

Levelt, W. J. M., Roelofs, A., and Meyer, A. S. (1999). A theory of lexical access in speech production. *Behavioral and Brain Sciences,* **22**: 1–75.

Lotto, L. and De Groot, A. M. B. (1998). Effects of learning method and word type on acquiring vocabulary in an unfamiliar language. *Language Learning,* **48**: 31–69.

Lucas, M. M. (1987). Frequency effects on the processing of ambiguous words in sentence context. *Language and Speech,* **30**: 25–46.

Lucas, T. H., McKhann, G. M., and Ojemann, G. A. (2004). Functional separation of languages in the bilingual brain: a comparison of electrical stimulation language mapping in

25 bilingual patients and 117 monolingual control patients. *Journal of Neurosurgery*, **101**: 449–57.

Marian, V., Spivey, M., and Hirsch, J. (2003). Shared and separate systems in bilingual language processing: converging evidence from eyetracking and brain imaging. *Brain and Language*, **86**: 70–82.

McElree, B., Jia, G., and Litvak, A. (2000). The time course of conceptual processing in three bilingual populations. *Journal of Memory and Language*, **42**: 229–54.

Meyer, D. E. and Ruddy, M. G. (1974). Bilingual word-recognition: organization and retrieval of alternative lexical codes. Paper presented to the Eastern Psychological Association, Philadelphia.

Neely, J. H. (1991). Semantic priming effects in visual word recognition: a selective review of current findings and theories. In D. Besner and G. W. Humphreys (eds.), *Basic Processes in Reading – Visual Word Recognition*. Hillsdale, NJ: Lawrence Erlbaum, pp. 264–337.

Ojemann, G. A. (1983). Neurosurgical management of epilepsy: a personal perspective in 1983. *Applied Neurophysiology*, **46**: 11–18.

Ojemann, G. A. and Whitacker, H. A. (1978). The bilingual brain. *Archives of Neurology*, **35**: 409–12.

Ojemann, G. A., Cawthon, D. F., and Lettich, E. (1990). Localization and physiological correlates of language and verbal memory in human lateral temporo-parietal cortex. In A. B. Scheibel and A. F. Wechsler (eds.), *Neurobiology of Higher Cognitive Function*. New York: Guilford Press, pp. 185–202.

Onifer, W. and Swinney, D. A. (1981). Accessing lexical ambiguity during sentence comprehension: effects of frequency of meaning and contextual bias. *Memory and Cognition*, **9**: 225–36.

Paradis, M. (1977). Bilingualism and aphasia. In H. Whitacker and H. A. Whitacker (eds.), *Studies in Neurolinguistics, Vol. 3*. New York: Academic Press, pp. 65–121.

Paradis, M. (2001). Bilingual and polyglot aphasia. In R. S. Berndt (ed.), *Handbook of Neuropsychology*, 2nd edition, *Vol. 3 Language and aphasia*. Elsevier Science: Amsterdam, pp. 69–91.

Paulmann, S., Elston-Güttler, K. E., Gunter, T. C., and Kotz, S. A. (2006). Is bilingual lexical access influenced by language context? *Neuroreport*, **17**(7): 727–31.

Pavlenko, A. (1999). New approaches to concepts in bilingual memory. *Bilingualism: Language and Cognition*, **2**: 209–30.

Perani, D., Dehaene, S., Grassi, F., Cohen, L., Cappa, S. F., Dupoux, E., Fazio, F., and Mehler, J. (1996). Brain processing of native and foreign languages. *Neuroreport*, **7**: 2439–44.

Perani, D., Paulesu, E., Galles, N., Dupoux, E., Dehaene, S., Bettinardi, V., Cappa, S. F., Fazio, F., and Mehler, J. (1998). The bilingual brain: proficiency and age of acquisition of the second language. *Brain*, **121**: 1841–2.

Perani, D., Abutalei, J., Paulesu, E., Brambati, S., Scifo, P., Cappa, S. F., and Fazio, F. (2003). The role of age of acquisition and language usage in early high-proficient bilinguals: an fMRI study during verbal fluency. *Human Brain Mapping*, **19**: 170–82.

Roelofs, A. (2000). Word meanings and concepts: what do the findings from aphasia and language specificity really say? *Bilingualism: Language and Cognition*, **3**: 25–7.

Rueschemeyer, S.-A., Fiebach, C., Kempe, V., and Friederici, A. D. (2005). Processing lexical semantic and syntactic information in first and second language: fMRI evidence from Russian and German. *Human Brain Mapping*, **25**: 266–86.

Scarborough, D. L., Gerard, L., and Cortese, C. (1984). Independence of lexical access in bilingual word recognition. *Journal of Verbal Learning and Verbal Behavior*, **23**: 84–99.

Schwanenflugel, P. J. and Rey, M. (1986). Interlingual semantic facilitation: evidence for a common representational system in the bilingual lexicon. *Journal of Memory and Language*, **25**: 605–18.

Seidenberg, M., Tanenhaus, M. K., Leiman, J. M., and Bienkowski, M. (1982). Automatic access of the meanings of ambiguous words in context: some limitations of knowledge-based processing. *Cognitive Psychology*, **14**: 489–537.

Smith, M. C. and Kirsner, K. (1982). Language and orthography as irrelevant features in colour–word and picture–word Stroop interference. *Quarterly Journal of Experimental Psychology, Section A – Human Experimental Psychology*, **34A**: 153–70.

Snodgrass, J. G. (1993). Translating vs. picture naming: Similarities and differences. In R. Schreuder and B. Weltens (eds.), *The Bilingual Lexicon*, Amsterdam/Philadelphia: John Benjamins, pp. 83–114.

Soares, C. and Grosjean, F. (1984). Bilinguals in a monolingual and a bilingual speech mode: the effect of lexical access. *Memory and Cognition*, **12**: 380–6.

Swinney, D. A. (1979). Lexical access during sentence comprehension: (re)consideration of context effects, *Journal of Verbal Learning and Verbal Behavior*, **18**: 545–69.

Thompson-Schill, S., D'Esposito, M., Aguirre, G., and Farah, M. (1997). Role of left inferior prefrontal cortex in retrieval of semantic knowledge: a reevaluation. *Proceedings of the National Academy of Science*, **94**: 14792–7.

Ullman, M. T. (2001). The neural basis of lexicon and grammar in first and second language: the declarative/procedural model. *Bilingualism: Language and Cognition*, **4**: 105–22.

Vaid, J. and Hull, R. (2002). Re-envisioning the bilingual brain using functional magnetic imaging: methodological and interpretative issues. In F. Fabbro (ed.), *Advances in Neurolinguistics of Bilingualism*. Udine: Forum, pp. 315–55.

Van den Brink, D., Brown, C. M., and Hagoort, P. (2001). Electrophysiological evidence for early contextual influences during spoken-word recognition: N200 versus N400. *Journal of Cognitive Neuroscience*, **13**: 967–85.

Van Hell, J. G. and De Groot, A. M. B. (1998a). Disentangling context availability and concreteness in lexical decision and word translation. *Quarterly Journal of Experimental Psychology, Section A – Human Experimental Psychology*, **51A**: 1, 41–63.

Van Hell, J. G. and De Groot, A. M. B. (1998b). Conceptual representation in bilingual memory: effects of concreteness and cognate status in word association. *Bilingualism: Language and Cognition*, **1**: 193–211.

Van Heste, T. (1999). Visual word recognition in bilinguals: selective and nonselective activation processes as a function of the experimental task, Unpublished Master's Thesis, University of Leuven.

Van Petten, C. and Kutas, M. (1990). Interactions between sentence context and word frequency in event-related brain potentials. *Memory and Cognition*, **18**: 380–93.

Wagner, A. D., Desmond, J. E., Demb, J. B., Glover, G. H., and Gabrieli, J. D. E. (1997). Semantic memory processes and left inferior prefrontal cortex: a functional MRI study of form specificity. *Journal of Cognitive Neurosicence*, **9**: 714–26.

Wartenburger, I., Heekeren, H., Abutalebi, J., Cappa, S. F., Vrillinger, A., and Perani, D. (2003). Early setting of grammatical processing in the bilingual brain. *Neuron*, **37**: 159–70.

Weber-Fox, C. M. and Neville, H. J. (1996). Maturational constraints on functional specializations for language processing: ERP and behavioral evidence in bilingual speakers. *Journal of Cognitive Neuroscience*, **8**: 231–56.

Weinreich, U. (1953). *Languages in Contact: Findings and problems.* The Hague: Mouton and Company.

Williams, J. N. (1994). The relationship between word meanings in the first and second language: evidence for a common, but restricted, semantic code. *European Journal of Cognitive Psychology*, **6**: 195–220.

Xue, G., Dong, Q., Jin, Z., Zhang, L., and Wang, Y. (2004). An fMRI study with semantic access in low proficiency second language processing in Chinese–English bilinguals. *Neuroreport*, **14**: 1557–62.

Part III

Applications of Models to Understanding Cognitive Dysfunction

5

Schizophrenia and semantic memory

Michal Assaf[1,2], Paul Rivkin[3], Michael A. Kraut[3], Vince Calhoun[1,2,3], John Hart Jr.[4] and Godfrey Pearlson[1,2,3]

[1]Institute of Living
[2]Yale University
[3]Johns Hopkins University
[4]University of Texas at Dallas

Schizophrenia is a severe, chronic, and disabling psychiatric illness that affects 1 percent of the population. It is often characterized by disorganized speech, delusions, hallucinations, disorganized or catatonic behavior, and negative symptoms such as flat affect and avolition (*Diagnostic and statistical Manual of Mental Disorders, 4th edn. − DSM-IV*). The symptoms related to disorganized and incoherent speech are also known as formal thought disorder (FTD). Although symptoms may vary from patient to patient and between different episodes of the illness in the same patient, 90 percent of the patients show FTD symptoms at some point during the course of their illness (Andreasen, 1979b). Even though these symptoms have been considered to be fundamental to schizophrenia since first described by Bleuler (Bleuler, 1911) and Kraepelin (Kraepelin *et al.*, 1919), the cognitive impairments associated with the neurobiology of FTD are still a matter of debate. One of the most influential theories to date suggests that FTD is strongly associated with impaired semantic memory processing (Spitzer, 1997; Goldberg *et al.*, 1998; Kerns & Berenbaum, 2002). In this chapter we will review the clinical and cognitive symptoms related to FTD, the evidence available that supports different aspects of semantic impairments in FTD, and recent data from our lab suggesting that a far-spreading activation theory within the semantic system is the core, underlying deficit resulting in FTD.

5.1 Formal thought disorder

As mentioned above, the symptoms of FTD have been considered by some investigators as pathognomonic to schizophrenia. For example, Bleuler, who first described the disease, reported these symptoms as "the associations lose their continuity ... In this way, thinking becomes illogical and often bizarre ... Furthermore, associations tend to proceed along new lines...two ideas are combined into one thought . . . clang-associations receive unusual significance as do indirect associations . . ." (Bleuler, 1911, p. 14). He referred to this group of symptoms as loose associations that point to a potential deficiency in the semantic system. However, others (e.g. Andreasen, 1979b; Sax *et al.*, 1995) note the occurrence of FTD in other psychiatric disorders, such as mania.

But it was not before 1979 that the first clinical assessment tool for FTD was published by Andreasen: the Thought, Language and Communication Scale (TLC; Andreasen, 1979a, 1986). This scale includes 18 items, such as poverty of speech and content; pressure of speech; derailment; circumstantiality; neologism; echolalia; blocking; incoherence, etc. Each item is scored on a 4 or 5 point rating scale based on a standardized interview that includes 10 minutes of free speech and series of abstract, concrete, impersonal, and personal questions. Andreasen (1979b) used this scale to distinguish between negative and positive FTD. This distinction is important since different patient groups might show either pattern of thought disorder, and also because the mechanisms that underlie these patterns are probably different. In this chapter, we will discuss mainly positive FTD.

The TLC provided the first standardized tool that quantified positive FTD severity which in turn enhanced FTD research. Several theories have been posited as to which cognitive domain, if disrupted, would result in the symptoms of FTD, including impairments in working memory, attention, semantic processing, language production, and/or executive functions (for review, see Kerns & Berenbaum, 2002). The most accepted theory is that FTD is strongly associated with impaired semantic processing (Spitzer, 1997; Goldberg *et al.*, 1998; Kerns & Berenbaum, 2002).

5.2 Semantic memory and formal thought disorder

As suggested earlier, the assumption that FTD is a disease of association was made as early as the concept of schizophrenia was introduced (Bleuler, 1911; Kraepelin *et al.*, 1919). Kraepelin demonstrated this concept initially using a free association paradigm (Spitzer & Mundt, 1994; Spitzer, 1997), with more recent studies suggesting a semantic disruption with FTD resulting from semantic priming studies (for review, see Spitzer, 1997). Normal semantic priming in healthy participants is usually demonstrated via a lexical decision task. In this task, a subject has to report if a letter string presented represents a real word ("tree") or a nonword ("gurk"). The semantic priming version of the task involves presenting a semantically related prime ("leaf") for a brief, subliminal period prior to presenting the target word, and if the target is a real word and related to the prime, then the lexical decision will be faster than without the prime. In normal individuals, a semantic priming effect of reduced reaction time in making a lexical decision has been commonly explained on the basis of an underlying semantic network being organized by interconnected units of related words (e.g. objects, features). An activation of one word unit activates all of the related units for a short period of time and thus the threshold for activation of all the related, interconnected words in this network decreases. Consequently, any activated word that is processed in this period of time is recognized faster. Manschreck *et al.* (1988) found that schizophrenic patients with FTD exhibited an increase in the semantic priming effect compared to healthy controls and non-FTD schizophrenic patients. This finding was explained by the suggestion that there is increased, automatic spreading of activation in the semantic network. According to this explanation, the magnitude of associational activation between units in the semantic network is greater (i.e. stronger) in FTD patients.

While the increased semantic priming was replicated by some studies (e.g. Spitzer *et al.*, 1993, 1994), others found no difference between FTD patients and healthy participants and even decreased semantic priming effect (e.g. Barch & Berenbaum, 1996; Aloia *et al.*, 1998; for review see Kerns & Berenbaum, 2002). These conflicting results have been accounted for by the theory of far-spreading activation suggested by Manfred Spitzer (1997). His work demonstrated that schizophrenia patients with FTD show increased indirect but not direct semantic priming effects at short-onset asynchronies (referring to the time between the prime and the target), and not at longer-onset asynchronies, when compared to non-FTD patients and healthy controls. Indirect priming refers to when the prime word is related to the target word by a third word not presented (e.g. milk−[white]−black). The far-spreading activation theory for FTD in schizophrenia accounts for this finding by suggesting that automatic semantic activation (evident by the short stimulus−onset asynchrony − SOA) occurs in more diffuse fashion, activating semantic units that are farther apart from the original activated prime word. At present, the underlying neural mechanism of this potential far-spreading activation within the semantic memory network has not yet been demonstrated.

5.3 Neuroimaging studies of FTD

Only a few studies to date, including one from our lab, have examined the brain abnormalities related to FTD using functional neuroimaging methods. However, studies from other labs have not explored the relationship of these brain abnormalities to semantic processes. In this section we will describe the results of these studies. We will then describe our research that focuses on brain abnormalities associated with semantic memory retrieval and FTD.

An early neuroimaging study used positron emission tomography (PET) to evaluate the relationship between regional blood flow and symptomatology of 30 schizophrenia patients during a resting state (Liddle *et al.*, 1992). This study showed that patients with disorganization syndrome, of which FTD is a primary symptom, had hypoperfusion of the right ventrolateral prefrontal cortex (VLPFC) and bilateral angular gyrus, and hyperperfusion of the anterior cingulate cortex (ACC) and dorsomedial thalamic nuclei. A second PET study (Kaplan *et al.*, 1993) measuring glucose metabolism showed an association between disorganization scores and glucose metabolism in left superior temporal and inferior parietal areas in 20 schizophrenia patients.

The studies that followed these early PET publications determined cerebral activity patterns during cognitive task performance in schizophrenia patients with FTD (McGuire *et al.*, 1998; Kircher *et al.*, 2001, 2002). McGuire *et al.* (1998) used H2 15O PET to measure brain activation in six males with schizophrenia while they were describing 12 ambiguous pictures. They found that FTD negatively correlated with activation in the ACC, right inferior frontal gyrus (IFG) and dorsolateral prefrontal cortex (DLPFC), and left superior temporal sulcus (STS) and insula. FTD positively correlated with activation in the area of parahippocampus and fusiform gyrus and the right caudate. Kircher *et al.*'s (2001, 2002) studies used functional magnetic resonance imaging (fMRI) to examine the neural correlates of continuous speech production in six thought-disordered schizophrenia patients versus healthy controls by eliciting speech output as subjects talked about Rorschach inkblots. They examined the relationship between the number of words spoken and blood-oxygen-level-dependent (BOLD) response, in a within-subject design. Patterns of speech production, i.e. the variances and patterns of fluctuation in the number of words produced, did not differ between the two groups. These studies demonstrated negative correlation between brain activity and FTD severity in the left superior and middle temporal gyri and a positive correlation in the cerebellar vermis, right caudate body, and precentral gyrus. These studies, albeit inconclusive, suggest a role of prefrontal areas, STS and inferior parietal lobule (IPL) in the pathophysiology of FTD.

5.4   Semantic object recall in schizophrenia

Based on the suggested role of semantic memory dysfunction in the pathophysiology of FTD, we examined whether a specific semantic memory operation is more relevant to this symptomatology. FTD is consistent with impaired connections between and within representational levels in semantic memory. To probe this, our group used a semantic memory task, the Semantic Object Recall from Features input Task (SORT), which required subjects to connect two features (e.g. "desert" and "humps") together to determine if the combination resulted in recall of a specific object (e.g. "camel"). Models of semantic object memory that support a hierarchical architecture define feature-level representations as beneath the object level. Thus a semantic memory task utilizing a bottom–up approach of features activating an object representation addresses the proposed dysfunction in FTD.

The SORT task that we employed has been investigated with neuroimaging and electrophysiological approaches, and has shown to engage two neural mechanisms for successful task performance. The first mechanism is a semantic search strategy or framework for the object to be recalled, which has been postulated to be mediated by a medial BA6 – dorsomedial nucleus of the thalamus interaction that results in a global cortical decrease in alpha electroencephalogram (EEG) power. The second is a "binding" process that links together the features of the object to be recalled, this being mediated by the pulvinar nucleus of the thalamus, which modulates a focal gamma EEG rhythm that synchronizes the firing of the neuronal elements that encode for the associated object features (see Kraut *et al.*, 2003). Therefore we suggest that a disruption in the process of object recall in semantic memory, which might lead to the positive symptom of FTD in schizophrenia, could result from two causes. These are (1) forming an inadequate framework or strategy to search for the correct object, or (2) dysfunctional synchronization of object features. To test this hypothesis we administered the SORT, and tasks that assess two other semantic object level operations, the Synonym Judgment Task and the Category Judgment Task. As mentioned above, during the SORT individuals assessed whether pairs of features/properties combined to result in recall of a specific object (bottom–up feature to object recall task that engages a frontal semantic selection operation and neural rhythm synchronization of cortical regions encoding object features). During the Synonym Judgment Task subjects were presented with one word and then had to choose from another pair of words the one whose meaning was closest to an exemplar (within-stratum task that assesses the ability to detect object-level equivalence in the lexical–semantic system). Finally, in the third task, the Category Judgment Task, individuals assessed whether two objects belonged to the same category (bottom–up semantic search for a category framework and hierarchical object-to-category membership decision).

We hypothesized that if the frontal lobe search component for target objects or neural synchronization mechanisms were dysfunctional, measures of positive FTD severity would correlate with performance decrements on the SORT only, as opposed to a generalized dysfunction on all semantic tasks. If there were a widespread semantic network dysfunction, as proposed by some models, then one would expect that any of the semantic memory operations that accessed the network would be equally likely to be disrupted and thus all tasks would be likely to be relatively equally impaired. A third possibility is that if one of the other processes in the category or synonym control tasks were selectively disrupted, then there would be an isolated association with FTD measures.

Twenty-one schizophrenia patients (10 males) from the psychiatry inpatient and outpatient clinics at Johns Hopkins Hospital were recruited to participate in this study. Participants' mean age ($\pm$SD) was 39.55 $\pm$ 10.07 with 12.5 $\pm$ 1.73 years of education. All subjects were receiving neuroleptic pharmacotherapy. Patients' symptoms were assessed by the Scale for the Assessment of Negative Symptoms (SANS) (Andreasen, 1984a) and the Scale for the Assessment of Positive Symptoms (SAPS) (Andreasen, 1984b). FTD severity was assessed by the SAPS positive formal thought disorder global rating scale. The patients also received the three semantic memory tasks described above.

Analysis of the standardized SAPS measure of thought disorder in relation to the semantic memory tasks shown in a regression analysis yielded a model in which 57.6 percent (adjusted R^2 for the regression model) of the variability of positive FTD was attributable to performance problems in semantic object recall test, Category Judgment Task, and Synonym Judgment Task assessments. Among these three candidate explanatory variables, only the standardized β coefficient for the semantic object recall test was significant ($\beta_a = -0.787$, $t = -4.015$, $p = 0.001$), whereas the Synonym Judgment Task ($\beta_s = 0.017$, $t = 0.107$, $p = 0.916$) and Category Judgment Task ($\beta_c = -0.027$, $t = -0.141$, $p = 0.889$) terms did not account for significant variability of positive FTD.

These findings demonstrate that positive FTD severity is substantially explained by performance on semantic object recall, whereas category and synonym judgment errors add no significant explanatory power to the model. This suggests that the FTD symptoms in schizophrenia may not extend from a disruption of the semantic network, but are secondary to selective dysfunction in specific components of semantic operations related to semantic object retrieval (Kraut *et al.*, 2002, 2003; Slotnick *et al.*, 2002; Assaf *et al.*, 2006b).

5.5 Neural correlates of semantic object recall in FTD

To further investigate the neural dysfunction that underlies the specific semantic deficit in FTD, we used fMRI during the performance of the SORT. We evaluated the association between brain activation related to semantic processing in schizophrenia and FTD symptom severity, as well as differences in signal change patterns between patients and matched healthy controls (Assaf *et al.*, 2006a). The fMRI version of the SORT included 16 recall (R) pairs, where two words were visually presented describing features of an object that combined to elicit an object that was not presented (e.g. "honey" and "stings", which evoke the object "bee"), and 16 no-recall (NR) pairs, where the words presented did not combine to recall such an object (e.g. "quacks" and "honey"; see Figure 5.1). Participants were instructed to push a button with their dominant index finger if the two words evoked a specific object and their dominant middle finger if they did not. To minimize stimulus-specific effects due to the words themselves, stimuli used in the NR pairs were permutations of words used in the R pairs. The order of the two pair types was pseudo-randomized and was consistent for all participants. Each pair was presented for 2.7 s and was not terminated by participants' button press, with 5.5 s inter-stimulus interval. (For complete imaging procedures see Assaf *et al.*, 2006a).

Sixteen chronic patients were recruited to the fMRI study: 14 chronic schizophrenia (12 paranoid, 2 undifferentiated) and 2 chronic schizoaffective subjects. Diagnoses were determined with the Structured Clinical Interview for *DSM-IV* Axis I Disorders (First *et al.*, 2002) and current symptoms assessed with the Positive and Negative Symptom Scale (PANSS; Kay *et al.*, 1987) and the Thought Disorder Index (TDI; Solovay *et al.*, 1986). TDI's total score and separate sum of positive, negative, and general items on the PANSS were used for statistical analyses. In addition, we calculated a disorganization score from the PANSS (Salokangas *et al.*, 2002) based on the summed scores of the following items: Conceptual Disorganization, Tension, Excitement and Mannerism oblique Posturing. PANSS ratings from one patient and TDI ratings from four patients

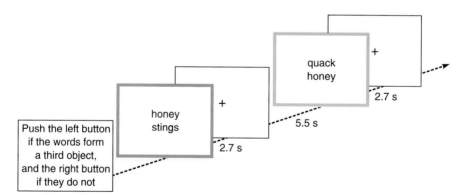

Figure 5.1.   Schematic representation of the object recall task. The task includes 16 recall pairs (R, orange square) and 16 no-recall pairs (NR, green square). The words pairs are presented for 2.7 s with a fixation cross of 5.5 s in between them. During the actual run the word pairs are presented in the center of a screen without a frame. Reprinted from Assaf *et al.* (2006a), with permission from Elsevier Science Inc. and Society of Biological Psychiatry.

were unavailable. Sixteen healthy controls, group-matched to patients on age, gender, race, and handedness, were also recruited. They had no current or past history of any axis I severe combined immunodeficiency (SCID) diagnosis and no first-degree family member with schizophrenia.

Analyses of performance accuracy and reaction times of the SORT revealed that schizophrenia patients showed a trend towards having more false positive responses than controls ($t = 1.98$, $p = 0.057$), i.e. they over-recalled NR pairs. They also tended to be slower when correctly responding to R pairs ($t = -1.92$, $p = 0.06$). The patients' number of over-recalled events tended to correlate positively with FTD severity on the TDI ($r = 0.52$, $p = 0.085$) and with positive symptom severity ($r = 0.46$, $p = 0.082$). No significant correlations were found between over-recalling and PANSS negative, general, or disorganization scores.

Analyses of brain activations showed a significant positive correlation between patients' FTD severity (as measured by the TDI) and brain activation during correctly recalled trials (R) in the rostral ACC (rACC, Talairach coordinates of maximum signal change: $x = -9$, $y = 38$, $z = 6$, $r = 0.70$, $p = 0.01$; Figure 5.2). A similar positive correlation in this area was found between FTD severity and brain activation during the false-positive trials (i.e. over-recalled trials) ($x = -3$, $y = 47$, $z = 6$, $r = 0.62$, $p = 0.05$). The activation of rACC during both correctly recalled and over-recalled trials showed no significant correlation with the PANSS scores.

A two-sample t-test of the R > NR contrast (this contrast explores greater activation during the correct R events than during the correct NR events) found that schizophrenia patients overactivated ($p < 0.05$) brain areas previously shown

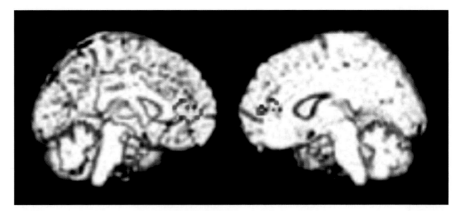

Figure 5.2. Correlation map of brain activation during correct recall trials with FTD severity in schizophrenia as measured by the TDI: n = 12, p < 0.05, k = 25. Reprinted from Assaf *et al.* (2006a), with permission from Elsevier Science Inc. and Society of Biological Psychiatry.

to be involved normally in this task (Kraut *et al.*, 2002, 2003; Assaf *et al.*, 2006b) and in other semantic processing tasks (Thompson-Schill *et al.*, 1997; Martin & Chao, 2001; Manns *et al.*, 2003) compared to healthy controls. These brain areas included bilateral dorsal and ventral ACC, pre-SMA (supplementary motor area), TOJ (temporo-occipital junction) (middle temporal gyms/middle occipital gyms – MTG/MOG), TP and parahippocampal complexes (PHC); right DLPFC; and left precentral gyrus (Figure 5.3). Right IFG also showed higher BOLD signal difference between R and NR events in schizophrenia compared to healthy controls; however, that was due to less activation during the "no-recall" trials rather than more activation during the recall trials, which was also the case in the other areas reported. The only area where schizophrenia patients activated less than healthy controls specific to the object-recall process was bilateral IPL (Figure 5.3).

The abnormal brain activations seen in the patient group during the performance of the SORT task can be related to three different cognitive functions: semantic memory (left IFG, MTG, TP and PHC), verbal working memory (DLPFC and IPL), and initiation and suppression of conflicting responses (ACC). Schizophrenia patients showed semantic memory network overactivation, possibly retrieving more distantly related semantic responses which create more potential responses "in the pipeline". Another plausible explanation is that, as in the findings in studies of older aging normals, schizophrenics need to recruit more brain regions than comparable controls to

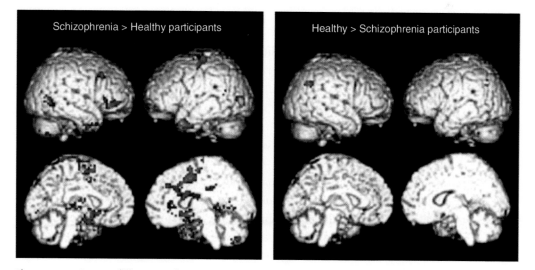

Figure 5.3.   Group differences brain maps contrasting correct recall with correct no-recall trials (Recall > No Recall). $n = 32$, $p < 0.05$, $k = 25$. Reprinted from Assaf *et al.* (2006a), with permission from Elsevier Science Inc. and Society of Biological Psychiatry.

maintain adequate performance on cognitive tasks. It is possible that the ACC activity in patients increases to handle this higher-volume input and to suppress the incorrect responses. Alternatively, the abnormal ACC activation may reflect inefficient semantic search initiation, leading to the abnormal activation of the semantic network.

Our results are generally in accord with the theory of far-spreading activation in schizophrenia. Behaviorally, patients retrieved more objects based on unrelated (distant) features and did so more slowly than healthy controls. Functionally, during the process of feature-based object retrieval from semantic memory, patients overactivated not only the normal semantic memory network, but also alternate semantic areas, not usually activated during this task (i.e. PHC) to retrieve objects from semantic memory. We conjecture that abnormalities in the verbal working memory network (as shown in the DLPFC and IPL) and inappropriate or inefficient suppression of these conflicting incorrect responses (as shown in the ACC) lead the patients to manifest overbinding in our task and potentially FTD symptoms in general.

This interpretation should be taken cautiously, since we found a direct relationship between brain activation and FTD symptoms only in the ACC. We failed to show this relationship with IPL, MTG, IFG, DLPFC, and PHC, areas that were reported previously to have functional correlations with FTD severity (Liddle *et al.*, 1992; Kaplan *et al.*, 1993; McGuire *et al.*, 1998; Kircher *et al.*, 2001, 2002). However, these two former studies approximated FTD by measuring symptoms of disorganization, and the other studies had small sample sizes of FTD subjects. Therefore the specificity of these past results of disrupted activation to FTD remains unclear.

In summary, FTD is a debilitating symptom that affects 90 percent of schizophrenic patients and undermines a patient's capacity to communicate. The most widely accepted hypothesis to date suggests that abnormalities in semantic memory processing are responsible for FTD. Although some studies have shown a relationship between brain activation in prefrontal, temporal and parietal areas and FTD, none has explored the relationship of these abnormalities to deficits in semantic memory. In our lab we showed that FTD is specifically associated with impaired object recall from features in semantic memory and not with other semantic processes (such as synonym and category judgment). We further demonstrated the neural abnormalities that underlie this semantic deficit. These abnormalities suggest an overactivation of semantic areas (left IFG, MTG, TP, and PHC), verbal working memory (DLPFC and IPL), and initiation and suppression of conflicting responses (ACC). These results are generally in accord with the hypothesis of far-spreading activation.

REFERENCES

Aloia, M. S., Gourovitch, M. L., Missar, D., Pickar, D., Weinberger, D. R., and Goldberg, T. E. (1998). Cognitive substrates of thought disorder, II: specifying a candidate cognitive mechanism. *American Journal of Psychiatry*, **155**(12): 1677–84.

American Psychiatric Association (1994). *Diagnostic and Statistical Manual of Mental Disorders: DSM-IV*, 4th edn. Washington, DC: American Psychiatric Association.

Andreasen, N. C. (1979a). Thought, language, and communication disorders. I. Clinical assessment, definition of terms, and evaluation of their reliability. *Archives of General Psychiatry*, **36**(12): 1315–21.

Andreasen, N. C. (1979b). Thought, language, and communication disorders. II. Diagnostic significance. *Archives of General Psychiatry*, **36**(12): 1325–30.

Andreasen, N. C. (1984a). *The Scale for the Assessment of Negative Symptoms (SANS)*. Iowa City: The University of Iowa.

Andreasen, N. C. (1984b). *The Scale for the Assessment of Positive Symptoms (SAPS)*. Iowa City: The University of Iowa.

Andreasen, N. C. (1986). Scale for the assessment of thought, language, and communication (TLC). *Schizophrenia Bulletin*, **12**(3): 473–82.

Assaf, M., Rivkin, P. R., Kuzu, C. H., Calhoun, V. D., Kraut, M. A., Groth, K. M., Yassa, M. A., Hart, J., and Pearlson, G. D. (2006a). Abnormal object recall and anterior cingulate overactivation correlate with formal thought disorder in schizophrenia. *Biological Psychiatry*, **59**(5): 452–9.

Assaf, M., Calhoun, V. D., Kuzu, C. H., Kraut, M. A., Rivkin, P. R., Hart, J., and Pearlson, G. D. (2006). Neural correlates of the object recall process in semantic memory. *Psychiatry Research: Neuroimaging*, **147**(2–3): 115–26.

Barch, D. M. and Berenbaum, H. (1996). Language production and thought disorder in schizophrenia. *Journal of Abnormal Psychology*, **105**(1): 81–8.

Bleuler, E. (1911/1950). *Dementia Praecox of the Group of Schizophrenias*, ed. J. T. Zinkin. New York: International Universities Press.

First, M. B., Spitzer, R. L., Gibbon, M., and Williams, J. B. W. (2002). *Structured Clinical Interview for DSM-IV-TR Axis I Disorders, Research Version, Patient Edition. (SCID-I/P)*. New York: Biometrics Research, New York State Psychiatric Institute.

Goldberg, T. E., Aloia, M. S., Gourovitch, M. L., Missar, D., Pickar, D., and Weinberger, D. R. (1998). Cognitive substrates of thought disorder, I: the semantic system. *American Journal of Psychiatry*, **155**(12): 1671–6.

Kaplan, R. D., Szechtman, H., Franco, S., Szechtman, B., Nahmias, C., Garnett, E. S., List, S., and Cleghorn, J. M. (1993). Three clinical syndromes of schizophrenia in untreated subjects: relation to brain glucose activity measured by positron emission tomography (PET). *Schizophrenia Research*, **11**(1): 47–54.

Kay, S. R., Fiszbein, A., and Opler, L. A. (1987). The positive and negative syndrome scale (PANSS) for schizophrenia. *Schizophrenia Bulletin*, **13**(2): 261–76.

Kerns, J. G. and Berenbaum, H. (2002). Cognitive impairments associated with formal thought disorder in people with schizophrenia. *Journal of Abnormal Psychology*, **111**(2): 211–24.

Kircher, T. T., Liddle, P. F., Brammer, M. J., Williams, S. C., Murray, R. M., and McGuire, P. K. (2001). Neural correlates of formal thought disorder in schizophrenia: preliminary findings from a functional magnetic resonance imaging study. *Archives of General Psychiatry*, **58**(8): 769–74.

Kircher, T. T., Liddle, P. F., Brammer, M. J., Williams, S. C., Murray, R. M., and McGuire, P. K. (2002). Reversed lateralization of temporal activation during speech production in thought disordered patients with schizophrenia. *Psychological Medicine*, **32**(3): 439–49.

Kraepelin, E., Barclay, R. M., and Robertson, G. M. (1919). *Dementia Praecox and Paraphrenia*. Edinburgh, Scotland: E & S Livingstone.

Kraut, M. A., Kremen, S., Segal, J. B., Calhoun, V., Moo, L. R., and Hart, J. Jr. (2002). Object activation from features in the semantic system. *Journal of Cognitive Neuroscience*, **14**(1): 24–36.

Kraut, M. A., Calhoun, V., Pitcock, J. A., Cusick, C., and Hart, J. Jr. (2003). Neural hybrid model of semantic object memory: implications from event-related timing using fMRI. *Journal of the International Neuropsychological Society*, **9**(7): 1031–40.

Liddle, P. F., Friston, K. J., Frith, C. D., Hirsch, S. R., Jones, T., and Frackowiak, R. S. (1992). Patterns of cerebral blood flow in schizophrenia. *British Journal of Psychiatry*, **160**: 179–86.

Manns, J. R., Hopkins, R. O., and Squire, L. R. (2003). Semantic memory and the human hippocampus. *Neuron*, **38**(1): 127–33.

Manschreck, T. C., Maher, B. A., Milavetz, J. J., Ames, D., Weisstein, C. C., and Schneyer, M. L. (1988). Semantic priming in thought disordered schizophrenic patients. *Schizophrenia Research*, **1**(1): 61–6.

Martin, A., and Chao, L. L. (2001). Semantic memory and the brain: structure and processes. *Current Opinion in Neurobiology*, **11**(2): 194–201.

McGuire, P. K., Quested, D. J., Spence, S. A., Murray, R. M., Frith, C. D., and Liddle, P. F. (1998). Pathophysiology of "positive" thought disorder in schizophrenia. *British Journal of Psychiatry*, **173**: 231–5.

Salokangas, R. K., Honkonen, T., Stengard, E., and Koivisto, A. M. (2002). Symptom dimensions and their association with outcome and treatment setting in long-term schizophrenia. Results of the DSP project. *Nordic Journal of Psychiatry*, **56**(5): 319–27.

Sax, K. W., Strakowski, S. M., McElroy, S. L., Keck, P. E. Jr., and West, S. A. (1995). Attention and formal thought disorder in mixed and pure mania, *Biological Psychiatry*, **37**: 420–3.

Slotnick, S. D., Moo, L. R., Kraut, M. A., Lesser, R. P., and Hart, J. Jr. (2002). Interactions between thalamic and cortical rhythms during semantic memory recall in human. *Proceedings of the National Academy of Sciences of the United States of America*, **99**(9): 6440–3.

Solovay, M. R., Shenton, M. E., Gasperetti, C., Coleman, M., Kestnbaum, E., Carpenter, J. T., and Holzman, P. S. (1986). Scoring manual for the Thought Disorder Index. *Schizophrenia Bulletin*, **12**(3): 483–96.

Spitzer, M., Braun, U., Hermle, L., and Maier, S. (1993). Associative semantic network dysfunction in thought-disordered schizophrenic patients: direct evidence from indirect semantic priming. *Biological Psychiatry*, **34**(12): 864–77.

Spitzer, M., Weisker, I., Winter, M., Maier, S., Hermle, L., and Maher, B. A. (1994). Semantic and phonological priming in schizophrenia. *Journal of Abnormal Psychology*, **103**(3): 485–94.

Spitzer, M. and Mundt, C. (1994). Interchanges between psychology and psychiatry: the continental tradition. *Current Opinion in Psychiatry*, **7**: 417–22.

Spitzer, M. (1997). A cognitive neuroscience view of schizophrenic thought disorder. *Schizophrenia Bulletin*, **23**(1): 29–50.

Thompson-Schill, S. L., D'Esposito, M., Aguirre, G. K., and Farah, M. J. (1997). Role of left inferior prefrontal cortex in retrieval of semantic knowledge: a reevaluation. *Proceedings of the National Academy of Sciences of the United States of America*, **94**(26): 14792–7.

Part IV

Representations of Nouns and Verbs vs. Objects and Actions

6

Effects of word imageability on semantic access: neuroimaging studies

Jeffrey R. Binder

Medical College of Wisconsin

The axiom that conceptual knowledge is grounded in perceptual experience has a long history in philosophy (Locke, 1690/1959; Hume, 1739/1975) and clinical neurology (Wernicke, 1874; Freud, 1891/1953; Geschwind, 1965), and has had considerable influence on modern neuroscience (e.g. Paivio, 1971; Allport, 1985; Damasio, 1989; Barsalou, 1999; Pulvermüller, 1999; Glenberg & Robertson, 2000; Martin *et al.*, 2000). This principle has been applied conspicuously, for example, in accounts of category-related knowledge deficits that postulate selective damage to modality-specific perceptual knowledge stores. Living things tend to have many salient, defining visual features, making access to these concepts highly reliant on knowledge about visual attributes. Conversely, tools and many other artifact concepts are distinguished on the basis of their functions, which could be partly encoded in motor programs and knowledge of the characteristic motion of artifacts (Warrington & McCarthy, 1987; Farah & McClelland, 1991; Martin *et al.*, 2000). Implicit in this account is the notion that conceptual knowledge is partially stored in perceptual and kinesthetic representations residing in or near the modality-specific sensory—motor systems through which these concrete object concepts were originally learned.

While many neuroimaging studies have tested this theory using comparisons between different types of concrete objects (see Martin & Chao, 2001; Bookheimer, 2002; Devlin *et al.*, 2002; Price & Friston, 2002; Thompson-Schill, 2003; Damasio *et al.*, 2004 for excellent reviews), another testable prediction of the theory involves the qualitative distinction between concrete and abstract concepts. Unlike concrete concepts, abstract concepts — such as *honesty, quantity, sense*, and *theory* — do not directly reference sensory—motor percepts. Although abstract concepts are ultimately grounded in experience, these experiences tend to involve complex human interactions unfolding over time and space rather than simple,

The three studies described here were supported by National Institutes of Health grants R01 NS33576, P01 MH51358, and M01 RR00058. My thanks to D. S. Sabsevitz, D. A. Medler, R. Desai, E. Liebenthal, L. L. Conant, and other colleagues in the Language Imaging Laboratory at MCW.

circumscribed perceptual events. Indeed, many researchers have distinguished abstract from concrete concepts on the basis of their *imageability*, a measure obtained by asking subjects to rate the ease with which a target concept can be "mentally visualized" (Paivio *et al.*, 1968). Abstract concepts are typically defined not in terms of readily visualized perceptual attributes but rather by reference to other verbal concepts, most of which are also abstract. If concrete concepts are stored partly within perceptual–motor systems, then these systems ought to be activated to a greater extent by concrete words than by abstract words.

The notion that neural processing of words is partly determined by imageability was first clearly articulated by Paivio as the "dual coding theory" (Paivio, 1971, 1986). Dual coding theory proposes that abstract concepts are encoded and stored in memory in the form of symbolic or "verbal" representations, whereas concrete concepts are dually encoded into memory as both verbal representations and "image" codes grounded in perceptual experience. From a neurobiological perspective, abstract nouns are hypothesized to rely on a verbal semantic system located in the language-dominant hemisphere, whereas concrete nouns access additional sensory–motor "image" codes located in both hemispheres. Much research supports the idea that conceptual processes are modulated by word imageability. For example, individuals respond more quickly and more accurately when making lexical decisions about concrete nouns than abstract nouns (James, 1975; Kroll & Merves, 1986; Kounios & Holcomb, 1994), and concrete nouns are better recalled on memory tests than abstract nouns (Paivio, 1971, 1986). Neurological patients often show performance advantages for concrete over abstract nouns (Goodglass *et al.*, 1969; Coltheart *et al.*, 1980; Roeltgen *et al.*, 1983; Katz & Goodglass, 1990; Franklin *et al.*, 1995) or the converse (Warrington, 1975, 1981; Warrington & Shallice, 1984; Breedin *et al.*, 1995; Marshall *et al.*, 1998). Other supporting evidence comes from divided visual field studies that have shown a concreteness advantage for words presented to the right hemisphere (left visual field) but not the left hemisphere (Day, 1979; Chiarello *et al.*, 1987; Deloche *et al.*, 1987), studies of patients with corpus callosum injuries (Zaidel, 1978; Coltheart *et al.*, 1980; Coslett & Saffran, 1989; Coslett & Monsul, 1994), and electrophysiological experiments (Kounios & Holcomb, 1994; Holcomb *et al.*, 1999; Kounios & Holcomb, 2000; Nittono *et al.*, 2002), all of which suggest more extensive processing of concrete words than abstract words in the right hemisphere.

6.1 Neuroimaging studies of concrete and abstract word processing

Despite prior behavioral, neuropsychological, and electrophysiological evidence, and despite intuitive differences between concrete and abstract concepts, functional neuroimaging studies on this topic have produced highly variable results (Table 6.1). Of the 15 studies comparing concrete and abstract words reported since 1997, six failed to find *any* areas with greater activation for concrete relative to abstract words (Kiehl *et al.*, 1999; Perani *et al.*, 1999b; Friederici *et al.*, 2000; Tyler *et al.*, 2001; Grossman *et al.*, 2002; Noppeney & Price, 2004). Two early experiments that did find positive imageability effects were potentially confounded by differences in the tasks used in the concrete and

Table 6.1. Activation peaks in 15 imaging studies comparing concrete and abstract noun processing

Study	Task Contrast	Concrete > Abstract		Abstract > Concrete	
		Region	x, y, z	Region	x, y, z
D' Esposito *et al.* (1997) n = 7 (fMRI)	Generate mental image to auditory CN vs. listen passively to AN	L Fusiform L Precentral L ant. Cingulate	−33, −48, −18 −45, −3, 31 −7, −3, 42	R SFG R Precuneus	19, 50, 24 4, −74, 35
Mellet *et al.* (1998) n = 8 (PET)	Generate mental image to auditory CN definitions vs. listen passively to AN definitions	L ITG/ Fusiform R ITG/ Fusiform L ITG L Precentral L MFG L SMG L Precentral	−44, −58, −22 −42, −32, −18 52, −50, −14 −52, −62, −6 −40, 4, 34 −28, 14, 30 −46, −38, 46 −42, −16, 38 −36, 4, 60	L STG R MTG R STG/STS	−60, −22, 12 58, 2, −18 54, −20, 6 52, −26, 18
Kiehl *et al.* (1999) n = 6 (fMRI)	Visual lexical decision (CN vs. AN blocks)[a]	−	−	R STG	56, 11, 0
Perani *et al.* (1999b) n = 14 (PET)	Visual lexical decision (CN vs. AN blocks)[a]	−	−	L IFG R IFG L STG R Temporal Pole	−44, 14, −4 52, 20, −12 −58, 8, −16 42, 16, −36

Table 6.1. *(cont.)* Activation peaks in 15 imaging studies comparing concrete and abstract noun processing

Study	Task Contrast	Concrete > Abstract		Abstract > Concrete	
		Region	x, y, z	Region	x, y, z
				R Angular	40, −70, 36
				R ant. Cingulate	6, 16, 40
				R Amygdala	30, −4, −8
Tyler *et al.* (2001) n = 9 (PET)	Lexical decision (CN vs. AN blocks)[a]	−	−	−	−
Fiebach *et al.* (2003) n = 12 (fMRI)	Visual lexical decision (CN vs. AN)	L Temporal Lobe[b]	−27, −41, 4	L IFG	−46, 23, 7
Binder *et al.* (2005a) n = 24 (fMRI)	Visual lexical decision (CN vs. AN)	L Angular	−37, −74, 26	L IFG	−46, 18, −4
		R Angular	52, −58, 22		−39, 15, 14
			54, −48, 33		−35, 27, 7
		R MTG	49, −49, 14		−48, 9, 25
		L post. Cingulate	−12, −56, 11		−48, 22, 17
			−9, −45, 13		−47, 33, 8
			−7, −37, 36	L Precentral	−48, −7, 40
		R post. Cingulate	5, −35, 38	L ant. STG	−44, 12, −16
			6, −68, 30		−54, 4, −9
		L Precuneus	−12, −62, 24		
			−3, −74, 31		
		R Precuneus	11, −54, 35		
			3, −62, 41		
		L MFG	−28, 25, 48		
			−38, 19, 42		
Binder *et al.* (2005b)[c] n = 24 (fMRI)	Name visual nouns varying in imageability	L Angular	−57, −54, 31	L IFG	−53, 10, 20
		R Angular	54, −57, 21		−46, 25, 13
			43, −60, 17	L Precentral	−41, −2, 27
			56, −48, 35		−47, −5, 41
			38, −75, 38	L IFS	−42, 10, 22
			55, −69, 35	L ant. Cingulate	−10, 8, 42
		R MTG	51, −16, −16	R ant. Cingulate	8, 12, 42
			55, −50, 4	L SMA	−5, 2, 52

Study	Task Contrast	Concrete > Abstract		Abstract > Concrete	
		Region	x, y, z	Region	x, y, z
		L Fusiform/ PHG	−28, −37, −10		
		L post. Cingulate	−8, −53, 32		
		R post. Cingulate	7, −51, 32		
			8, −53, 21		
		L SFS	−27, 49, 2		
		R SFS	24, 18, 41		
			18, 41, 24		
		R MFG	37, 20, 42		
Jessen *et al.* (2000) n = 14 (fMRI)	Memorize visual CN vs. memorize visual AN	L Angular R Angular L Prefrontal L Precuneus	−39, −69, 36 42, −63, 42 −42, 42, 9 −3, −57, 45	L IFG R Occipital	−57, 30, 3 33, −78, 12
Wise *et al.* (2000) n = 18 (PET)	Reading, hearing, and semantic similarity judgment on words varying in imageability	L Fusiform	−31, −40, −18 −35, −50, −14	L STG	not reported
Friederici *et al.* (2000) n = 14 (fMRI)	Concreteness decision on visual words	−	−	L IFG R Thalamus	−46, 21, 25 4, −18, 15
Grossman *et al.* (2002) n = 16 (fMRI)	"Pleasant" or "not pleasant" decision on visual names of animals, implements, and abstract nouns	−	−	*[Abs > Implem]* L post. MTG/STS *[Abs > Anim]* L post. ITG L Prefrontal R med. Frontal R post. STG	−60, −32, 12 −52, −68, 4 −24, 44, 12 16, 36, −4 56, −32, 16
Noppeney and Price (2004) n = 15 (fMRI)	Semantic relatedness decision on visual CN & AN word triads	−	−	L IFG L Temporal Pole L post. MTG	−54, 21, −6 −51, 18, −27 −51, 9, −24 −60, −42, −6

Table 6.1. *(cont.)* Activation peaks in 15 imaging studies comparing concrete and abstract noun processing

Study	Task Contrast	Concrete > Abstract		Abstract > Concrete	
		Region	x, y, z	Region	x, y, z
Whatmough et al. (2004) n = 15 (PET)	Semantic similarity decision on visual CN & AN word pairs	L Fusiform	−44, −57, −21	R Fusiform/ PHG	21, −54, −6
Sabsevitz et al. (2005)[c] n = 28 (fMRI)	Semantic similarity decision on visual CN & AN word triads	L Angular	−28, −79, 36 −31, −66, 31	L IFG	−43, 22, −5 −50, 15, 9
		R Angular	36, −60, 32 42, −69, 31	L medial SFG	−9, 49, 33
				L ant. STS	−49, 6, −14
		L PHG	−27, −22, −20	L STS	−46, −29, −3
			−25, −37, −12	L post. MTG	−59, −47, 3
		R Hippocampus	21, −5, −14		
		L ITG	−57, −49, −14		
		L post. Cingulate	−14, −54, 15		
		R post. Cingulate	6, −52, 9		
		L SFG	−19, 8, 52		
		L MFG	−37, 27, 19		
		R MFG	28, 10, 46 45, 31, 14		
		L Orbital Frontal	−22, 26, −9		
		R Orbital Frontal	27, 26, −7		

Abbreviations: AN = abstract noun; ant. = anterior; CN = concrete noun; IFG = inferior frontal gyrus; IFS = inferior frontal sulcus; ITG = inferior temporal gyrus; L = left; MTG = middle temporal gyrus; PHG = parahippocampal gyrus; post. = posterior; R = right; SFG = superior frontal gyrus; SFS = superior frontal sulcus; SMA = supplementary motor area; STG = superior temporal gyrus; STS = superior temporal sulcus.

[a]These studies used a block design that combined activation from words and nonwords in each condition.

[b]The authors report this focus as near the collateral sulcus, but it is probably in the posterior hippocampus.

[c]Only representative peaks are given for these studies; see the original articles for a complete list.

abstract conditions (D'Esposito *et al.*, 1997; Mellet *et al.*, 1998). The authors of these earlier studies were interested in processes involved in explicit visual imagery; thus subjects were asked to form conscious mental images of the concrete items but to simply listen passively to the abstract items. Both studies reported greater activation in the left fusiform gyrus (and elsewhere) for the mental imagery condition, but the study design leaves open the question of whether this activation represents access to concepts or additional activation of an explicit visual image not necessary for concept retrieval.

Among the nine studies demonstrating positive effects of imageability, four failed to find such effects in the right hemisphere (D'Esposito *et al.*, 1997; Wise *et al.*, 2000; Fiebach & Friederici, 2003; Whatmough *et al.*, 2004). This is significant because, as mentioned above, behavioral and electrophysiological evidence supports the proposal, posited by dual-coding theory, that concrete concepts are processed bilaterally, while abstract concepts are processed mainly in the language-dominant hemisphere. This theory predicts that positive imageability effects will occur primarily in the right hemisphere. Most functional imaging studies, in contrast, suggest that concrete noun processing is strongly left-lateralized. Of the 15 studies summarized in Table 6.1, only five have shown right-hemisphere areas with stronger responses to concrete words than abstract words (Mellet *et al.*, 1998; Jessen *et al.*, 2000; Binder *et al.*, 2005a, 2005b; Sabsevitz *et al.*, 2005).

A critical review of the published studies suggests a number of potential reasons why imageability effects may have been missed. Three of the negative studies, for example, used lexical decision tasks in which blocks of concrete and abstract words were mixed together with nonwords (Kiehl *et al.*, 1999; Perani *et al.*, 1999b; Tyler *et al.*, 2001). Recent event-related functional magnetic resonance imaging (fMRI) experiments demonstrate marked differences between the neural responses to words and nonwords during lexical decision (Binder *et al.*, 2003, 2005a; Rissman *et al.*, 2003; Ischebeck *et al.*, 2004); thus this mixing of words and nonwords within blocks may have masked differences between the concrete and abstract words. In another negative study (Noppeney & Price, 2004), many items were included in the concrete word list that were of questionable concreteness (e.g. *pop*, *transparent*, *music*, *picking*). In two other studies, the image analysis was confined to brain regions activated by all words, a procedure that eliminates from consideration areas with a strong dependence on concreteness (Friederici *et al.*, 2000; Grossman *et al.*, 2002). Finally, as with much of the functional neuroimaging literature, many of the negative studies used relatively small sample sizes (6 to 16 participants), which may have limited detection of small but reliable imageability effects.

Results for abstract concepts have been somewhat more consistent. Several studies showed stronger activation for abstract items in left perisylvian regions, including the left superior temporal lobe (Mellet *et al.*, 1998; Perani *et al.*, 1999b; Wise *et al.*, 2000; Noppeney & Price, 2004; Binder *et al.*, 2005a; Sabsevitz *et al.*, 2005) and/or left inferior frontal lobe (Perani *et al.*, 1999b; Friederici *et al.*, 2000; Jessen *et al.*, 2000; Fiebach & Friederici, 2003; Noppeney & Price, 2004; Binder *et al.*, 2005a, 2005b; Sabsevitz *et al.*, 2005). A few studies found abstract word activations in homologous right superior temporal or inferior frontal regions (Mellet *et al.*, 1998; Kiehl *et al.*, 1999; Perani *et al.*, 1999b; Sabsevitz *et al.*, 2005).

The following sections describe in more detail three recent event-related fMRI experiments in which word imageability was manipulated during visual lexical decision, semantic decision, and word naming tasks. In these experiments, my colleagues and I attempted to resolve some of the inconsistencies in the imaging literature by using relatively large samples of participants and large numbers of items to ensure reliable activation patterns, by careful matching of concrete and abstract items on all possible nuisance variables, and by matching as closely as possible the task demands for the concrete and abstract conditions. The results were remarkably consistent across studies and provide clear support for some of the basic tenets of the dual-coding model.

6.2 Imageability effects during lexical decision

Discrimination of words from very word-like nonwords (pseudowords) requires access to word-specific knowledge. In previous studies using such tasks, concrete, imageable words were more rapidly recognized than abstract words (James, 1975; Kroll & Merves, 1986; Kounios & Holcomb, 1994), suggesting either that concrete words arouse qualitatively distinct semantic codes not accessed by abstract words (e.g. image-based codes: Paivio, 1971) or activate the same kinds of semantic codes more efficiently (Schwanenflugel, 1991). The facilitatory effect of semantic access on performance can be understood by viewing lexical decision as a signal detection task in which participants combine orthographic, phonological, and semantic information in whatever way most efficiently and accurately classifies stimuli as words or nonwords (Balota & Chumbley, 1984; Waters & Seidenberg, 1985; Stone & Van Orden, 1993; Grainger & Jacobs, 1996). When words and nonwords are closely matched on orthographic and phonological characteristics, access to semantic information plays a dominant role in determining performance.

The lexical decision task thus provides a convenient procedure for ensuring and confirming (through behavioral measures) access to semantic knowledge while also offering the potential for controlled manipulation of stimulus characteristics in fMRI experiments. In this lexical decision study (Binder *et al.*, 2005a), brain responses to concrete and abstract words were compared using event-related fMRI. Individual trial-by-trial response time (RT) measurements were used in the analysis to separate effects of word imageability from general effects of task difficulty on attention and other executive systems.

6.2.1 Methods

The stimuli were 50 English concrete nouns (e.g. *cabin, leaf, pigeon*), 50 abstract nouns (e.g. *dogma, plea, hybrid*), and 100 word-like nonwords (e.g. *dinant, grak, rulam*). The concrete and abstract words were matched on word frequency, and all sets were matched on letter and phoneme length, position-specific bigram frequency, and orthographic neighborhood size. Concrete and abstract words were defined using imageability and concreteness ratings from the Medical Research Council (MRC) lexical database (www.psy.uwa.edu.au/mrcdatabase/uwa_mrc.htm). Items were presented in random order for lexical decision and separated by a variable inter-stimulus interval. The participants were 24 healthy, right-handed adults. A 1.5 Tesla MRI device was used to acquire 528 blood-oxygenation-level-dependent (BOLD) image volumes on each participant, which were then analyzed using event-related deconvolution techniques available in the AFNI software package (http://afni.nimh.nih.gov/afni). This method creates statistical parametric maps showing the magnitude of the hemodynamic response to each trial type (concrete, abstract, nonword) at each image voxel. Error trials were removed from the analysis. Individual-item RT values for correct trials were included as a regressor in the model, resulting in a statistical parametric map of coefficients for this regressor at each image voxel. Individual parameter maps were then combined in a group-level random effects analysis.

6.2.2 Results

Behavioral data showed the expected advantage for concrete over abstract words. Responses to concrete words were faster (740 vs. 773 ms, $p < 0.0001$) and more accurate (2.07 vs. 6.14 percent error, $p = 0.001$) than responses to abstract words. These results confirm that participants accessed semantic information in discriminating the words from nonwords.

Concrete and abstract words activated a number of common areas in the left hemisphere relative to nonwords (Figure 6.1), including the angular gyrus, middle and inferior temporal gyri, and dorsal prefrontal cortex. In marked contrast to the abstract words, which produced activation only in the left-hemisphere, the concrete words activated several right-hemisphere areas, including the right angular gyrus, superior frontal gyrus, and posterior cingulate gyrus. Additional areas activated only by the concrete words included the left posterior cingulate gyrus and precuneus, left hippocampus, and left parahippocampus. Several areas

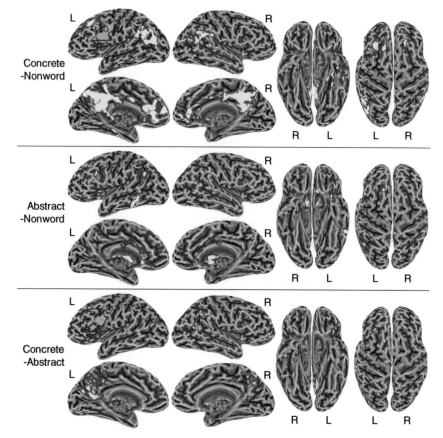

Figure 6.1.   FMRI maps showing group differences in brain activity during processing of concrete words, abstract words, and nonwords in a visual lexical decision task. Left and right lateral and medial views of the "inflated" brain surface are shown on the left half of the figure, ventral and dorsal views on the right half. All maps are thresholded at a corrected map-wise $p < 0.05$. **(Top)** Concrete words vs. nonwords. **(Middle)** Abstract words vs. nonwords. **(Bottom)** Concrete words vs. abstract words. In all cases, warm colors indicate stronger activation for concrete words; cool colors indicate stronger activation for abstract words.

showed stronger activation by nonwords compared to concrete words, including the left inferior and dorsolateral frontal lobe, left premotor cortex, left supplementary motor area, and left dorsal temporal pole. These differences were much less evident in the abstract—nonword contrast, suggesting a greater degree of similarity in the processing of abstract words and nonwords.

The direct contrast between concrete and abstract words showed stronger activation by concrete words bilaterally in the angular gyrus, posterior cingulate gyrus, and precuneus; and in the left dorsal prefrontal cortex (Figure 6.1). Stronger activation by abstract words occurred solely in left-hemisphere regions, including the inferior frontal gyrus, premotor cortex, and dorsal temporal pole. Most of these regions had also been activated by nonwords compared to concrete words.

Finally, extensive and widespread brain regions showed positive correlations with RT (Figure 6.2), including the inferior frontal lobe, premotor cortex, anterior insula, anterior cingulate gyrus, supramarginal gyrus, intraparietal sulcus, anterior thalamus, and midbrain bilaterally. Other areas sensitive to RT included the left ventral temporo-occipital junction, left primary sensorimotor area, left ventro-medial occipital lobe, and right dorsolateral frontal cortex. Activations in the posterior cingulate gyri bilaterally were negatively correlated with RT.

6.2.3 Discussion

The word−nonword contrasts shown in Figure 6.1 provide clear evidence for bilateral processing of concrete concepts and much more unilateral, left-hemisphere processing of abstract concepts. Regions engaged particularly by concrete words included the angular gyrus, posterior cingulate gyrus, and precuneus bilaterally. These regions have been linked with semantic processing in many prior imaging studies (Démonet *et al.*, 1992; Price *et al.*, 1997; Binder *et al.*, 1999, 2003; Roskies *et al.*, 2001; Scott *et al.*, 2003). Other regions in the left lateral temporal lobe (middle and inferior temporal gyri) were activated by both concrete and abstract words compared to nonwords, but did not appear to be modulated by concreteness in the direct contrast, suggesting equivalent levels of activation for both word types. Still other regions, including the left inferior frontal lobe and superior temporal pole, were activated more strongly by abstract than concrete words.

These results are quite consistent with one general claim of dual-coding theory, that concrete concepts are represented bihemispherically while abstract concepts are represented primarily in the left hemisphere. According to dual-coding theory,

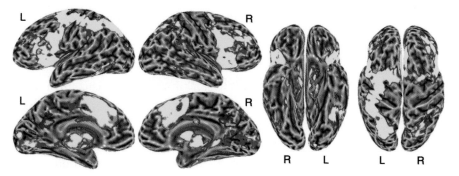

Figure 6.2. Effects of response time (RT) on brain activity during a visual lexical decision task. Warm colors indicate stronger activation as RT increases; cool colors indicate stronger activation as RT decreases.

the additional activation of angular gyrus and posterior medial areas by concrete words is due to activation of "image"-based representations, though an equally plausible alternative is that concrete concepts simply have more complex, richer featural representations that are not necessarily image-based. Left lateral temporal lobe regions, which were activated equivalently by concrete and abstract words, may represent the "verbal" semantic system posited by dual-coding theory, which is hypothesized to represent knowledge about both concrete and abstract concepts. Notably, none of these "semantic" areas showed sensitivity to RT, ruling out the possibility that their activation was related to differences in difficulty between the concrete and abstract items. This would be an unlikely proposition in the first place, given that most of the semantic regions were activated more strongly by concrete words, yet the behavioral measures indicate that processing of concrete words was easier than abstract words.

The left inferior frontal and superior temporal activations favoring abstract words confirm several previous reports (Mellet *et al.*, 1998; Perani *et al.*, 1999b; Jessen *et al.*, 2000; Wise *et al.*, 2000; Fiebach & Friederici, 2003; Noppeney & Price, 2004), but the interpretation of these results is difficult. Because these regions are also preferentially activated by nonwords, it is unlikely that they are involved in processing semantic information per se. Their activation by abstract words rather appears to reflect the weaker semantic representations associated with these words. In the case of abstract words, the lexical decision response may depend less on activation of conceptual information and more on retrieval of associated words, resulting in greater activation of left perisylvian areas subserving phonological working memory and lexical retrieval. In the case of nonwords, there is no associated semantic representation, and the inferior frontal region is consequently activated by the attempted retrieval of associated words. It is notable that many of these inferior frontal regions were also robustly modulated by task difficulty, as measured by RT. Therefore it is possible that some of the inferior frontal gyrus activation by abstract words and nonwords simply reflects domain-general processes such as attention and response selection.

6.3   Imageability effects during semantic decision

A somewhat surprising result of the lexical decision study is that the ventral temporal lobe was not modulated by imageability. The ventral visual pathway has been a particular focus of interest in testing the "sensory–motor hypothesis" of conceptual representation. As discussed earlier, many neuroimaging studies have shown activation in ventral occipital and temporal locations during the processing of living things relative to other concepts (e.g. Perani *et al.*, 1995, 1999a; Damasio *et al.*, 1996, 2004; Martin *et al.*, 1996; Mummery *et al.*, 1996; Cappa *et al.*, 1998;

Chao *et al.*, 1999; Moore & Price, 1999; Thompson-Schill *et al.*, 1999b; Grossman *et al.*, 2002; Emmorey *et al.*, 2003). The ventral position of these activations has usually been interpreted as related to the salient visual properties of animals and other living things. Several other studies have shown activation along the ventral visual pathway during retrieval of specific visual attribute knowledge (Martin *et al.*, 1995; Mummery *et al.*, 1998; Chao & Martin, 1999; Thompson-Schill *et al.*, 1999b; Kellenbach *et al.*, 2001; Kan *et al.*, 2003) and during explicit mental imagery tasks (D'Esposito *et al.*, 1997; Howard *et al.*, 1998; Mellet *et al.*, 1998; Ishai *et al.*, 2000; Kosslyn & Thompson, 2000; O'Craven & Kanwisher, 2000). These findings have led to proposals that the ventral temporal lobe, and particularly the fusiform gyrus, stores conceptual knowledge related to the visual attributes of concrete objects. Because abstract concepts have few, if any, visual attributes, this hypothesis also predicts stronger activation of the ventral temporal lobe by concrete than abstract words.

In fact, several studies have demonstrated activation of the ventral temporal lobe by concrete over abstract words (D'Esposito *et al.*, 1997; Mellet *et al.*, 1998; Wise *et al.*, 2000; Fiebach & Friederici, 2003; Whatmough *et al.*, 2004). Wise *et al.* (2000) observed a positive correlation between activation in the left mid-fusiform gyrus and word imageability during reading, listening, and semantic decision tasks. Fiebach and Friederici (2003) found activation in the left ventral temporal lobe, very close to the site of activation seen by Wise et al., for concrete nouns relative to abstract nouns during an event-related lexical decision study. Finally, Whatmough *et al.* (2004) observed greater activation in the left lateral fusiform gyrus for concrete compared to abstract words during a semantic decision task. In contrast to these positive results, however, most studies comparing concrete and abstract words failed to show modulation of the ventral temporal lobe by word imageability (Kiehl *et al.*, 1999; Perani *et al.*, 1999b; Friederici *et al.*, 2000; Jessen *et al.*, 2000; Tyler *et al.*, 2001; Grossman *et al.*, 2002; Noppeney & Price, 2004; Binder *et al.*, 2005a).

One explanation for the lack of ventral temporal activation in the lexical decision study is that the lexical decision task may not make sufficient demands on retrieval of visual attribute knowledge. Perhaps explicit use of visual perceptual knowledge is required to activate this region. We tested this possibility in the following fMRI study (Sabsevitz *et al.*, 2005) by using an explicit semantic decision task designed to ensure deep semantic processing. Participants were required to make semantic similarity judgments on a large number of concrete and abstract noun triads. In addition to the imageability factor, task difficulty was manipulated by varying the degree to which the words in a triad were similar or different in meaning. This factorial design allowed general effects of task difficulty to be distinguished from imageability effects.

6.3.1 Methods

The stimuli were 240 visual word triads, each presented in a pyramid arrangement with a sample word (e.g. *cheetah*) positioned at the top center of the display and two choice words (e.g. *tiger, wolf*) on either side of the bottom of the display. Triads were composed of either concrete nouns or abstract nouns. Participants were instructed to select the choice word that was most similar in meaning to the sample. To create the triads, similarity ratings for a large number of concrete and abstract word pairs were first collected from 99 college students. These scores were then used to compute similarity difference (SD) scores for word triads that measured the difference in similarity rating between the sample and each choice word. SD scores ranged from 0, reflecting no difference in the degree of similarity between the choices and the sample, to 9, indicating a large difference. Finally, SD scores were used to create easy (SD scores from 4 to 8) and hard (SD scores from 0 to 3) trials using either concrete or abstract words.

Stimulus presentation and image acquisition were similar to the lexical decision study. Trials were presented in a randomized, event-related manner with variable inter-stimulus intervals. Participants were 28 healthy, right-handed adults. Analyses of the fMRI data, including deconvolution of hemodynamic responses for multiple regressors, followed by group-level random effects analyses, were identical to those used in the lexical decision study.

3.2 Results

The behavioral data showed the expected large effect of task difficulty on both RT (easy, 1951 ms; hard, 2303 ms; $p < 0.0001$) and accuracy (easy, 98.8 percent correct; hard, 86.9 percent correct; $p < 0.0001$). There were no main effects of concreteness, and no interactions between the concreteness and difficulty factors.

A direct comparison between the concrete and abstract conditions showed potent effects of word imageability in several cortical regions (Figure 6.3). Many of these effects were virtually identical to those observed in the lexical decision study, including stronger activation for the concrete condition in the angular gyrus, dorsal prefrontal cortex, and posterior cingulate region bilaterally. In addition, however, greater activation for concrete words was observed at several other sites, including the inferior frontal sulcus (dorsolateral prefrontal cortex) and orbital frontal cortex bilaterally. Of particular note is a major focus of greater activation for concrete words centered on the collateral sulcus in the ventral inferior temporal cortex. This activation was more extensive in the left hemisphere and included the anterior-medial fusiform gyrus, parahippocampal gyrus, and anterior hippocampus.

Activation associated with abstract words was also similar to that seen in the lexical decision study, involving cortex in the left interior frontal gyms (IFG) (pars

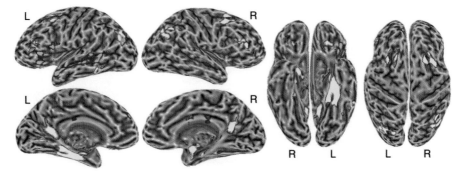

Figure 6.3.   Differences in brain activity during processing of concrete words and abstract words in a
semantic decision task. Warm colors indicate stronger activation for concrete words; cool
colors indicate stronger activation for abstract words.

opercularis, triangularis, and orbitalis) and dorsal temporal pole. In addition,
however, the temporal lobe activation spread back along the entire horizontal
length of the left superior temporal sulcus and into the posterior middle temporal
gyrus. A much smaller area of activation involved the right superior temporal
sulcus.

Irrespective of imageability, harder trials produced greater activation in many of
the same bilateral regions that had been positively modulated by RT in the lexical
decision study, including the anterior cingulate gyrus, rostral aspects of the IFG
and adjacent inferior frontal sulcus, anterior insula, premotor cortex, anterior
thalamus, and midbrain. A small focus was also found in the left superior parietal
lobe at the anterior aspect of the intraparietal sulcus. As shown in the composite
map of Figure 6.4, overlap between the regions modulated by the concreteness and
task difficulty factors was minimal. The only regions of significant overlap were in
the left pars triangularis of the IFG, where a large focus modulated by difficulty was
sandwiched between and partially overlapped a ventral abstract word focus and
a rostral concrete word focus, and in a small portion of the left parietal lobe near
the intraparietal sulcus.

6.3.3   Discussion

These data largely replicate the results from the lexical decision study and provide strong confirmatory evidence that particular cortical regions are involved in
processing information associated with concrete, imageable concepts. These
regions include the angular gyrus, dorsal prefrontal cortex, and posterior
cingulate cortex bilaterally. In contrast, abstract words produce greater activation
in the left IFG and dorsal temporal pole. These modulations of neural activity are
unlikely to have been caused by differences in general attentional, working
memory, selection, or decision demands. There were no significant differences in

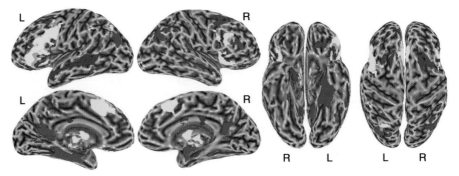

Figure 6.4.   Composite map showing areas modulated by word imageability and task difficulty during a semantic decision task. Red = stronger activation for concrete words than abstract words; blue = stronger activation for abstract words than concrete words; yellow = stronger activation for difficult trials than easy trials; green and orange = overlap between areas modulated by imageability and difficulty.

RT or accuracy between these conditions, and error trials were removed from the analysis. Moreover, a strong manipulation of task difficulty, produced by varying the degree of semantic similarity between sample and choice items, had no effect on activation in these regions, with the exception of the left inferior frontal gyrus.

In addition to this replication, the semantic decision study provides firm evidence for the involvement of ventral and medial temporal areas in processing of concrete concepts. As discussed earlier, the lexical decision results were notable for a lack of concreteness effects in this region. This prior negative result could be due to the nature of the lexical decision task, which does not require explicit retrieval of visual–perceptual knowledge. In contrast, the similarity judgment task used in the semantic decision experiment makes much greater demands on retrieval of visual attribute knowledge, which is required for judging similarity. The sensitivity of the fusiform gyrus and surrounding areas to word imageability during an explicit semantic task but not during lexical decision is reminiscent of an observation by Kan *et al.* (2003), who found activation of the left fusiform gyrus during a concept-property verification task (e.g. judge whether "cake–frosting" is a correct pairing of a concept with a property) relative to a perceptual baseline task. Notably, this activation occurred only when the false trials contained highly associated words (e.g. "stapler–paper"), thus necessitating explicit access to visual property knowledge for correct task performance, and not when the false trials contained unassociated words that could be rejected using an associative strategy. The robust modulation of this region by word imageability in the current study provides strong additional evidence that explicit retrieval of knowledge about imageable concepts involves modality-specific, higher visual association cortex, consistent with several earlier reports (D'Esposito *et al.*, 1997; Mellet *et al.*, 1998; Wise *et al.*, 2000; Fiebach & Friederici, 2003; Whatmough *et al.*, 2004).

Activation associated with abstract concepts extended much farther posteriorly in the left temporal lobe in the semantic decision study compared to lexical decision. The left IFG and anterior temporal regions activated by abstract words in the lexical decision study were probably not related to processing of conceptual knowledge per se, since these areas were also activated by nonwords (Figure 6.1). It is possible, however, that the more posterior temporal regions activated in the semantic decision study, which included the posterior middle temporal gyrus, could represent a "verbal" conceptual system of the sort proposed by dual-coding theory. Abstract nouns have less access to perceptually based representations and are therefore more dependent on word associations for retrieval of meaning. Processing abstract nouns for meaning might therefore be expected to activate the verbal semantic system to a greater degree than concrete nouns. Two previous studies using semantic decision tasks showed similar posterior temporal foci that responded more to abstract than concrete nouns (Grossman *et al.*, 2002; Noppeney & Price, 2004).

The effects of task difficulty corroborate and extend the RT findings of the lexical decision study. In both experiments, increasing task difficulty activated a bilateral network of brain regions previously linked with attention, arousal, working memory, decision, and response monitoring processes. This network includes the anterior cingulate gyrus, IFG and premotor cortex, anterior insula, intraparietal sulcus, anterior thalamus, and midbrain reticular activating system (see e.g. Falkenstein *et al.*, 1991; Gehring *et al.*, 1993; Paulesu *et al.*, 1993; Dehaene *et al.*, 1994; Taylor *et al.*, 1994; Awh *et al.*, 1996; Fiez, 1997; Jonides *et al.*, 1997; Badgaiyan & Posner, 1998; Carter *et al.*, 1998; Smith *et al.*, 1998; Botvinick *et al.*, 1999; D'Esposito *et al.*, 1999; Gitelman *et al.*, 1999; LaBar *et al.*, 1999; Thompson-Schill *et al.*, 1999a; Honey *et al.*, 2000; Kastner & Ungerleider, 2000; Adler *et al.*, 2001; Braver *et al.*, 2001; Menon *et al.*, 2001; Sturm & Willmes, 2001; Ullsperger & von Cramon, 2001; Barde & Thompson-Schill, 2002; Corbetta & Shulman, 2002; van Veen & Carter, 2002; Wager & Smith, 2003; Binder *et al.*, 2004). A remarkable finding in both studies is the almost complete lack of overlap between those regions modulated by task difficulty and those modulated by imageability, with the exception of the left inferior frontal gyrus (Figure 6.4). There are at least two reasons why a larger interaction between these factors might have been expected. First, more difficult trials might intuitively be expected to require more 'extensive' semantic processing, such as retrieval of a greater number of concept attributes (see, e.g. Whatmough *et al.*, 2004 for assumptions along these lines). Second, longer decision times might require that the activation of semantic knowledge be sustained for a longer period of time while a decision is reached. These intuitions notwithstanding, the lack of difficulty effects in brain areas modulated by imageability implies that activation of semantic codes in these putative semantic regions occurs in a relatively "all or none" fashion. That is, once the semantic representation of a concept is activated, further maintenance and manipulation of that semantic information in working memory does not appreciably increase the level of neural activation in the semantic memory store itself.

6.4 Imageability effects during word naming

A final experiment (Binder *et al.*, 2005b) addressed the controversial issue of whether and to what extent semantic information is accessed during word naming (i.e. reading aloud). This task is often considered to require minimal semantic access (Van Order *et al.*, 1990; Carello *et al.*, 1992), and empirical studies of word imageability effects on word naming latency have produced relatively small and inconsistent results (Brown & Watson, 1987; Strain *et al.*, 1995; Monaghan & Ellis, 2002; Strain *et al.*, 2002; Shibahara *et al.*, 2003; Balota *et al.*, 2004). Semantic access is a critical feature of some parallel distributed accounts of word naming that propose computation of phonology based on activation of sublexical orthographic and semantic information (Seidenberg & McClelland, 1989; Plaut *et al.*, 1996; Harm & Seidenberg, 2004). Activation of semantic codes, according to such models, is particularly important for generating the phonological representation for exception words (e.g. *wand, sweat, plaid, caste, spook, threat*) and unique words (e.g. *aisle, choir, fruit, heir, corps, scheme*) that violate "pronunciation rules". Semantic information should also be more critical for naming low-frequency words for which the mapping from orthography to phonology is less practiced. In support of this framework, Strain and colleagues (1995) demonstrated an imageability effect (faster responses for concrete than abstract words) during naming of low-frequency exception words but not high-frequency exception or regular words.

In contrast to such distributed accounts, whole-word theories of word naming, such as versions of the dual-route model (Marshall & Newcombe, 1973; Meyer *et al.*, 1974; Morton & Patterson, 1980; Coltheart *et al.*, 1993, 2001), postulate a separate lexical mechanism for exception word naming in which whole-word phonological representations are accessed from a lexicon. The orthographic and phonological lexicons in most such models contain no semantic information and so should not be affected by semantic variables such as imageability. A main aim of this fMRI study, therefore, was to assess whether any brain regions would be modulated by imageability during word naming.

Unlike most previous fMRI studies, imageability was treated as a continuous rather than a dichotomous variable, and effects of this variable were analyzed using linear regression.

6.4.1 Methods

The stimuli included 160 low-to-medium-frequency nouns and 80 pronounceable pseudowords. Imageability ratings, taken from the MRC database and from norms published by Bird *et al.* (2001) and Cortese and Fugett (2004), ranged from 140 to 659 with a relatively flat distribution. The imageability ratings were uncorrelated with letter length, phoneme length, mean positional bigram frequency, orthographic neighborhood count, or word frequency.

The participants were 24 healthy, right-handed adults. Items were presented in random order for reading aloud. Scanning was performed using a "clustered acquisition" (or "sparse imaging") technique in which a single image volume was acquired every 7 s, with a 5 s interval of silence between each acquisition. One stimulus was presented and one spoken response produced during each 5 s silent interval. The silent interval allowed a clear recording of the spoken response to be collected along with vocal RT measurements. The lexical category (word vs. nonword), imageability, and RT for the preceding trial were coded for each image volume. Error trials were removed from the analysis. Other aspects of the data analysis were similar to the lexical decision and semantic decision studies.

6.4.2 Results

For the sake of brevity, the current discussion focuses only on imageability effects during word naming. There were also effects of RT strikingly similar to those observed in the lexical decision study, differences between words and nonwords, and differences between regular and exception words (see Binder *et al.*, 2005b for a full description). The imageability effects are shown in Figure 6.5. Positive correlations (stronger activation for more imageable words) were observed in many of the same areas identified in the lexical decision and semantic decision studies, including the angular gyrus (R > L), dorsal prefrontal cortex, and posterior cingulate region bilaterally. There was a small focus in the left ventromedial temporal cortex, centered on the collateral sulcus. Negative correlations (stronger activation for less imageable words) occurred in the left IFG and adjacent premotor cortex, and in the anterior cingulate gyrus bilaterally.

6.4.3 Discussion

The results provide further confirmation that word imageability affects neural processing. In the context of a word naming task, these effects suggest that semantic information plays a role in accessing phonology from print. While a

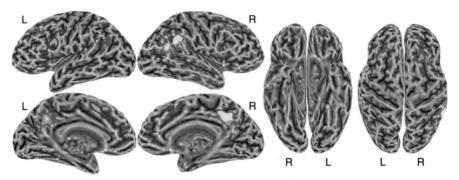

Figure 6.5.   Modulation of brain activity by imageability during a word naming task. Warm colors indicate stronger activation as imageability increases; cool colors indicate stronger activation as imageability decreases. (Reprinted from Binder *et al.*, 2005b with permission from Elsevier Inc.)

semantic contribution is not necessarily incompatible with lexicon-based models of reading, it is a specific, central feature of the distributed, single-mechanism model developed by Seidenberg, McClelland, Plaut, and colleagues (Seidenberg & McClelland, 1989; Plaut *et al.*, 1996; Harm & Seidenberg, 2004). Activation of a semantic representation offers an alternative theoretical mechanism by which a distributed code can provide word-specific information for computing unique spelling-to-sound mappings, as seems to be required for naming words that violate pronunciation rules.

6.5   Summary and conclusions

The combined results of these experiments offer compelling evidence for modulation of the semantic system by imageability. These effects are unlikely to be due to non-specific differences in task requirements, task difficulty, or processing time between the concrete and abstract word conditions, for several reasons. Task instructions were constant throughout all of the experiments. Error trials were excluded from the analyses, removing any differences in accuracy across conditions. Most importantly, explicit regression analyses demonstrated that the effects of variation in response latency occurred in brain regions associated with domain-general attention, arousal, working memory, decision, and response monitoring processes, and not in areas that were modulated by imageability. The main exception to this was the left inferior frontal gyrus, which showed stronger responses to abstract than concrete items and was also sensitive to task difficulty.

Figure 6.6 shows a composite figure created by superimposing activated areas from the imageability contrasts in each study on an inflated cortical surface.

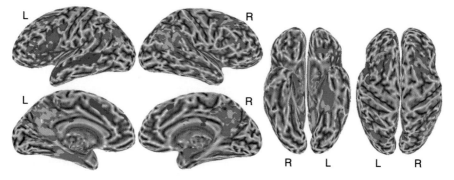

Figure 6.6.   Composite map showing areas modulated by word imageability during lexical decision, semantic decision, and word naming tasks. Warm colors indicate stronger activations for concrete words in one or more studies; cool colors indicate stronger activations for abstract words in one or more studies.

Four brain regions show *stronger activation for highly imageable compared to abstract words:*

1. *Posterior parieto-occipital cortex*, including the angular gyrus (BA 39) and adjacent lateral occipital cortex (BA 19). Imageability effects are typically bilateral, though with some rightward lateralization.

2. *Ventral-medial temporal cortex*, including middle and anterior aspects of the fusiform gyrus, parahippocampus, and hippocampus. Imageability effects occur bilaterally but are clearly left-lateralized in this region. The magnitude of the effect appears to depend on the "depth of processing" required by the task.

3. *Posterior cingulate region*, including the posterior cingulate gyrus (BA 23, 31), retrosplenial cortex and cingulate isthmus (BA 26, 29, 30), and ventral precuneus (BA 7/31). Imageability effects occur bilaterally and symmetrically.

4. *Dorsal prefrontal cortex*, including dorsal aspects of the superior frontal gyrus (BA 8, 9) and adjacent posterior middle frontal gyrus (BA 8). This region is centered on the superior frontal sulcus and lies just anterior to the frontal eye field. Imageability effects are bilateral and symmetrical.

These four regions are frequently implicated in semantic processing (Binder & Price, 2001). For example, these areas show stronger activation during semantic than phonological tasks (Démonet *et al.*, 1992; Price *et al.*, 1997; Mummery *et al.*, 1998; Binder *et al.*, 1999; Roskies *et al.*, 2001; Scott *et al.*, 2003). They are also activated more by words than nonwords during lexical decision (Binder *et al.*, 2003, 2005a; Ischebeck *et al.*, 2004). Some of these brain areas, notably the hippocampus, parahippocampus, and retrosplenial cortex, are also known to be involved in episodic memory encoding. It seems likely that concrete nouns are encoded more "deeply" than abstract nouns given their multimodal representation, and thus activate the episodic memory encoding system to a greater degree. Indeed, dual-coding theory was originally motivated by the finding that concrete words are better encoded into episodic memory than abstract words during semantic tasks (Paivio, 1971). Greater activation of the hippocampus, parahippocampus, and posterior cingulate gyrus for concrete words provides a plausible anatomical substrate for this effect.

In addition to these consistent foci, stronger activation for concrete relative to abstract words was found occasionally in the right middle temporal gyrus (BA 21), rostral parts of the IFG (BA 45 and 46), orbital frontal cortex (BA 11), and left inferior temporal gyrus (BA 20/37).

In contrast to the bilateral pattern of activation elicited by concrete concepts, processing of abstract concepts appears to be strongly left-lateralized. This left lateralization was evident both in a contrast with a pseudoword baseline (Figure 6.1) and in the contrasts between abstract and concrete words. Two general regions consistently show *stronger activation for abstract than imageable words:*

1. Left inferior frontal gyrus, including the pars orbitalis (BA 47), triangularis (BA 45), and opercularis (BA 44), with some extension posteriorly into the precentral gyrus (BA 6). As mentioned earlier, there are several reasons why this preference for abstract words may not reflect semantic processing per se. Much of this region was also sensitive to RT and manipulation of task difficulty across the studies. Furthermore, this region also responds more strongly to nonwords than to concrete words (Figure 6.1). We have therefore interpreted the preference for abstract words in this region as resulting from increased demands on phonological working memory, lexical search, attention, and response selection mechanisms during processing of abstract relative to imageable concepts.

2. Left anterior superior temporal gyrus, particularly the dorsal aspect of the temporal pole (BA 38). In the semantic decision study, this activation spread much farther posteriorly along the superior temporal sulcus and into the posterior middle temporal gyrus, similar to results from two previous semantic decision experiments (Grossman *et al.*, 2002; Noppeney & Price, 2004).

A final result worth emphasis is the fact that in the lexical decision study, both concrete and abstract words activated regions in the left lateral temporal lobe relative to nonwords (Figure 6.1), yet these regions were not differentially activated in the direct contrast between concrete and abstract words. Thus this region was activated by meaningful (word) relative to meaningless (nonword) stimuli, suggesting a role in semantic processing, but was activated equivalently by concrete and abstract words (see Whatmough *et al.*, 2004 for similar results). We have tentatively interpreted this pattern as consistent with the behavior of a "verbal" semantic system, which, according to dual-coding theory, participates in the processing of both concrete and abstract concepts (Paivio, 1971, 1986). Activation of this region, however, appears to show an interaction between imageability and task demands. While it was equally activated by concrete and abstract words during lexical decision, the superior aspect of the left lateral temporal cortex, including the superior temporal sulcus and the posterior middle temporal gyrus, was engaged more strongly by abstract words than concrete words during the more difficult semantic decision task (Figure 6.3). Together, these results suggest that the role of the left lateral temporal lobe is to process conceptual information that is verbally encoded, and that such information, while elicited during processing of all words, is particularly crucial for comprehension of abstract concepts. The close proximity of this region to left perisylvian temporal, parietal, and inferior frontal areas that are believed to play a role in lexical phonological retrieval (Indefrey & Levelt, 2000) is consistent with such a hypothesis.

Relative to concrete concepts, there has been scarcely any empirical investigation of the organizational principles underlying abstract concepts. Much research has focused on the developmental and ontological bases for concrete concept category formation. Taxonomic groupings of concrete objects arise naturally from structure in the perceptual environment, exemplified by the fact that attributes are not randomly distributed but instead are intercorrelated across objects (e.g. *wings* occur with *feathers* more often than with *fur*) (Berlin *et al.*, 1966; Rosch *et al.*, 1976). Concrete object categories form during human development from gradual accumulation of knowledge about shared and distinctive physical attributes and from acquisition of conceptual primitives such as animacy, agency, causation, containment, and partition (Gelman, 1990; Mandler, 1992; Caramazza & Shelton, 1998; Mareschal, 2000). These principles, however, simply do not apply well to abstract concepts such as *value, regret*, and *fate*. Instead, abstract concepts appear to be learned primarily through linguistic experience. That is, the many senses of *value* are gradually built up in the conceptual system through verbal association of this word with other words, such as *money, desirable, worth, good, principle, prize, utility, quantity*, etc. Rather than being organized according to hierarchical categories defined by perceptual attribute conjunctions, abstract concepts thus seem to be organized primarily as verbal associative networks (Breedin *et al.*, 1995; Crutch & Warrington, 2005).

The leftward lateralization of this verbal associative system is consistent with a number of behavioral and electrophysiological studies suggesting left lateralization of abstract word processing (Day, 1979; Chiarello *et al.*, 1987; Deloche *et al.*, 1987; Kounios & Holcomb, 1994, 2000; Holcomb *et al.*, 1999; Nittono *et al.*, 2002) and with the fact that aphasic patients with stroke in the left perisylvian region generally show greater processing deficits for words with low imageability (Goodglass *et al.*, 1969; Coltheart *et al.*, 1980; Roeltgen *et al.*, 1983; Katz & Goodglass, 1990; Franklin *et al.*, 1995). Beyond this close association with the left perisylvian language system, however, little is currently known about the neural processing of abstract concepts. This state of affairs is perhaps a reflection of the fact that abstract semantics remains a topic that has attracted surprisingly little theoretical interest. There may be organizational principles that govern the representation of abstract concepts, such as the functional domain to which they apply (e.g. concepts related to emotion, cognition, communication, states of being, time, etc.), but coherent theories along these lines must await further research.

Abstract concepts tend to be acquired at a later age than concrete concepts (Gilhooly & Logie, 1980), so it is important to consider this variable as a potential confound in studies of imageability effects. Several authors have argued that effects of concreteness and imageability observed in behavioral studies can be explained by differences in the age of acquisition of concrete and abstract words, that is, by differences in familiarity rather than semantic quality (Gernsbacher, 1984; Coltheart *et al.*, 1988; Monaghan & Ellis, 2002). While age of acquisition is undoubtedly a potent factor influencing speed of processing in a variety of word recognition tasks, there also is clear theoretical (Jones, 1985; Plaut & Shallice, 1993; Plaut *et al.*, 1996) and empirical (Strain *et al.*, 1995, 2002; Shibahara *et al.*, 2003) justification for the claim that imageability effects are at least partly independent from general effects of familiarity. The main hypothesis of the studies outlined in this chapter is that imageability determines (along with other semantic factors) the type of semantic knowledge that is engaged by a word; this hypothesis predicts effects of imageability even when age of acquisition and other measures of familiarity (frequency, meaningfulness) are controlled. On the other hand, imageability and familiarity are, to a degree, two sides of the same "semantic coin": concepts with which one is more familiar — by virtue of earlier acquisition or more frequent use — are also likely to have richer semantic representations. Future projects teasing apart the effects of these intercorrelated phenomena on word recognition processes should provide much new insight into the neural representation of semantic knowledge.

REFERENCES

Adler, C. M., Sax, K. W., Holland, S. K., Schmithorst, V., Rosenberg, L., and Strakowski, S. M. (2001). Changes in neuronal activation with increasing attention demand in healthy volunteers: An fMRI study. *Synapse*, **42**: 266–72.

Allport, D. A. (1985). Distributed memory, modular subsystems and dysphasia. In S. K. Newman and R. Epstein (eds.), *Current Perspectives in Dysphasia.* Edinburgh: Churchill Livingstone, pp. 207–44.

Awh, E., Jonides, J., Smith, E. E., Schumacher, E. H., Koeppe, R. A., and Katz, S. (1996). Dissociation of storage and rehearsal in verbal working memory: evidence from positron emission tomography. *Psychological Science*, **7**: 25–31.

Badgaiyan, R. D. and Posner, M. I. (1998). Mapping the cingulate cortex in response selection and monitoring. *Neuroimage*, **7**: 255–60.

Balota, D. A. and Chumbley, J. I. (1984). Are lexical decisions a good measure of lexical access? The role of word frequency in the neglected decision stage. *Journal of Experimental Psychology: Human Perception and Performance*, **10**: 340–57.

Balota, D. A., Cortese, M. J., Sergent-Marshall, S. D., Spiele, D. H., and Yap, M. J. (2004). Visual word recognition of single-syllable words. *Journal of Experimental Psychology: General*, **133**: 283–316.

Barde, L. H. F. and Thompson-Schill, S. L. (2002). Models of functional organization of lateral prefrontal cortex in verbal working memory: Evidence in favor of the process model. *Journal of Cognitive Neuroscience*, **14**: 1054–63.

Barsalou, L. W. (1999). Perceptual symbol systems. *Behavioral Brain Science*, **22**: 577–660.

Berlin, B., Breedlove, D. E., and Raven, P. H. (1966). Folk taxonomies and biological classification. *Science*, **154**: 273–5.

Binder, J. R. and Price, C. J. (2001). Functional imaging of language. In R. Cabeza and A. Kingstone (eds.), *Handbook of Functional Neuroimaging of Cognition.* Cambridge, MA: MIT Press, pp. 187–251.

Binder, J. R., Frost, J. A., Hammeke, T. A., Bellgowan, P. S. F., Rao, S. M., and Cox, R. W. (1999). Conceptual processing during the conscious resting state: a functional MRI study. *Journal of Cognitive Neuroscience*, **11**: 80–93.

Binder, J. R., McKiernan, K. A., Parsons, M., Westbury, C. F., Possing, E. T., Kaufman, J. N., and Buchanan, L. (2003). Neural correlates of lexical access during visual word recognition. *Journal of Cognitive Neuroscience*, **15**: 372–93.

Binder, J. R., Liebenthal, E., Possing, E. T., Medler, D. A., and Ward, B. D. (2004). Neural correlates of sensory and decision processes in auditory object identification. *Nature Neuroscience*, **7**: 295–301.

Binder, J. R., Westbury, C. F., Possing, E. T., McKiernan, K. A., and Medler, D. A. (2005a). Distinct brain systems for processing concrete and abstract concepts. *Journal of Cognitive Neuroscience*, **17**: 905–17.

Binder, J. R., Medler, D. A., Desai, R., Conant, L. L., and Liebenthal, E. (2005b). Some neurophysiological constraints on models of word naming. *Neuroimage*, **27**: 677–93.

Bird, H., Franklin, S., and Howard, D. (2001). Age of acquisition and imageability ratings for a large set of words, including verbs and function words. *Behavior Research Methods, Instruments, & Computers*, **33**: 73–9.

Bookheimer, S. Y. (2002). Functional MRI of language: new approaches to understanding the cortical organization of semantic processing. *Annual Review of Neuroscience*, **25**: 151–88.

Botvinick, M., Nystrom, L. E., Fissel, K., Carter, C. S., and Cohen, J. D. (1999). Conflict monitoring versus selection-for-action in anterior cingulate cortex. *Nature*, **402**: 179–81.

Braver, T. S., Barch, D. M., Gray, J. R., Molfese, D. L., and Snyder, A. (2001). Anterior cingulate cortex and response conflict: Effects of frequency, inhibition and errors. *Cerebral Cortex*, **11**: 825–36.

Breedin, S. D., Saffran, E. M., and Coslett, H. B. (1995). Reversal of a concreteness effect in a patient with semantic dementia. *Cognitive Neuropsychology*, **11**: 617–60.

Brown, G. D. and Watson, F. L. (1987). First in, first out: word learning age and spoken frequency as predictors of word familiarity and word naming latency. *Memory and Cognition*, **15**: 208–16.

Cappa, S. F., Perani, D., Schnur, T., Tettamanti, M., and Fazio, F. (1998). The effects of semantic category and knowledge type on lexical–semantic access: A PET study. *Neuroimage*, **8**: 350–9.

Caramazza, A. and Shelton, J. R. (1998). Domain-specific knowledge systems in the brain: the animate–inanimate distinction. *Journal of Cognitive Neuroscience*, **10**: 1–34.

Carello, C., Turvey, M. T., and Lukatela, G. (1992). Can theories of word recognition remain stubbornly nonphonological? In R. Frost and L. Katz (eds.), *Orthography, Phonology, Morphology, and Meaning: Advances in psychology*. Amsterdam: North-Holland, pp. 211–26.

Carter, C. S., Braver, T. S., Barch, D. M., Botvinick, M. M., Noll, D., and Cohen, J. D. (1998). Anterior cingulate cortex, error detection, and the online monitoring of performance. *Science*, **280**: 747–9.

Chao, L. L. and Martin, A. (1999). Cortical regions associated with perceiving, naming, and knowing about colors. *Journal of Cognitive Neuroscience*, **11**: 25–35.

Chao, L. L., Haxby, J. V., and Martin, A. (1999). Attribute-based neural substrates in temporal cortex for perceiving and knowing about objects. *Nature Neuroscience*, **2**: 913–19.

Chiarello, C., Senehi, J., and Nuding, S. (1987). Semantic priming with abstract and concrete words: differential asymmetry may be postlexical. *Brain and Language*, **31**: 302–14.

Coltheart, M., Patterson, K., and Marshall, J. (1980). *Deep Dyslexia*. London: Routledge & Kegan Paul.

Coltheart, M., Curtis, B., Atkins, P., and Haller, M. (1993). Models of reading aloud: dual-route and parallel-distributed-processing approaches. *Psychological Review*, **100**: 589–608.

Coltheart, M., Rastle, K., Perry, C., Langdon, R., and Ziegle, J. (2001). DRC: a dual route cascaded model of visual word recognition and reading aloud. *Psychological Review*, **108**: 204–56.

Coltheart, V., Laxon, V. J., and Keating, C. (1988). Effects of word imageability and age of acquisition on children's reading. *British Journal of Psychology*, **79**: 1–12.

Corbetta, M. and Shulman, G. L. (2002). Control of goal-directed and stimulus-driven attention in the brain. *Nature Review Neuroscience*, **3**: 201–15.

Cortese, M. J. and Fugett, A. (2004). Imageability ratings for 3,000 monosyllabic words. *Behavior Research Methods, Instruments, and Computers*, **36**: 384–7.

Coslett, H. B. and Saffran, E. M. (1989). Evidence for preserved reading in "pure alexia". *Brain*, **112**: 327–59.

Coslett, H. B. and Monsul, N. (1994). Reading with the right hemisphere: evidence from transcranial magnetic stimulation. *Brain and Language*, **46**: 198–211.

Crutch, S. J. and Warrington, E. K. (2005). Abstract and concrete concepts have structurally different representational frameworks. *Brain*, **128**: 615–27.

D'Esposito, M., Detre, J. A., Aguirre, G. K., Stallcup, M., Alsop, D. C., Tippet, L. J., and Farah, M. J. (1997). A functional MRI study of mental image generation. *Neuropsychologia*, **35**: 725–30.

D'Esposito, M., Postle, B. R., Ballard, D., and Lease, J. (1999). Maintenance versus manipulation of information held in working memory: an event-related fMRI study. *Brain and Cognition*, **41**: 66–86.

Damasio, A. R. (1989). Time-locked multiregional retroactivation: a systems-level proposal for the neural substrates of recall and recognition. *Cognition*, **33**: 25–62.

Damasio, H., Grabowski, T. J., Tranel, D., Hichwa, R. D., and Damasio, A. R. (1996). A neural basis for lexical retrieval. *Nature*, **380**: 499–505.

Damasio, H., Tranel, D., Grabowski, T., Adolphs, R., and Damasio, A. (2004). Neural systems behind word and concept retrieval. *Cognition*, **92**: 179–229.

Day, J. (1979). Visual half-field word recognition as a function of syntactic class and imageability. *Neuropsychologia*, **17**: 515–19.

Dehaene, S., Posner, M. I., and Tucker, D. M. (1994). Localization of a neural system for error detection and compensation. *Psychological Science*, **5**: 303–5.

Deloche, G., Seron, X., Scius, G., and Segui, J. (1987). Right hemisphere language processing: lateral difference with imageable and nonimageable ambiguous words. *Brain and Language*, **30**: 197–205.

Démonet, J.-F., Chollet, F., Ramsay, S., Cardebat, D., Nespoulous, J.-L., Wise, R., Rascol, A., and Frackowiak, R. (1992). The anatomy of phonological and semantic processing in normal subjects. *Brain*, **115**: 1753–68.

Devlin, J. T., Russell, R. P., Davis, M. H., Price, C. J., Moss, H. E., Jalal Fadili, M., *et al.* (2002). Is there an anatomical basis for category-specificity? Semantic memory studies with PET and fMRI. *Neuropsychologia*, **40**: 54–75.

Emmorey, K., Grabowski, T., McCullough, S., Damasio, H., Ponto, L. L. B., Hichwa, R. D., and Bellugi, U. (2003). Neural systems underlying lexical retrieval for sign language. *Neuropsychologia*, **41**: 85–95.

Falkenstein, M., Hohnsbein, J., Hoormann, J., and Blanke, L. (1991). Effects of crossmodal divided attention on late ERP components: II. Error processing in choice reaction tasks. *Electroencephalography and Clinical Neurophysiology*, **78**: 447–55.

Farah, M. J. and McClelland, J. L. (1991). A computational model of semantic memory impairment: Modality specificity and emergent category specificity. *Journal of Experimental Psychology General*, **120**: 339–57.

Fiebach, C. J. and Friederici, A. D. (2003). Processing concrete words: fMRI evidence against a specific right-hemisphere involvement. *Neuropsychologia*, **42**: 62–70.

Fiez, J. A. (1997). Phonology, semantics and the role of the left inferior prefrontal cortex. *Human Brain Mapping*, **5**: 79–83.

Franklin, S., Howard, D., and Patterson, K. (1995). Abstract word anomia. *Cognitive Neuropsychology*, **12**: 549—66.

Freud, S. (1891/1953). *On Aphasia: A critical study*. Madison, NY: International Universities Press.

Friederici, A. D., Opitz, B., and von Cramon, D. Y. (2000). Segregating semantic and syntactic aspects of processing in the human brain: an fMRI investigation of different word types. *Cerebral Cortex*, **10**: 698—705.

Gehring, W. J., Goss, B., Coles, M. G. H., Meyer, D. E., and Donchin, E. (1993). A neural system for error detection and compensation. *Psychological Science*, **4**: 385—90.

Gelman, R. (1990). First principles organize attention to and learning about relevant data: number and the animate—inanimate distinction as examples. *Cognitive Science*, **14**: 79—106.

Gernsbacher, M. A. (1984). Resolving 20 years of inconsistent interactions between lexical familiarity and orthography, concreteness, and polysemy. *Journal of Experimental Psychology: General*, **113**: 256—81.

Geschwind, N. (1965). Disconnection syndromes in animals and man. *Brain*, **88**: 237—94, 585—644.

Gilhooly, K. J. and Logie, R. H. (1980). Age of acquisition, imagery, concreteness, familiarity and ambiguity measures for 1944 words. *Behaviour Research Methods and Instrumentation*, **12**: 395—427.

Gitelman, D. R., Nobre, A. C., Parrish, T. B., LaBar, K. S., Kim, Y. H., Meyer, J. R., and Mesulam, M. M. (1999). A large-scale distributed network for covert spatial attention: further anatomical delineation based on stringent behavioural and cognitive controls. *Brain*, **122**: 1093—106.

Glenberg, A. M. and Robertson, D. A. (2000). Symbol grounding and meaning: a comparison of high-dimensional and embodied theories of meaning. *Journal of Memory and Language*, **43**: 379—401.

Goodglass, H., Hyde, M. R., and Blumstein, S. (1969). Frequency, picturability and availability of nouns in aphasia. *Cortex*, **5**: 104—19.

Grainger, J. and Jacobs, A. M. (1996). Orthographic processing in visual word recognition: a multiple read-out model. *Psychological Review*, **103**: 518—65.

Grossman, M., Koenig, P., DeVita, C., Glosser, G., Alsop, D., Detre, J., and Gee, J. (2002). The neural basis for category-specific knowledge: an fMRI study. *Neuroimage*, **15**: 936—48.

Harm, M. W. and Seidenberg, M. S. (2004). Computing the meanings of words in reading: cooperative division of labor between visual and phonological processes. *Psychological Review*, **111**: 662—720.

Holcomb, P. J., Kounios, J., Anderson, J. E., and West, W. C. (1999). Dual-coding, context availability, and concreteness effects in sentence comprehension: an electrophysiological investigation. *Journal of Experimental Psychology: Learning, Memory, and Cognition*, **25**: 721—42.

Honey, G. D., Bullmore, E. T., and Sharma, T. (2000). Prolonged reaction time to a verbal working memory task predicts increased power of posterior parietal cortical activation. *NeuroImage*, **12**: 495—503.

Howard, R. J., Ffytche, D. H., Barnes, J., McKeefry, D., Ha, Y., Woodruff, P. W., Bullmore, E. T., Simons, A., and Williams, S. C. R. (1998). The functional anatomy of imagined and perceived colour. *Neuroreport*, **9**: 1019–23.

Hume, D. (1739/1975). *A Treatise of Human Nature*. London: Oxford University Press.

Indefrey, P. and Levelt, W. J. M. (2000). The neural correlates of language production. In M. S. Gazzaniga (ed.), *The New Cognitive Neurosciences*. Cambridge, MA: MIT Press, pp. 845–65.

Ischebeck, A., Indefrey, P., Usui, N., Nose, I., Hellwig, F., and Taira, M. (2004). Reading in a regular orthography: an fMRI study investigating the role of visual familiarity. *Journal of Cognitive Neuroscience*, **16**: 727–41.

Ishai, A., Ungerleider, L. G., and Haxby, J. V. (2000). Distributed neural systems for the generation of visual images. *Neuron*, **28**: 979–90.

James, C. T. (1975). The role of semantic information in lexical decisions. *Journal of Experimental Psychology: Human Perception and Performance*, **104**: 130–6.

Jessen, F., Heun, R., Erb, M., Granath, D. O., Klose, U., Papassotiropoulos, A., and Grodd, W. (2000). The concreteness effect: Evidence for dual-coding and context availability. *Brain and Language*, **74**: 103–12.

Jones, G. V. (1985). Deep dyslexia, imageability, and ease of predication. *Brain and Language*, **24**: 1–19.

Jonides, J., Schumacher, E. H., Smith, E. E., Lauber, E., Awh, E., Minoshima, S., and Koeppe, R. A. (1997). The task-load of verbal working memory affects regional brain activation as measured by PET. *Journal of Cognitive Neuroscience*, **9**: 462–75.

Kan, I. P., Barsalou, L. W., Solomon, K. O., Minor, J. K., and Thompson-Schill, S. L. (2003). Role of mental imagery in a property verification task: fMRI evidence for perceptual representations of conceptual knowledge. *Cognitive Neuropsychology*, **20**: 525–40.

Kastner, S. and Ungerleider, L. G. (2000). Mechanisms of visual attention in the human cortex. *Annual Review of Neuroscience*, **23**: 315–41.

Katz, R. B. and Goodglass, H. (1990). Deep dysphasia: Analysis of a rare form of repetition disorder. *Brain and Language*, **39**: 153–85.

Kellenbach, M. L., Brett, M., and Patterson, K. (2001). Large, colourful or noisy? Attribute- and modality-specific activations during retrieval of perceptual attribute knowledge. *Cognitive, Affective, and Behavioral Neuroscience*, **1**: 207–21.

Kiehl, K. A., Liddle, P. F., Smith, A. M., Mendrek, A., Forster, B. B., and Hare, R. D. (1999). Neural pathways involved in the processing of concrete and abstract words. *Human Brain Mapping*, **7**: 225–33.

Kosslyn, S. M. and Thompson, W. L. (2000). Shared mechanisms in visual imagery and visual perception: insights from cognitive neuroscience. In M. S. Gazzaniga (ed.), *The New Cognitive Neurosciences*, 2nd edn. Cambridge, MA: MIT Press, pp. 975–85.

Kounios, J. and Holcomb, P. J. (1994). Concreteness effects in semantic processing: ERP evidence supporting dual-encoding theory. *Journal of Experimental Psychology: Learning, Memory and Cognition*, **20**: 804–23.

Kounios, J. and Holcomb, P. J. (2000). Concreteness effects in semantic processing: ERP evidence supporting dual-coding theory. *Journal of Experimental Psychology: Language, Memory and Cognition*, **20**: 804–23.

Kroll, J. F. and Merves, J. S. (1986). Lexical access for concrete and abstract words. *Journal of Experimental Psychology: Learning, Memory and Cognition*, **12**: 92–107.

LaBar, K. S., Gitelman, D. R., Parrish, T. B., and Mesulam, M. M. (1999). Neuroanatomic overlap of working memory and spatial attention networks: a functional MRI comparison within subjects. *Neuroimage*, **10**: 695–704.

Locke, J. (1690/1959). *An Essay Concerning Human Understanding*. New York: Dover.

Mandler, J. M. (1992). How to build a baby: II. Conceptual primitives. *Psychological Review*, **99**: 587–604.

Mareschal, D. (2000). Infant object knowledge: current trends and controversies. *Trends in Cognitive Science*, **4**: 408–16.

Marshall, J., Pring, T., Robson, J., and Chiat, S. (1998). When ottoman is easier than chair: an inverse frequency effect in jargon aphasia. *Brain and Language*, **65**: 78–81.

Marshall, J. C. and Newcombe, F. (1973). Patterns of paralexia: a psycholinguistic approach. *Journal of Psycholinguist Research*, **2**: 175–99.

Martin, A. and Chao, L. L. (2001). Semantic memory in the brain: Structure and processes. *Current Opinion in Neurobiology*, **11**: 194–201.

Martin, A., Haxby, J. V., Lalonde, F. M., Wiggs, C. L., and Ungerleider, L. G. (1995). Discrete cortical regions associated with knowledge of color and knowledge of action. *Science*, **270**: 102–5.

Martin, A., Wiggs, C. L., Ungerleider, L. G., and Haxby, J. V. (1996). Neural correlates of category-specific knowledge. *Nature*, **379**: 649–52.

Martin, A., Ungerleider, L. G., and Haxby, J. V. (2000). Category-specificity and the brain: The sensory-motor model of semantic representations of objects. In M. S. Gazzaniga (ed.), *The New Cognitive Neurosciences*, 2nd edn. Cambridge, MA: MIT Press, pp. 1023–36.

Mellet, E., Tzourio, N., Denis, M., and Mazoyer, B. (1998). Cortical anatomy of mental imagery of concrete nouns based on their dictionary definition. *Neuroreport*, **9**: 803–8.

Menon, V., Adleman, N. E., White, C. D., Glover, G. H., and Reiss, A. L. (2001). Error-related brain activation during a Go/NoGo response inhibition task. *Human Brain Mapping*, **12**: 131–43.

Meyer, D. E., Schvaneveldt, R. W., and Ruddy, M. G. (1974). Functions of graphemic and phonemic codes in visual word recognition. *Memory and Cognition*, **2**: 309–21.

Monaghan, J. and Ellis, A. W. (2002). What exactly interacts with spelling–sound consistency in word naming? *Journal of Experimental Psychology: Learning, Memory, and Cognition*, **28**: 183–206.

Moore, C. J. and Price, C. J. (1999). A functional neuroimaging study of the variables that generate category specific object processing differences. *Brain*, **122**: 943–62.

Morton, J. and Patterson, K. (1980). A new attempt at an interpretation, or, an attempt at a new interpretation. In M. Coltheart, K. Patterson, and J. C. Marshall (eds.), *Deep Dyslexia*. London: Routledge & Kegan Paul, pp. 91–118.

Mummery, C. J., Patterson, K., Hodges, J. R., and Wise, R. J. S. (1996). Generating "tiger" as an animal name or a word beginning with T: differences in brain activation. *Proceedings of the Royal Society of London B*, **263**: 989–95.

Mummery, C. J., Patterson, K., Hodges, J. R., and Price, C. J. (1998). Functional neuroanatomy of the semantic system: divisible by what? *Journal of Cognitive Neuroscience*, **10**: 766–77.

Nittono, H., Suehiro, M., and Hori, T. (2002). Word imageability and N400 in an incidental memory paradigm. *International Journal of Psychophysiology*, **44**: 219–29.

Noppeney, U. and Price, C. J. (2004). Retrieval of abstract semantics. *Neuroimage*, **22**: 164–70.

O'Craven, K. M. and Kanwisher, N. (2000). Mental imagery of faces and places activates corresponding stimulus-specific brain regions. *Journal of Cognitive Neuroscience*, **12**: 1013–23.

Paivio, A. (1971). *Imagery and Verbal Processes.* New York: Holt, Rinehart & Winston.

Paivio, A. (1986). *Mental Representations: A dual-coding approach.* New York: Oxford University Press.

Paivio, A., Yuille, J. C., and Madigan, S. A. (1968). Concreteness, imagery, and meaningfulness values for 925 nouns. *Journal of Experimental Psychology Monograph Supplement*, **76**: 1–25.

Paulesu, E., Frith, C. D., and Frackowiak, R. S. J. (1993). The neural correlates of the verbal component of working memory. *Nature*, **362**: 342–5.

Perani, D., Cappa, S. F., Bettinardi, V., Bressi, S., Gorno-Tempini, M., Matarrese, M., and Fazio F. (1995). Different neural systems for the recognition of animals and man-made tools. *Neuroreport*, **6**: 1637–41.

Perani, D., Schnur, T., Tettamanti, M., Gorno-Tempini, M., Cappa, S. F., and Fazio, F. (1999a). Word and picture matching: a PET study of semantic category effects. *Neuropsychologia*, **37**: 293–306.

Perani, D., Cappa, S. F., Schnur, T., Tettamanti, M., Collina, S., Rosa, M. M., and Fazio, F. (1999b). The neural correlates of verb and noun processing. A PET study. *Brain*, **122**: 2337–44.

Plaut, D. C. and Shallice, T. (1993). Deep dyslexia: a case study of connectionist neuropsychology. *Cognitive Neuropsychology*, **10**: 377–500.

Plaut, D. C., McClelland, J. L., Seidenberg, M. S., and Patterson, K. (1996). Understanding normal and impaired word reading: computational principles in quasi-regular domains. *Psychological Review*, **103**: 45–115.

Price, C. J. and Friston, K. J. (2002). Functional imaging studies of category specificity. In E. M. E. Forde and G. Humphreys (eds.), *Category Specificity in Brain and Mind.* Hove, UK: Psychology Press, pp. 427–48.

Price, C. J., Moore, C. J., Humphreys, G. W., and Wise, R. J. S. (1997). Segregating semantic from phonological processes during reading. *Journal of Cognitive Neuroscience*, **9**: 727–33.

Pulvermüller, F. (1999). Words in the brain's language. *Behavioral Brain Science*, **22**: 253–336.

Rissman, J., Eliassen, J. C., and Blumstein, S. E. (2003). An event-related fMRI investigation of implicit semantic priming. *Journal of Cognitive Neuroscience*, **15**: 1160–75.

Roeltgen, D. P., Sevush, S., and Heilman, K. M. (1983). Phonological agraphia: Writing by the lexical–semantic route. *Neurology*, **33**: 755–65.

Rosch, E., Mervis, C. B., Gray, W. D., Johnson, D. M., and Boyes-Braem, D. (1976). Basic objects in natural categories. *Cognitive Psychology*, **8**: 382–439.

Roskies, A. L., Fiez, J. A., Balota, D. A., Raichle, M. E., and Petersen, S. E. (2001). Task-dependent modulation of regions in the left inferior frontal cortex during semantic processing. *Journal of Cognitive Neuroscience*, **13**: 829–43.

Sabsevitz, D. S., Medler, D. A., Seidenberg, M., and Binder, J. R. (2005). Modulation of the semantic system by word imageability. *Neuroimage*, **27**: 188–200.

Schwanenflugel, P. (1991). Why are abstract concepts hard to understand? In P. Schwanenflugel (ed.), *The Psychology of Word Meanings*. Hillsdale, NJ: Erlbaum, pp. 223–50.

Scott, S. K., Leff, A. P., and Wise, R. J. S. (2003). Going beyond the information given: a neural system supporting semantic interpretation. *Neuroimage*, **19**: 870–6.

Seidenberg, M. S. and McClelland, J. L. (1989). A distributed, developmental model of word recognition and naming. *Psychological Review*, **96**: 523–68.

Shibahara, N., Zorzi, M., Hill, M. P., Wydell, T., and Butterworth, B. (2003). Semantic effects in word naming: evidence from English and Japanese Kanji. *Quarterly Journal of Experimental Psychology*, **56A**: 263–86.

Smith, E. E., Jonides, J., Marshuetz, C., and Koeppe, R. A. (1998). Components of verbal working memory: Evidence from neuroimaging. *Proceedings of the National Academy of Sciences USA*, **95**: 876–82.

Stone, G. O. and Van Orden, G. C. (1993). Strategic control of processing in word recognition. *Journal of Experimental Psychology: Human Perception and Performance*, **19**: 744–74.

Strain, E., Patterson, K., and Seidenberg, M. S. (1995). Semantic effects in single-word naming. *Journal of Experimental Psychology: Learning, Memory, and Cognition*, **21**: 1140–54.

Strain, E., Patterson, K., and Seidenberg, M. S. (2002). Theories of word naming interact with spelling–sound consistency. *Journal of Experimental Psychology: Learning, Memory, and Cognition*, **28**: 207–14.

Sturm, W. and Willmes, K. (2001). On the functional neuroanatomy of intrinsic and phasic alertness. *Neuroimage*, **14**: S76–84.

Taylor, S. F., Kornblum, S., Minoshima, S., Oliver, L. M., and Koeppe, R. A. (1994). Changes in medial cortical blood flow with a stimulus–response compatibility task. *Neuropsychologia*, **32**: 249–55.

Thompson-Schill, S. L. (2003). Neuroimaging studies of semantic memory: inferring "how" from "where". *Neuropsychologia*, **41**: 280–92.

Thompson-Schill, S. L., D'Esposito, M., and Kan, I. P. (1999a). Effects of repetition and competition on activity in left prefrontal cortex during word generation. *Neuron*, **23**: 513–22.

Thompson-Schill, S. L., Aguirre, G. K., D'Esposito, M., and Farah, M. J. (1999b). A neural basis for category and modality specificity of semantic knowledge. *Neuropsychologia*, **37**: 671–6.

Tyler, L. K., Russell, R., Fadili, J., and Moss, H. E. (2001). The neural representation of nouns and verbs: PET studies. *Brain*, **124**: 1619–34.

Ullsperger, M. and von Cramon, D. Y. (2001). Subprocesses of performance monitoring: a dissociation of error processing and response competition revealed by event-related fMRI and ERPs. *Neuroimage*, **14**: 1387–401.

Van Order, G. C., Pennington, B. F., and Stone, G. O. (1990). Word identification in reading and the promise of subsymbolic psycholinguistics. *Psychological Review*, **97**: 488–522.

van Veen, V. and Carter, C. S. (2002). The anterior cingulate as a conflict monitor: fMRI and ERP studies. *Physiology and Behavior*, **77**: 477–82.

Wager, T. D. and Smith, E. E. (2003). Neuroimaging studies of working memory: a meta-analysis. *Cognitive, Affective, and Behavioral Neuroscience*, **3**: 255–74.

Warrington, E. K. (1975). The selective impairment of semantic memory. *Quarterly Journal of Experimental Psychology*, **27**: 635–57.

Warrington, E. K. (1981). Concrete word dyslexia. *British Journal of Psychology*, **72**: 175–96.

Warrington, E. K. and Shallice, T. (1984). Category specific semantic impairments. *Brain*, **107**: 829–54.

Warrington, E. K. and McCarthy, R. A. (1987). Categories of knowledge. Further fractionations and an attempted integration. *Brain*, **110**: 1273–96.

Waters, G. S. and Seidenberg, M. S. (1985). Spelling–sound effects in reading: time course and decision criteria. *Memory and Cognition*, **13**: 557–72.

Wernicke, C. (1874). *Der aphasische Symptomenkomplex*. Breslau: Cohn & Weigert.

Whatmough, C., Verret, L., Fung, D., and Chertkow, H. (2004). Common and contrasting areas of activation for abstract and concrete concepts: an H2 15O PET study. *Journal of Cognitive Neuroscience*, **16**: 1211–26.

Wise, R. J. S., Howard, D., Mummery, C. J., Fletcher, P., Leff, A., Büchel, C., and Scott, S. K. (2000). Noun imageability and the temporal lobes. *Neuropsychologia*, **38**: 985–94.

Zaidel, E. (1978). Auditory language comprehension in the right hemisphere following commissurotomy and hemispherectomy: a comparison with child language and aphasia. In A. Caramazza and E. B. Zurif (eds.), *Language Acquisition and Language Breakdown: Parallels and divergences*. Baltimore, MD: The Johns Hopkins University Press, pp. 229–75.

7

The neural systems processing tool and action semantics

Uta Noppeney

Max-Planck-Institute for Biological Cybernetics

This chapter discusses the contributions of functional imaging to our under-standing of how action and tool concepts are represented and processed in the human brain. Section 7.1 introduces cognitive models of semantic organization. Section 7.2 provides a brief overview of functional imaging approaches to identify brain regions that have specialized for processing action and tool representations. Section 7.3 discusses the relationship between the visuomotor system and semantic processing of actions. Section 7.4 investigates the effects of action type and visual experience on action-selective responses. Section 7.5 characterizes the neural systems engaged in tool processing and how they are modulated by task and stimulus modality. Section 7.6 delineates future directions that may enable us to characterize the neural mechanisms that mediate tool and action-selective brain responses.

7.1 Cognitive models of semantic organization

Since the seminal work of Warrington and Shallice (1984), double dissociations of semantic deficits have been established between tools and animals (for review, see Gainotti *et al.*, 1995; Warrington & Shallice, 1984; Capitani *et al.*, 2003; Gainotti & Silveri, 1996; Farah *et al.*, 1996; Hillis & Caramazza, 1991; Sacchett & Humphreys, 1992; Warrington & McCarthy, 1987). These double dissociations persist even when attempts are made to control general processing differences due to confounding variables such as familiarity, visual complexity, or word frequency (Farah *et al.*, 1996; Sartori *et al.*, 1993). They appear, therefore, to reflect some sort of semantic organization at the neuronal level.

Many cognitive models have been offered to explain these category-specific deficits.

For instance, the *category-specific model* (Caramazza & Shelton, 1998) postulates distinct neuronal systems that have specialized in processing items from different semantic categories (e.g. animals or artifacts) due to evolutionary pressures.

Here, a functional segregation of different semantic categories may have emerged to allow for rapid identification and classification of animals as potential predators and plants as a source of food.

In contrast, the *conceptual structure account* (Tyler & Moss, 2001; Tyler *et al.*, 2000) assumes a unitary distributed conceptual system that is structured according to correlations among semantic features (i.e. the degree to which semantic features co-occur in the environment). Selective semantic deficits are explained by differences in the structure of concepts across categories. Artifacts are defined by few and more distinctive features. In contrast, living items are characterized by many overlapping shared and highly intercorrelated features but only relatively few distinctive features. Hence living items may place increased demands on integration and differentiation processes.

This chapter is framed within the *feature-based account* of semantic memory (Warrington & Shallice, 1984), also referred to as the *sensorimotor theory* (Martin *et al.*, 2000). This approach assumes that conceptual knowledge is represented in a large distributed network, indexing a range of semantic features (e.g. visual, auditory, action, functional properties; Allport, 1985). Although category-specificity is not the underlying organizational principle, an apparent category structure emerges because concepts rely differentially on sensory, action, and verbally learnt knowledge. In particular, category-specific semantic deficits for living and nonliving items are explained by their differential associations with sensory and action features: while sensory features are important for distinguishing between living items, action semantics plays a critical role in the representation of inanimate items (especially tools) (Warrington & Shallice, 1984; Shallice, 1988). Hence loss of sensory or action knowledge differentially disrupts the semantic representation of animate or inanimate objects respectively.

In terms of brain architecture, sensory (e.g. visual, auditory) and action (e.g. hand action, body motion) features have been related to the input and output channels within the human brain (Martin *et al.*, 2000; Martin & Chao, 2001). While sensory features may be subserved by brain regions close to or even overlapping with areas involved in perception (e.g. visual association areas), action semantics is hypothesized to be related to motor output regions as well as to brain areas involved in motion/action perception. Thus the neural systems representing/processing sensory or action semantic features are (1) related to or (2) even identical with the regions that are engaged when the particular type of semantic knowledge is acquired during sensory–motor experience. In case (1), there might be "semantic regions" that are selective for a particular type of semantic feature because of their afferent or efferent connections to sensory–motor regions. In case (2), "sensory–motor regions" themselves can sustain semantic representations or processes. From a cognitive perspective,

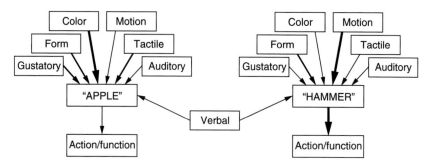

Figure 7.1. The feature-based model of semantic memory. Illustration of the animate–non-animate distinction. Arrow width indicates the contribution of a semantic feature to a particular semantic concept.

the function of a so-called "sensory–motor region" would then depend on the particular task context. From a neuronal perspective, it would depend on the brain regions it is interacting with. For instance, motion area V5 might be involved in motion processing when being activated via forward (bottom–up) connections from early visual areas but in semantic processes when being activated via backward (top–down) connections from semantic retrieval regions. Here, a so-called "sensory–motor" region would be engaged in both sensory/motor processing and higher cognitive functions such as semantic processing (Figure 7.1).

7.2 Overview of functional imaging approaches

Over the past decade, a large corpus of functional imaging studies has investigated the neural systems processing semantic concepts — in particular action and tool representations. These studies have primarily manipulated one or several of the following factors:

1. *Semantic content of the stimuli:* To identify brain responses that are selective for action or tool semantics, we need to compare different semantic features or object categories. For this, studies have compared action semantics with sensory or abstract features (e.g. hand action vs. color words (Martin *et al.*, 1995; Noppeney *et al.*, 2005) or tools with other object categories (for review see Price & Friston, 2002; Joseph, 2001).

2. *Stimulus modality and material:* Stimuli have been presented as written words, spoken words, sounds or pictures that were either static or moving. Manipulations of stimulus material (e.g. verbal vs. nonverbal) and modality (e.g. visual vs. auditory) have been used for the following purposes:
   • It is often difficult to equate stimuli from different categories with respect to all their characteristic dimensions such as word frequency, familiarity, word length, structural complexity, imageability, and low-level visual or

auditory features. Identifying category-selective activations that are observed irrespective of changes in stimulus modality or material is a means to remove — at least — the low-level stimulus confounds. Common activations can be identified using a conjunction analysis (Price & Friston, 1997; Nichols *et al.*, 2005; Friston *et al.*, 2005). For instance, this procedure allows one to test the joint hypothesis that an area is activated for (i) tool words relative to animal words and (ii) tool pictures relative to animal pictures.

- At least in some frameworks (Humphreys & Forde, 2001), "semantics" has been operationally defined as representations that can be activated irrespective of (i) the input modality and (ii) the stimulus material. By contrast, structural processing (i.e. structural encoding or object identification) is influenced by input modality and stimulus material. Hence manipulations of stimulus material or modality allow one to dissociate category-selective responses at the perceptual/structural and the semantic level. Category-selective activations at the semantic level are observed irrespective of stimulus material. Category-selective activations at the structural level are enhanced for nonverbal (i.e. pictures, movies, or sounds) relative to verbal material. In other words, semantic processes are identified by a conjunction analysis, whereas structural processes are revealed by an interaction between category and stimulus material.

3. *Task*: To engage subjects in processing tool and action semantics, various tasks have been used that can be classified as implicit (e.g. reading, listening, viewing) and explicit (decision or generation) semantic tasks. Task manipulations may serve the following purposes:
- Task instructions during explicit semantic tasks are used to direct the subject's attention to particular semantic aspects. Task instructions are a means to induce processing of different semantic features while holding the stimuli constant (e.g. semantic decisions on tool stimuli with the task instructions: "Do you twist this object?" = action features vs. "Is the object bigger than a kiwi?" = visual features; (Phillips *et al.*, 2002b; Noppeney & Price, 2002). Task manipulations permit the comparison between, e.g. action and nonaction features, while controlling completely for stimulus confounds. However, they are susceptible to task-induced or strategic confounds. For instance, real life-size judgments may require the comparison between two objects, while action judgments induce motor imagery. Furthermore, task manipulations may underestimate or miss activation differences between different features because of implicit processing. Implicit processing refers to the fact that the human brain processes many linguistic and object attributes automatically irrespective of the explicit task demands (e.g. the Stroop effect; MacLeod, 1991). Hence, despite task-induced attentional shifts to specific

semantic properties of an object, the entire semantic system might be activated in a highly connected fashion – thus reducing activation differences between action and nonaction semantics.

- Functional attributions such as the "action semantic area" or "tool area" raise the fundamental issue whether category-selective responses are a function of the stimulus or whether the selectivity arises from an interaction between stimulus and cognitive set (i.e. a stimulus-selective operation). In other words, the specificity or selectivity of evoked brain responses may be understood in terms of the nature of the stimulus being operated upon (i.e. tools vs. animals), or in terms of the cognitive operation induced by the stimulus in a particular context. Empirically, this question can be answered by manipulating both the category of the stimulus (e.g. animals vs. tools) and the cognitive set or task in a multifactorial fashion and looking for either a main effect of stimulus category or the interaction between category and task. For instance, the interaction between category (animals vs. tools) and task (implicit/shallow vs. explicit/deep semantic encoding) may provide insight into the role of cognitive set (or attentional effects) in tool-selective activations. Furthermore, tool-selective activations that are observed only during explicit semantic tasks may result from task-induced strategies such as motor imagery, which are not required for implicit tool processing.
- Comparing "sensory–motor" and semantic tasks may enable us to address the question whether "sensorimotor" regions may indeed play an essential role in both sensory–motor functions and semantic processing. For instance, comparing action execution, imagery, semantic action retrieval, and reading action words may allow us to investigate whether the premotor cortex is engaged in action processing ranging from execution to implicit action semantics during reading. Similarly, comparing perception of moving stimuli and reading motion words may enable us to decide whether area MT/V5 or the superior temporal sulcus (STS) is engaged in motion perception and semantics.

4. *Additional factors*: Introducing additional factors such as priming (Chao *et al.*, 2002) or awareness (Fang & He, 2005) may permit a further dissociation of brain regions based on their characteristic response patterns.

7.3   The visuomotor system and action semantics

7.3.1   The visuomotor system

The feature-based account (Martin *et al.*, 2000) proposes that the neural substrates underlying action and tool semantics are anatomically and functionally related to brain regions taking part in a visuomotor action system encompassing the left ventral premotor cortex (BA6), the parietal cortex, and the left posterior middle temporal gyrus (LPMT).

Neurophysiological studies in non-human primates have suggested that the frontoparietal circuitry may play a role in (1) visuomotor transformations and (2) action matching, imitation and understanding (Rizzolatti & Luppino, 2001).

1. Visuomotor transformations such as visual searching or grasping are thought to be mediated through interactions between the ventral premotor cortex and an anterior intraparietal area (AIP) that receives visual input and is connected with inferior temporal cortex (IT) (Rizzolatti & Craighero, 2004). In both AIP and ventral premotor cortex (in particular in the posterior bank of the ventral limb of the arcuate sulcus) canonical neurons have been found that fire when the monkey sees and grasps an object. In AIP, these visual-dominant neurons respond selectively to visual presentation of a particular class of three-dimensional objects (Murata *et al.*, 2000). Hence it has been suggested that AIP extracts and selects the relevant three-dimensional features. These visual object properties (or affordances) may subsequently activate congruent motor prototypes in the ventral premotor cortex and thus enable the appropriate action for a particular object (e.g. object grasping).

2. Action understanding may be sustained by a ventral premotor area (F5c, on the cortical convexity) and an anterior inferior parietal area (7b/PF) that is connected with the superior temporal sulcus (STS). In F5c and PF, neurons with mirror properties have been identified, i.e. these neurons discharge when the monkey makes a particular action and observes another individual making a similar action (Fogassi & Luppino, 2005; Fogassi *et al.*, 2005; Rizzolatti & Luppino, 2001; Rizzolatti *et al.*, 2002; Rizzolatti & Craighero, 2004). This action-selectivity depends primarily on the final goal of the action rather than particular kinematic characteristics. Thus mirror neuron discharges are also observed when (i) the kinematics is altered (Fogassi & Luppino, 2005; Fogassi *et al.*, 2005), (ii) the final hand–object interaction is hidden (Umilta *et al.*, 2001) and (iii) only the sound of a particular action is presented (Kohler *et al.*, 2002). This F5–PF mirror neuron circuitry has been proposed to form the basis for action/intention understanding and imitation learning (Arbib & Bota, 2003; Rizzolatti & Arbib, 1998).

A recent fMRI study in the macaque has identified and further characterized multiple action representations with different degrees of abstraction within the frontal lobe (Nelissen *et al.*, 2005). In particular, it has dissociated (i) caudal F5c, which responds in context-dependent fashion and is activated only when the agent is fully visible (e.g. the person together with the arm picking up the object),

(ii) rostral F5ab (in the depth of the ventral limb of the arcuate sulcus), which is also activated by observation of an isolated arm and even an artificial device (though less effective), and (iii) 45B, which is activated not only by actions but also by graspable objects. There has been some controversy over the homology between monkey and human mirror neuron areas. Based on cytoarchitectonic and electrophysiological analyses, homologies have been suggested between human ventral premotor BA6 and caudal F5c in the macaque. Similarly, F5a (as designated by Nelissen *et al.*, 2005) may be the homologue of human BA44 (see Petrides *et al.*, 2005 for further discussion). PF and AIP may be related to the anterior inferior parietal cortex in humans. In line with this conjecture, human functional imaging studies have implicated the ventral premotor cortex and the anterior parietal cortex (supramarginal gyrus/AIP) in action observation, simulation, imitation and execution (Rizzolatti *et al.*, 2002; Buccino *et al.*, 2001, 2004a, 2004b; Rushworth *et al.*, 2001, 2003; Grezes *et al.*, 2003; Johnson-Frey *et al.*, 2003; Iacoboni *et al.*, 1999, 2005).

7.3.2   The neural systems of action semantics

Consistent with the feature-based account, a series of functional imaging studies have reported increased activation in the ventral premotor and the anterior inferior parietal cortex for retrieval of action semantics using verbal and nonverbal stimuli. Activation in the left ventral premotor cortex has been observed for generation of semantically related action words relative to naming of an object (Warburton *et al.*, 1996; Grafton *et al.*, 1997). While these results may be confounded by internal verbalization and thus phonological retrieval, the seminal study by Martin *et al.* (1995) has revealed increased left premotor activation for generating an action associated with an object relative to its color (*ibid.*). Surprisingly, a recent study has shown selective activation along the (pre)motor cortex in a somatotopic fashion for action words referring to face, arm, or leg actions (e.g. lick, pick, kick) in a passive reading task (Hauk *et al.*, 2004; Tettamanti *et al.*, 2005). Similarly, anterior inferior parietal activation has been observed for semantic decisions on action relative to nonaction words and for retrieval of an object's action relative to its function (Kellenbach *et al.*, 2003; Noppeney *et al.*, 2005; Tettamanti *et al.*, 2005).

In addition to AIP and ventral premotor areas, the left posterior middle temporal region (LPMT) has been associated consistently with action semantics. As LPMT is just anterior (or overlapping) to motion area MT/V5, its role in action semantics might be engendered by its functional relation to action/motion perception mediated by afferents from area MT/V5. Thus LPMT is activated for observing grasping movements relative to static objects (Perani *et al.*, 2001; Rizzolatti *et al.*, 1996), hands (Grezes *et al.*, 1998) or random motion

(Bonda *et al.*, 1996; Beauchamp *et al.*, 2002). Obviously, these activation differences may be due to specific kinematic characteristics of the stimuli at the perceptual level. However, LPMT activation was also increased for static pictures or sentences with implied motion/action relative to similar stimuli that did not imply motion (Kourtzi & Kanwisher, 2000; Ruby & Decety, 2001; Senior *et al.*, 2000). Moreover, in semantic decision or generation tasks, LPMT is activated for retrieval of action (e.g. "Do you twist this object?") relative to retrieval of visual semantics (e.g. "Is the object bigger than a kiwi?"), when the stimuli are written words or pictures referring to real-world objects (Martin *et al.*, 1995; Phillips, Noppeney, Humphreys, & Price, 2002b). Similarly, LPMT activation is increased for semantic tasks on spoken or written words (or sentences) referring to action/motion (e.g. "twist", "run") relative to visual (e.g. "red"), auditory (e.g. "pop"), or abstract (e.g. "idea") semantic features (Noppeney *et al.*, 2005; Wallentin *et al.*, 2005). Collectively, these studies demonstrate that LPMT is more engaged in action semantics relative to a range of other semantic types regardless of stimulus material (e.g. written words, sentences, or pictures) or modality (auditory or visual, e.g. spoken or written words). Hence the activations cannot be attributed to low-level stimulus characteristics. Instead, these results characterize LPMT as a multimodal semantic region associated with action processing.

7.4 Effects of action type and visual experience

7.4.1 The distinction between hand manipulations and whole-body movements

"Actions" can be classified as hand manipulations or whole-body movements. A distinction between these two categories can be drawn at the perceptual and at the semantic level. At the perceptual level, hand manipulations are often characterized by simple motion trajectories. For instance, the movement for using a saw is primarily a simple translation movement. By contrast, whole-body movements are described by complex motion trajectories. Thus humans can independently move different body parts that are connected by articulated joints. At the semantic level, hand manipulations are transitive actions and more strongly associated with tools and utensils. In contrast, whole-body movements are intransitive actions and primarily linked with humans and animals. Based on these distinctions, the question arises whether regions within or beyond the action retrieval system respond more to hand manipulations than to whole-body movements. At the perceptual level, this question has been addressed (Beauchamp *et al.*, 2002) by comparing activations during observation of (i) natural simple tool movements (e.g. sawing), (ii) artificial simple tool movements (e.g. a rotating saw),

(iii) natural complex human movements (e.g. running) and (iv) artificial simple human movements (e.g. a rotating human). While the right superior temporal sulcus (STS) showed an enhanced response to whole-body movements, LPMT responded preferentially to hand movements — though this effect was very small. Using words rather than pictures, a recent study (Noppeney et al., 2005) aimed to identify regions that responded selectively to particular action types, i.e. hand actions or whole-body movements at the semantic level. Although AIP and LPMT showed enhanced responses for action relative to nonaction words, they did not distinguish between hand manipulations and whole-body movements. However, an area in the right STS, anterior to the region that responded selectively to movies of whole-body movements, exhibited increased activation for whole-body movements relative to hand actions (see also James & Gauthier, 2003). In summary, studies of action observation and semantic retrieval provide converging evidence that LPMT activation is commonly increased for both hand manipulation and whole-body movements. So far, there is only weak evidence that hand manipulations further enhance LPMT activation relative to whole-body movements at the perceptual level.

7.4.2 The distinction between manipulation and functional knowledge: knowing "how" and knowing "what for"

Tools or objects can be characterized by the motion features of an associated hand action (i.e. knowing "how" = manipulation knowledge) and by their function (i.e. knowing "what for" or the context of usage = functional knowledge). Although a particular type of manipulation can sometimes be associated with a specific function (e.g. a saw and a knife are associated with similar actions and have similar functions), the mapping between manipulation and functional properties is many to many. For instance, a piano and a record player subserve similar functions but are manipulated differently, while a piano and a typewriter fulfill different functions but are manipulated similarly. Neuropsychological studies (Buxbaum et al., 2000; Sirigu et al., 1991) have reported patients who could match items on the basis of their function but not on the basis of how they are manipulated and vice versa. This double dissociation suggests that the neural substrates of function and manipulation knowledge may be anatomically segregated and one might hypothesize that ventral premotor, AIP or LPMT respond to manipulation more than functional knowledge. Consistent with this notion, no increased activation (Cappa et al., 1998; Mummery et al., 1998; Thompson-Schill et al., 1999) has been reported in any of these regions for retrieval of functional relative to visual semantics. A recent study directly compared retrieval of (i) an action associated with a manipulable object (e.g. "Does using a saw involve a twisting or a turning movement?"), (ii) a function of a manipulable object (e.g. "Is a saw used to put a substance on another object?") and (iii) a function of a non-manipulable object (e.g. a traffic light). This experimental design revealed distinct activation patterns in the cortical regions of the visuomotor action system: in LPMT and ventral premotor cortex, activations were significantly increased for manipulable relative to non-manipulable objects. Only a small non-significant increase was observed for retrieval of action relative to functional knowledge (see Gerlach *et al.*, 2002b for converging results in the ventral premotor cortex). In contrast, in AIP, activation was increased for (i) manipulable objects relative to non-manipulable objects and (ii) action decisions relative to function decisions (see Boronat *et al.*, 2005 for similar results). Thus, while AIP showed an effect of stimulus (manipulable vs. nonmanipulable objects) and task (action vs. function retrieval), LPMT and the ventral premotor cortex showed only an effect of stimulus.

These results suggest that activation in the visuomotor system is primarily driven by action knowledge. Furthermore, in LPMT and the ventral premotor cortex, this action-selective response is automatically/implicitly invoked by manipulable objects irrespective of the specific task instructions. In contrast, in AIP it is modulated by the particular task demands.

7.4.3   The influence of sensory experience on action-selective LPMT response

The "sensorimotor theory" hypothesizes that semantic information is represented in a distributed neuronal network encoding semantic features (e.g. visual, auditory, action), which are anatomically linked to the sensory (or motor) areas that are active when the features (e.g. motion, color) are experienced (Allport, 1985; Barsalou *et al.*, 2003; Martin *et al.*, 2000; Warrington & McCarthy, 1987). Thus the functional anatomy of semantic memory is predicated on the organization of sensory systems. From this perspective, one might expect that sensory deprivation leading to the restructuring of sensory systems will also modify the neural systems underlying semantic representations. In particular, one might hypothesize that visual deprivation, which enforces action experience via somatosensory—motor associations rather than visual motion perception, reduces the action-selective response in LPMT. Contrary to this conjecture, in both blind and sighted subjects, LPMT activation increased for semantic decisions on spoken words referring to actions relative to words referring to visual, auditory, or motion features (Noppeney *et al.*, 2003). This remarkable resilience of LPMT action-selectivity to early visual deprivation might be explained by multimodal response characteristics of LPMT. For instance, action-selectivity may depend on connections to motor areas. Alternatively, the semantic system develops not only due to experiential factors but also to innately specified neurobiological mechanisms.

7.5   Tool-selective responses

7.5.1   Tool-selectivity in the visuomotor action system

The feature-based theory predicates category-specific effects on anatomical segregation for different types of semantics. In particular, it explains tool-selective effects by the association between tools and actions. In support of this hypothesis, many studies have consistently reported tool-selective activation in one or several regions of the visuomotor action system: the left premotor cortex (Mecklinger *et al.*, 2002; Chao & Martin, 2000; Grabowski *et al.*, 1998; Grafton *et al.*, 1997; Martin *et al.*, 1996; Devlin *et al.*, 2002; Gerlach *et al.*, 2000, 2002a; Kraut *et al.*, 2002), the left posterior middle temporal (Chao *et al.*, 1999; Damasio *et al.*, 1996; Mummery *et al.*, 1998; Perani *et al.*, 1999; Devlin *et al.*, 2002; Cappa *et al.*, 1998; Chao & Martin, 2000; Chao *et al.*, 2002; Martin *et al.*, 1996; Moore & Price, 1999; Mummery *et al.*, 1996; Phillips *et al.*, 2002a; Lewis *et al.*, 2005) and AIP (Chao & Martin, 2000; Noppeney *et al.*, 2006; Devlin *et al.*, 2002; Chao *et al.*, 2002; Cappa *et al.*, 1998). These tool-selective activations have been observed irrespective of stimulus modality (e.g. sounds or pictures) or material (e.g. pictures or written words). Surprisingly, tool-selective responses in parietal cortex have been observed even without accompanying conscious knowledge. Thus, during binocular rivalry, tool pictures that subjects are unaware of due to inter-ocular suppression still elicit enhanced activations in the dorsal pathway (Fang & He, 2005). Taken together with the research on action semantics, these studies suggest that semantic category (e.g. tools vs. animals) and semantic feature (e.g. action vs. visual) may modulate the neural responses in overlapping brain systems. Tool-selective responses can thus be mediated by their association with action features and an apparent category-specific organization may emerge from a feature-based brain architecture.

Indeed, independently manipulating stimulus-category (i.e. tools vs. fruits; (Phillips *et al.*, 2002b) and task instructions (i.e. attention to action vs. visual features) in a 2×2 factorial design revealed that the tool and the action-selective effects influence LPMT in an additive fashion: Tools relative to fruits activated LPMT irrespective of whether action or visual semantics is retrieved. Conversely, retrieval of action relative to visual knowledge activated LPMT regardless of whether tools or fruits are presented (see Figure 7.2, top and bottom left). Thus, even when the stimuli were fruits, LPMT was more active when subjects made a semantic decision on an appropriate action (i.e. "Can you peel it by hand?") than on its real life size (i.e. "Is it bigger than a lemon?"). This pattern of results was replicated in a follow-up study (Contreras, 2002), where subjects made semantic judgments on visual or action features that referred to animals or tools.

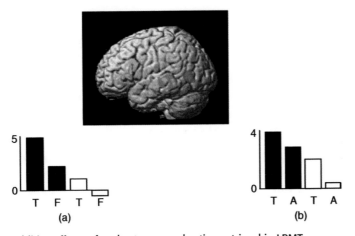

Figure 7.2. Additive effects of tool category and action retrieval in LPMT
Top: Activation patterns for action > visual semantics ($p < 0.05$ corr.) masked with action semantics > baseline ($p < 0.001$ uncorr.)
(a) Data from Phillips *et al.* (2002b). Subjects were presented pictures or written words of tools or fruits made a decision on and their action or visual properties. Parameter estimates at the peak coordinate of action > visual semantics ($x = -56$, $y = -60$, $z = 0$). T = Tools, F = Fruits; Black = Action, White = Visual.
(b) Data from Contreras (2002). In the activation conditions, subjects were presented with two written words referring to an object's properties (e.g. WEIGH and MEASURE) followed by three potential written object names (e.g. SCALES, MIRROR, BED). The properties were visual, action, or functional attributes and the objects were household items or animals. Subjects decided which of the three objects was described by the two properties. Parameter estimates for each semantic condition relative to baseline are shown at the peak coordinate of action > visual semantics ($x = -62$, $y = -58$, $z = 2$). T = Tools, A = Animals; Black = Action, White = Visual.

Again, tools relative to animals and action relative to visual features increased LPMT activation in an additive fashion (see Figure 7.2, bottom). Similarly, AIP activation was increased for (i) manipulable objects relative to nonmanipulable objects and (ii) action relative to function decisions (Kellenbach *et al.*, 2003).

So far, we have emphasized the consistency of tool-selective activations across studies in regions of the visuomotor action system. However, most studies have reported tool-selective responses only in a subset of these regions. Furthermore, manipulating task context (e.g. explicit vs. implicit semantic task) and object category (e.g. tools vs. animals) in a multifactorial design has demonstrated that tool-selective activations in the dorsal visuomotor systems are profoundly context-sensitive and primarily detected for explicit semantic tasks (Noppeney *et al.*, 2006). The question therefore emerges whether or not these action-selective activations are truly essential for "daily" semantic processing. In the first case, they may simply be too small during implicit semantic tasks and may only be detected during explicit semantic tasks when being amplified by attentional top—down modulation. In the second case, they might reflect particular task-induced strategies such as action imagery, which are not necessarily involved in semantic processing. Transient lesion methods such as transcranial magnetic stimulation (TMS) may help us to distinguish between these two possibilities: for instance, applying TMS to LPMT or ventral premotor cortex should be associated with impaired semantic processing and comprehension only if LPMT makes a critical functional contribution to action retrieval.

In conclusion, consistent with the feature-based account, tools that are more strongly linked with action features than animals, fruits, or nonmanipulable objects activate regions within the visuomotor action system. However, these tool-selective responses are profoundly context-sensitive and primarily observed for explicit semantic tasks. These semantic content—task context interactions may represent attentional top—down modulation or task-induced strategies such as action imagery. Future studies using transient lesion methods may enable us to clarify whether regions of the visuomotor system make essential functional contributions to our "daily" semantic processing.

7.5.2   Dorsoventral dissociation of tool-selective activations

In addition to activations in the visuomotor action system, tool-selective responses have also been found within the ventral occipitotemporal cortex: within the fusiform, activations have been found medially for tools and laterally for animals. Three recent studies have dissociated the functional roles of the dorsal visuomotor system and the ventral occipitotemporal cortex in tool processing based on their distinct response patterns using the following manipulations:

The first study (Chao *et al.*, 2002) manipulated semantic category (animals vs. tools) and visual experience (primed vs. unprimed) and demonstrated a priming-induced response reduction nonselectively for tools and animals in the medial fusiform, but selectively for tools in LPMT. This unselective priming effect in the occipitotemporal area suggests that the "fusiform tool region" responds to both categories similarly.

The second study (Beauchamp *et al.*, 2003) manipulated (i) semantic type (i.e. human motion vs. tool motion) and (ii) stimulus display (real objects vs. point light display) in a factorial design and showed a tool motion selective response in LPMT irrespective of stimulus display but in the medial fusiform primarily for real objects. Again, this suggests that LPMT is responsive to tools irrespective of stimulus modality, whereas the medial fusiform is driven by pictures of objects.

The third study (Noppeney *et al.*, 2006) factorially manipulated (i) semantic category (tools vs. animals), (ii) task (explicit vs. implicit semantic one-back-task) and (iii) stimulus modality/material (pictures, spoken or written words) (Figure 7.3). Furthermore, it combined functional imaging with effective connectivity analyses (i.e. dynamic causal modeling) to investigate the neural mechanisms that mediate the tool-selective responses in multiple cortical regions. This approach dissociated two distinct mechanisms that engender tool-selectivity: in the ventral occipitotemporal cortex, category-selectivity was modality-dependent, primarily observed for pictures and mediated by bottom–up effects. In the dorsal visuomotor system, it was task-dependent, observed primarily for explicit semantic tasks and mediated by increased top–down influences of task-related prefrontal activity.

Collectively, the regionally distinct activation and connectivity patterns in the dorsal visuomotor system and the ventral occipitotemporal cortex suggest that these two category-selective systems may support different cognitive operations: the tool-selectivity in occipitotemporal regions is strongly influenced by stimulus-bound factors such as modality (pictures vs. words), display (real objects vs. point

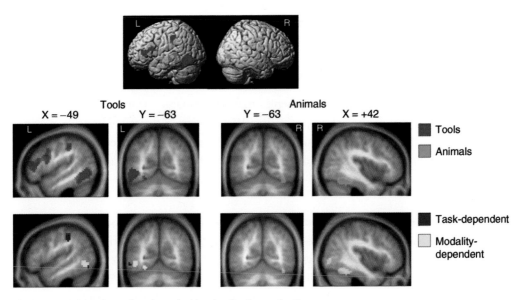

Figure 7.3.   Overview of tool- and animal-selective activations
Top: Main effects of category: tool- and animal-selective activation patterns. Height threshold: $p < 0.05$ corrected.
Bottom: Main effects of category and category × task/modality interactions. Red: Tools > Animals; Green: Animals > Tools; Blue: Tools > Animals for Semantic Decision > Implicit task; Yellow: (i) Tools > Animals for Pictures > Words or (ii) Animals > Tools for Pictures > Words. Height threshold: $p < 0.001$ uncorrected for illustration purposes.

lights) or perceptual priming. These regions may therefore be engaged in structural processing of tools. In contrast, tool-selective responses in regions of the visuomotor system were modulated by the task context and only observed for explicit semantic tasks. These regions might therefore play a role in strategic semantic processing. These results converge with neuropsychological studies that revealed category-selective impairments at multiple levels ranging from structural to semantic (Humphreys & Forde, 2001).

In conclusion, tool-selectivity lies in the interaction of semantic content with either (i) stimulus-bound factors such as modality (= ventral occipito-temporal system) or (ii) task (= dorsal visuomotor system). From a cognitive perspective, category-selective responses therefore reflect either stimulus-bound structural processing or task-induced semantic operations. In terms of neural mechanisms, category-selective brain responses emerge from the patterns of interactions among brain regions. The two distinct classes of category-selectivity can be explained by differential top–down and bottom–up influences for task and modality-dependent category-selective effects respectively. Thus both functional imaging and neuropsychology suggest that some sort of category-selective organization may be realized at both structural and semantic processing levels.

7.6 Conclusions and future directions

This section revisits several themes that have emerged from functional imaging studies of tool and action processing. We will first evaluate the positive evidence for the feature-based account of semantic memory and then conclude by briefly highlighting future directions to investigate the neural mechanisms of tool and action processing.

7.6.1 The feature-based model of semantic memory: action and tool semantics

The feature-based model of semantic memory has primarily emerged from neuropsychology. It was developed to account for category-selective impairments of semantic memory (Shallice, 1988; Warrington & Shallice, 1984; Warrington & McCarthy, 1987). Rather than assuming a category-specific organization, it explains category-specific deficits by (1) a functional segregation for different types of semantic features and (2) differential contributions of semantic features to distinct object categories. Translated into functional imaging, the feature-based model of semantic memory postulates that (1) there are brain regions with selective responses to different types of semantic features and (2) these brain regions overlap with those that show a category-selective response. In particular, we would expect that tools and action features show increased activation in identical brain regions. More closely related to the functional brain architecture, it has been suggested that the neural substrates underlying semantic features are (1) related to or (2) even identical with the regions that were engaged when the particular type of semantic knowledge was acquired during primary sensory–motor experience (Martin *et al.*, 2000; Martin & Chao, 2001). Functional imaging studies of tools and action semantics provide at least partial evidence for the feature-based model: semantic processing of tools and action features increased activation the left posterior middle temporal gyrus (LPMT), the anterior inferior parietal sulcus and ventral premotor cortex, which have previously been implicated in action imagery, observation, and execution. Activation in this visuo-motor system was observed irrespective of stimulus material or modality. Hence, in the case of action semantics, the functional imaging results show the expected congruency of (1) feature: action semantics, (2) category: tools, and (3) sensorimotor region: visuomotor system.

However, some studies have highlighted that tool-selective activations are profoundly sensitive to the context as defined by the task type (e.g. repetition, semantic decision) and the specific task instructions (e.g. different instructions used for action retrieval). Therefore semantic segregation needs to be considered within different task contexts. For this, multifactorial designs are required that allow us to (1) dissociate context-independent from context-sensitive effects and (2) characterize the interactions between semantic type and task context. This approach may reveal "tool or action selectivity" as a semantic type/category by task interaction whereby the tool/action-selective role of a brain area is defined and modulated by the specific task context. Investigating the retrieval of action semantics in a series of task contexts and redefining tool/action selectivity as stimulus by task interaction may enable us to further characterize the particular functional contributions of different regions to tool and action processing.

7.6.2   The neural mechanisms underlying tool and action semantics

In terms of neural mechanisms, task–stimulus interactions are consistent with the well-established notion that functional specialization emerges from changes in the interactions among brain areas that serve different functions (McIntosh, 2000; Mesulam, 1990; Horwitz, 2003). Accordingly, the functional role played by any neuronal system is defined by its interactions with other neuronal systems. Although it is widely acknowledged that semantics is represented and processed in a distributed network (Martin & Chao, 2001; Barsalou *et al.*, 2003; Pulvermüller, 2005; Noppeney, 2004), only few studies have investigated semantic processing formally from the perspective of functional integration (Noppeney *et al.*, 2003; Mechelli *et al.*, 2003; Noppeney *et al.*, 2006). Studies combining functional imaging with effective connectivity analyses will allow us to investigate how regionally semantic-selective responses emerge from interactions among brain regions and to address the predictions made by the "sensorimotor" theory of semantics. In particular, we can test whether identical brain regions sustain sensory–motor functions and semantic processing depending on their connectivity pattern. For instance, we can investigate whether V5/MT is activated via forward connections from early visual areas during action observation, but via backward connections from prefrontal regions during semantic processing of action words.

7.6.3   Multimodal integration during action and tool categorization

Previous research has focused on the cortical regions that showed selective responses to modality-specific features such as color, motion or sounds. Obviously, multiple modality-specific features collectively characterize objects such as tool and action concepts. Thus the question emerges where, when, and how the human brain integrates sensory features into tool or action concepts. In particular, one might investigate whether there are particular regions that are specialized for multisensory integration. Only few functional imaging studies have investigated cross-modal integration at the semantic level using actions and tools characterized by one or multiple modality-specific features. By presenting auditory and visual tool features separately and together, and manipulating their semantic congruency, a recent fMRI study (Beauchamp *et al.*, 2004) has revealed a cross-modal integration effect in the left intraparietal and superior temporal sulci. Clearly, further studies are needed to investigate the neural mechanisms that solve the "binding" problem of semantic features during processing of tool and action semantics.

In conclusion, future functional imaging studies investigating tool and action semantics will need to (1) redefine tool and action selectivity as stimulus–task interactions using multifactorial designs, (2) determine the underlying neural mechanisms by combining functional imaging with modeling approaches, e.g. dynamic causal modeling, and (3) investigate how modality-specific features are integrated into tool and action concepts.

REFERENCES

Allport, D. A. (1985). Distributed memory, modular subsystems and dysphasia. In S. K. Newman and R. Epstein (eds.), *Current Perspectives in Dysphasia*. Edinburgh: Churchill Livingstone, pp. 32–60.

Arbib, M. and Bota, M. (2003). Language evolution: neural homologies and neuroinformatics. *Neural Networks*, **16**: 1237−60.

Barsalou, L. W., Simmons, W. K., Barbey, A. K., and Wilson, C. D. (2003). Grounding conceptual knowledge in modality-specific systems. *Trends in Cognitive Sciences*, **7**: 84−91.

Beauchamp, M. S., Lee, K. E., Haxby, J. V., and Martin, A. (2002). Parallel visual motion processing streams for manipulable objects and human movements. *Neuron*, **34**: 149−59.

Beauchamp, M. S., Lee, K. E., Haxby, J. V., and Martin, A. (2003). FMRI responses to video and point-light displays of moving humans and manipulable objects. *Journal of Cognitive Neuroscience*, **15**: 991−1001.

Beauchamp, M. S., Lee, K. E., Argall, B. D., and Martin, A. (2004). Integration of auditory and visual information about objects in superior temporal sulcus. *Neuron*, **41**: 809−23.

Bonda, E., Petrides, M., Ostry, D., and Evans, A. (1996). Specific involvement of human parietal systems and the amygdala in the perception of biological motion. *Journal of Neuroscience*, **16**: 3737−44.

Boronat, C. B., Buxbaum, L. J., Coslett, H. B., *et al.* (2005). Distinctions between manipulation and function knowledge of objects: evidence from functional magnetic resonance imaging. *Brain Research Cognitive Brain Research*, **23**: 361−73.

Buccino, G., Binkofski, F., Fink, G. R., *et al.* (2001). Action observation activates premotor and parietal areas in a somatotopic manner: an fMRI study. *European Journal of Neuroscience*, **13**: 400−4.

Buccino, G., Lui, F., Canessa, N., *et al.* (2004a). Neural circuits involved in the recognition of actions performed by nonconspecifics: an FMRI study. *Journal of Cognitive Neuroscience*, **16**: 114−26.

Buccino, G., Vogt, S., Ritzl, A., *et al.* (2004b). Neural circuits underlying imitation learning of hand actions: an event-related fMRI study. *Neuron*, **42**: 323−34.

Buxbaum, L., Veramonti, T., and Schwartz, M. (2000). Function and manipulation tool knowledge in apraxia: Knowing "what for" but not "how". *Neurocase*, **6**: 83−97.

Capitani, E., Laiacona, M., Mahon, B., and Caramazza, A. (2003). What are the facts of category-specific deficits? A critical review of the clinical evidence. *Cognitive Neuropsychology*, **20**: 213−62.

Cappa, S. F., Perani, D., Schnur, T., Tettamanti, M., and Fazio, F. (1998). The effects of semantic category and knowledge type on lexical−semantic access: a PET study. *Neuroimage*, **8**: 350−9.

Caramazza, A. and Shelton, J. R. (1998). Domain-specific knowledge systems in the brain: the animate−inanimate distinction. *Journal of Cognitive Neuroscience*, **10**: 1−34.

Chao, L. L. and Martin, A. (2000). Representation of manipulable man-made objects in the dorsal stream. *Neuroimage*, **12**: 478−84.

Chao, L. L., Haxby, J. V., and Martin, A. (1999). Attribute-based neural substrates in temporal cortex for perceiving and knowing about objects. *Nature Neuroscience*, **2**: 913−19.

Chao, L. L., Weisberg, J., and Martin, A. (2002). Experience-dependent modulation of category-related cortical activity. *Cerebral Cortex*, **12**: 545−51.

Contreras, V. (2002). Category-specific effects: segregation of semantic knowledge and degree of feature processing in the brain. Thesis/Dissertation.

Damasio, H., Grabowski, T. J., Tranel, D., Hichwa, R. D., and Damasio, A. R. (1996). A neural basis for lexical retrieval. *Nature*, **380**: 499–505.

Devlin, J. T., Moore, C. J., Mummery, C. J., *et al.* (2002). Anatomic constraints on cognitive theories of category specificity. *Neuroimage*, **15**: 675–5.

Fang, F. and He, S. (2005). Cortical responses to invisible objects in the human dorsal and ventral pathways. *Nature Neuroscience*, **8**: 1380–5.

Farah, M. J., McMullen, P. A., and Meyer, M. M. (1996). The living–nonliving dissociation is not an artefact: giving an a priori implausible hypothesis a strong test. *Cognitive Neuropsychology*, **13**: 137–54.

Fogassi, L., Ferrari, P. F., Gesierich, B., Rozzi, S., Chersi, F., and Rizzolatti, G. (2005). Parietal lobe: from action organization to intention understanding. *Science*, **308**: 662–7.

Fogassi, L. and Luppino, G. (2005). Motor functions of the parietal lobe. *Current Opinion in Neurobiology*, **15**: 626–31.

Friston, K. J., Penny, W. D., and Glaser, D. E. (2005). Conjunction revisited. *Neuroimage*, **25**: 661–7.

Gainotti, G., Giustolisi, L., Daniele, A., and Silveri, M. C. (1995). Neuroanatomical correlates of category-specific semantic disorders: a critical survey. *Memory*, **3**: 247–64.

Gainotti, G. and Silveri, M. C. (1996). Cognitive and anatomical locus of lesion in a patient with a category-specific semantic impairment for living beings. *Cognitive Neuropsychology*, **13**: 357–89.

Gerlach, C., Law, I., Gade, A., and Paulson, O. B. (2000). Categorization and category effects in normal object recognition. A PET study. *Neuropsychologia*, **38**: 1693–703.

Gerlach, C., Law, I., Gade, A., and Paulson, O. B. (2002a). The role of action knowledge in the comprehension of artifacts – a PET study. *Neuroimage*, **15**: 143–52.

Gerlach, C., Law, I., and Paulson, O. B. (2002b). When action turns into words. Activation of motor-based knowledge during categorization of manipulable objects. *Journal of Cognitive Neuroscience*, **14**: 1230–9.

Grabowski, T. J., Damasio, H., and Damasio, A. R. (1998). Premotor and prefrontal correlates of category-related lexical retrieval. *Neuroimage*, **7**: 232–43.

Grafton, S. T., Fadiga, L., Arbib, M. A., and Rizzolatti, G. (1997). Premotor cortex activation during observation and naming of familiar tools. *Neuroimage*, **6**: 231–6.

Grezes, J., Armony, J. L., Rowe, J., and Passingham, R. E. (2003). Activations related to "mirror" and "canonical" neurones in the human brain: an fMRI study. *Neuroimage*, **18**: 928–37.

Grezes, J., Costes, N., and Decety, J. (1998). Top–down effect of strategy on the perception of human biological motion: a PET investigation. *Cognitive Neuropsychology*, **15**: 553–82.

Hauk, O., Johnsrude, I., and Pulvermüller, F. (2004). Somatotopic representation of action words in human motor and premotor cortex. *Neuron*, **41**: 301–7.

Hillis, A. E. and Caramazza, A. (1991). Category-specific naming and comprehension impairment: a double dissociation. *Brain*, **114**: 2081–94.

Horwitz, B. (2003). The elusive concept of brain connectivity. *Neuroimage*, **19**: 466–70.

Humphreys, G. W. and Forde, E. M. (2001). Hierarchies, similarity, and interactivity in object recognition: "category-specific" neuropsychological deficits. *Behavioral Brain Science*, **24**: 453–76.

Iacoboni, M., Molnar-Szakacs, I., Gallese, V., Buccino, G., Mazziotta, J. C., and Rizzolatti, G. (2005). Grasping the intentions of others with one's own mirror neuron system. *Public Library of Science Biology*, **3**: e79.

Iacoboni, M., Woods, R. P., Brass, M., Bekkering, H., Mazziotta, J. C., and Rizzolatti, G. (1999). Cortical mechanisms of human imitation. *Science*, **286**: 2526–8.

James, T. W. and Gauthier, I. (2003). Auditory and action semantic features activate sensory-specific perceptual brain regions. *Current Biology*, **13**: 1792–6.

Johnson-Frey, S. H., Maloof, F. R., Newman-Norlund, R., Farrer, C., Inati, S., and Grafton, S. T. (2003). Actions or hand–object interactions? Human inferior frontal cortex and action observation. *Neuron*, **39**: 1053–8.

Joseph, J. E. (2001). Functional neuroimaging studies of category specificity in object recognition: a critical review and meta-analysis. *Cognitive, Affective and Behavioral Neuroscience*, **1**: 119–36.

Kellenbach, M., Brett, M., and Patterson, K. (2003). Actions speak louder than functions. The importance of manipulability and action in tool representation. *Journal of Cognitive Neuroscience*, **15**: 30–46.

Kohler, E., Keysers, C., Umilta, M. A., Fogassi, L., Gallese, V., and Rizzolatti, G. (2002). Hearing sounds, understanding actions: action representation in mirror neurons. *Science*, **297**: 846–8.

Kourtzi, Z. and Kanwisher, N. (2000). Activation in human MT/MST by static images with implied motion. *Journal of Cognitive Neuroscience*, **12**: 48–55.

Kraut, M. A., Moo, L. R., Segal, J. B., and Hart, J., Jr. (2002). Neural activation during an explicit categorization task: category- or feature-specific effects? *Brain Research: Cognitive Brain Research*, **13**: 213–20.

Lewis, J. W., Brefczynski, J. A., Phinney, R. E. Janik, J. J., and DeYoe, E. A. (2005). Distinct cortical pathways for processing tool versus animal sounds. *Journal of Neuroscience*, **25**: 5148–58.

MacLeod, C. M. (1991). Half a century of research on the Stroop effect: an integrative review. *Psychological Bulletin*, **109**: 163–203.

Martin, A. and Chao, L. L. (2001). Semantic memory and the brain: structure and processes. *Current Opinion in Neurobiology*, **11**: 194–201.

Martin, A., Haxby, J. V., Lalonde, F. M., Wiggs, C. L., and Ungerleider, L. G. (1995). Discrete cortical regions associated with knowledge of color and knowledge of action. *Science*, **270**: 102–5.

Martin, A, Ungerleider, L. G., and Haxby, J. V. (2000). Category-specificity and the brain: the sensory/motor model of semantic representations of objects. In M. S. Gazzaniga (ed.), *The Cognitive Neurosciences*. Cambridge, MA: MIT Press, pp. 1023–37.

Martin, A., Wiggs, C. L., Ungerleider, L. G., and Haxby, J. V. (1996). Neural correlates of category-specific knowledge. *Nature*, **379**: 649–52.

McIntosh, A. R. (2000). Towards a network theory of cognition. *Neural Networks*, **13**: 861–70.

Mechelli, A., Price, C. J., Noppeney, U., and Friston, K. J. (2003). A dynamic causal modeling study on category effects: bottom−up or top−down mediation? *Journal of Cognitive Neuroscience*, **15**: 925−34.

Mecklinger, A., Gruenewald, C., Besson, M., Magnie, M. N., and von Cramon, D. Y. (2002). Separable neuronal circuitries for manipulable and non-manipulable objects in working memory. *Cerebral Cortex*, **12**: 1115−23.

Mesulam, M. M. (1990). Large-scale neurocognitive networks and distributed processing for attention, language, and memory. *Annals of Neurology*, **28**: 597−613.

Moore, C. J. and Price, C. J. (1999). A functional neuroimaging study of the variables that generate category-specific object processing differences. *Brain*, **122**: 943−62.

Mummery, C. J., Patterson, K., Hodges, J. R., and Price, C. J. (1998). Functional neuroanatomy of the semantic system: divisible by what? *Journal of Cognitive Neuroscience*, **10**: 766−77.

Mummery, C. J., Patterson, K., Hodges, J. R., and Wise, R. J. (1996). Generating "tiger" as an animal name or a word beginning with T: differences in brain activation. *Proceedings of the Royal Society, London, B: Biological Sciences*, **263**: 989−95.

Murata, A., Gallese, V., Luppino, G., Kaseda, M., and Sakata, H. (2000). Selectivity for the shape, size, and orientation of objects for grasping in neurons of monkey parietal area AIP. *Journal of Neurophysiology*, **83**: 2580−601.

Nelissen, K., Luppino, G., Vanduffel, W., Rizzolatti, G., and Orban, G. A. (2005). Observing others: multiple action representation in the frontal lobe. *Science*, **310**: 332−6.

Nichols, T., Brett, M., Andersson, J., Wager, T., and Poline, J. B. (2005). Valid conjunction inference with the minimum statistic. *Neuroimage*, **25**: 653−60.

Noppeney U. (2004). The feature-based model of semantic memory. In R. Frackowiak, K. Friston, C. D. Frith, *et al.* (eds.), *Human Brain Function*. London: Elsevier, pp. 533−47.

Noppeney, U. and Price, C. J. (2002). A PET study of stimulus- and task-induced semantic processing. *Neuroimage*, **15**: 927−35.

Noppeney, U., Friston, K., and Price, C. (2003). Effects of visual deprivation on the organisation of the semantic system. *Brain*, **126**: 1620−7.

Noppeney, U., Josephs, O., Kiebel, S., Friston, K., and Price, C. (2005). Action selectivity in parietal and temporal cortex. *Brain Research: Cognitive Brain Research*, **25**: 641−9.

Noppeney, U., Price, C. J., Penny, W. D., and Friston, K. J. (2006). Two distinct neural mechanisms for category-selective responses. *Cerebral Cortex*, **16**: 437−45.

Perani, D., Fazio, F., Borghese, N. A., *et al.* (2001). Different brain correlates for watching real and virtual hand actions. *Neuroimage*, **14**: 749−58.

Perani, D., Schnur, T., Tettamanti, M., Gorno-Tempini, M., Cappa, S. F., and Fazio, F. (1999). Word and picture matching: a PET study of semantic category effects. *Neuropsychologia*, **37**: 293−306.

Petrides, M., Cadoret, G., and Mackey, S. (2005). Orofacial somatomotor responses in the macaque monkey homologue of Broca's area. *Nature*, **435**: 1235−8.

Phillips, J. A., Humphreys, G. W., Noppeney, U., and Price, C. J. (2002a). The neural substrates of action retrieval: an examination of semantic and visual routes to action. *Vision and Cognition*, **9**(4): 662−84.

Phillips, J. A., Noppeney, U., Humphreys, G. W., and Price, C. J. (2002b). Can segregation within the semantic system account for category-specific deficits? *Brain*, **125**: 2067–80.

Price, C. and Friston, K. (2002). Functional imaging studies of category specificity. In E. M. Forde and G. W. Humphreys (eds.), *Category Specificity in Brain and Mind*. Hove, Sussex: Psychology Press, pp. 427–45.

Price, C. J. and Friston, K. J. (1997). Cognitive conjunction: a new approach to brain activation experiments. *Neuroimage*, **5**: 261–70.

Pulvermüller, F. (2005). Brain mechanisms linking language and action. *Nature Reviews Neuroscience*, **6**: 576–82.

Rizzolatti, G. and Arbib, M. A. (1998). Language within our grasp. *Trends in Neuroscience*, **21**: 188–94.

Rizzolatti, G. and Craighero, L. (2004). The mirror-neuron system. *Annual Review of Neuroscience*, **27**: 169–92.

Rizzolatti, G., Fadiga, L., Matelli, M., *et al.* (1996). Localization of grasp representations in humans by PET: 1. Observation versus execution. *Experimental Brain Research*, **111**: 246–52.

Rizzolatti, G., Fogassi, L., and Gallese, V. (2002). Motor and cognitive functions of the ventral premotor cortex. *Current Opinion in Neurobiology*, **12**: 149–54.

Rizzolatti, G. and Luppino, G. (2001). The cortical motor system. *Neuron*, **31**: 889–901.

Ruby, P. and Decety, J. (2001). Effect of subjective perspective taking during simulation of action: a PET investigation of agency. *Nature Neuroscience*, **4**: 546–50.

Rushworth, M. F., Ellison, A., and Walsh, V. (2001). Complementary localization and lateralization of orienting and motor attention. *Nature Neuroscience*, **4**: 656–61.

Rushworth, M. F., Johansen-Berg, H., Gobel, S. M., and Devlin, J. T. (2003). The left parietal and premotor cortices: motor attention and selection. *Neuroimage*, **20** Suppl 1: S89–100.

Sacchett, C. and Humphreys, G. W. (1992). Calling a squirrel a squirrel but a canoe a wigwam: a categry-specific deficit for artifactual objects and body parts. *Cognitive Neuropsychology*, **5**: 3–25.

Sartori, G., Job, R., and Miozzo, M. (1993). Category-specific naming impairments? Yes. *Quarterly Journal of Experimental Psychology*, **46A**: 489–504.

Senior, C., Barnes, J., Giampietro, V., *et al.* (2000). The functional neuroanatomy of implicit-motion perception or representational momentum. *Current Biology*, **10**: 16–22.

Shallice, T. (1988). *From Neuropsychology to Mental Structure*. Cambridge: Cambridge University Press.

Sirigu, A., Duhamel, J. R., and Poncet, M. (1991). The role of sensorimotor experience in object recognition. A case of multimodal agnosia. *Brain*, **114**: 2555–73.

Tettamanti, M., Buccino, G., Saccuman, M. C., *et al.* (2005). Listening to action-related sentences activates fronto-parietal motor circuits. *Journal of Cognitive Neuroscience*, **17**: 273–81.

Thompson-Schill, S. L., Aguirre, G. K., D'Esposito, M., and Farah, M. J. (1999). A neural basis for category and modality specificity of semantic knowledge. *Neuropsychologia*, **37**: 671–6.

Tyler, L. K. and Moss, H. E. (2001). Towards a distributed account of conceptual knowledge. *Trends Cognitive Science*, **5**: 244–52.

Tyler, L. K., Moss, H. E., Durrant-Peatfield, M. R., and Levy, J. P. (2000). Conceptual structure and the structure of concepts: a distributed account of category-specific deficits. *Brain and Language*, **75**: 195–231.

Umilta, M. A., Kohler, E., Gallese, V., *et al.* (2001). I know what you are doing. a neurophysiological study. *Neuron*, **31**: 155–65.

Wallentin, M., Lund, T. E., Ostergaard, S., Ostergaard, L., and Roepstorff, A. (2005). Motion verb sentences activate left posterior middle temporal cortex despite static context. *Neuroreport*, **16**: 649–52.

Warburton, E., Wise, R. J., Price, C. J., *et al.* (1996). Noun and verb retrieval by normal subjects. Studies with PET. *Brain*, **119**: 159–79.

Warrington, E. K. and McCarthy, R. A. (1987). Categories of knowledge. Further fractionations and an attempted integration. *Brain*, **110**: 1273–96.

Warrington, E. K. and Shallice, T. (1984). Category specific semantic impairments. *Brain*, **107**: 829–54.

The semantic representation of nouns and verbs

Kevin Shapiro[1,2], Argye E. Hillis[3], and Alfonso Caramazza[1]

[1]Harvard University
[2]Harvard Medical School
[3]Johns Hopkins University

That which we call a rose
By any other name would smell as sweet.

William Shakespeare, *Romeo and Juliet*, Act II, Scene 2

8.1 Introduction

What's in a name? For cognitive science, the question is more than rhetorical. Rather, it gets to the heart of what we know — and do not know — about how words are stored and retrieved by the human brain, and there are several competing ideas about how it should be approached. The question becomes even more complex when one considers that not all words are names, or nouns; a complete theory of lexical semantics should also account for the meaning of verbs, adjectives, and other so-called "content" words, associated with what many have argued are fundamentally different types of concepts (O'Grady, 1997). Where can we begin?

8.2 Sensory/functional approaches

One school of thought holds that there are roughly two kinds of semantic knowledge associated with the lexical entry for any given word. On the one hand, there is information that derives directly from the senses, including features representing an object's smell, color, size, and propensity to have sharp thorns. On the other hand, there is everything else — for example, the same item's monetary and sentimental value, where it can typically be found, and whether it is suitable for consumption as jam. The latter sort of information is often (somewhat imprecisely) called "associative" or "functional." Accordingly, this method of partitioning the lexicon has been called the sensory/functional theory (SFT) of semantic knowledge.

The SFT was originally motivated by a series of remarkable observations about the neurobiology of language production (Warrington & McCarthy, 1983, 1987; Warrington & Shallice, 1984). In particular, it was noted that certain patients with acquired brain damage had difficulty naming animals, but less difficulty naming artifacts, while other patients presented with the reverse pattern of impairment. According to the proponents of the SFT, this dissociation can be explained if one posits that names of animals are strongly associated with sensory or perceptual semantic features (shape, size, color, characteristic sound, etc.), while names of artifacts are more associated with functional features. On this hypothesis, a "selective" deficit in naming animals, for example, is attributable to a cortical lesion affecting areas important for the representation of sensory knowledge. Conversely, a lesion affecting the representation of functional or associative knowledge should disproportionately impair the naming of artifacts.

8.2.1   Imageability and concreteness

How well the SFT and related theories can account for all cases of category-specific deficits involving object names remains controversial (Caramazza & Mahon, 2003). Moreover, it is not immediately clear how the SFT can be applied to understand the representation of words that do not refer to concrete objects, including more than 90 percent of the words in this chapter so far. Bird *et al.* (Bird, Howard, & Franklin, 2000) made an attempt to extend the SFT to include the class of verbs, positing that they differ from nouns in two ways. First, verbs have a higher ratio of functional to sensory features than do nouns. Second, verbs have fewer semantic features overall than do nouns − a proposition that Bird *et al.* equate with the notion of lower "imageability." From the two prongs of this hypothesis, which we have called the extended sensory/functional theory or ESFT (Shapiro & Caramazza, 2001), there follow two strong predictions: first, that verb impairments should always pattern with impairments in naming artifacts; and second, that deficits in noun naming should always be accompanied by a proportionately greater deficit in verb naming.

We have argued elsewhere (Shapiro & Caramazza, 2001) that the assumptions on which the ESFT is based are theoretically untenable, and that its predictions are empirically invalid. Indeed, some case series have shown that the manipulation of imageability affects performance on noun and verb production tasks only for a subset of patients (Berndt, Haendiges, & Burton, 2002; Luzzatti *et al.*, 2002) suggesting that the ESFT is not adequate to explain many cases of impairment in noun or verb naming. This argument is illustrated most dramatically by considering the behavior of several patients with deficits in noun or verb production that are confined entirely to one modality of output.

If verb production were impaired in a patient because of damage to areas of the cerebral cortex important for semantic processing, we would expect this problem to manifest in both writing and speech. Caramazza and Hillis (1991), however, reported two patients with ischemic cerebral infarcts who presented with complementary deficits in verb production: SJD, who could not write verbs well but could produce them in speech, and HW, who could produce verbs in written naming but was impaired in oral naming of the same verbs. In both cases, the disparities were not merely relative; production was at ceiling (or nearly so) for verbs in the spared modality, and for nouns in both modalities. A similar pattern has also been documented in patient MML, who suffered from a neurodegenerative disorder known as primary progressive aphasia. Her ability to produce verbs in speech progressively declined over the course of two years, while oral and written production of nouns and written production of verbs remained virtually unaffected (Hillis, Tuffiash, & Caramazza, 2002).

The stark dissociations in these three patients strongly suggest that, in at least some instances, selective verb production difficulties do not arise because of a deficit in the fund of semantic knowledge. A fourth patient, KSR, shows that the same is true for noun production. KSR made more errors with nouns than verbs in oral production, but made more errors with verbs than nouns in written production (Rapp & Caramazza, 2003) — demonstrating not only that selective deficits in noun and verb naming need not arise from damage to the semantic system, but also that they cannot be explained by appealing to the lesser imageability of words in one or the other category, as posited by the ESFT.

Indeed, such patients pose problems not only for the ESFT, but also for other hypotheses about noun and verb representation that hold that these categories can be differentiated along the semantic dimension of concreteness or image-ability. For example, Marshall *et al.* (Marshall, Chiat, & Robson, 1996a; Marshall, Pring, & Chiat, 1996b) proposed that the production of concrete nouns depends on access to visual or perceptual information, while the production of verbs and abstract nouns depends more on access to thematic information. Like the ESFT, this hypothesis distinguishes nouns from verbs primarily in terms of the amount of concrete or sensory semantic knowledge with which words of each category are associated. Unlike the ESFT, however, it allows for the possibility of selective deficits in noun production. The patient studied by Marshall *et al.*, RG, was in fact worse at naming nouns than verbs, and displayed a *reverse* concreteness effect within the category of nouns.

Patients such as HW, SJD, MML, and KSR (all with modality-specific deficits disproportionately affecting verbs or nouns) seem to provide evidence that this kind of hypothesis is not sufficient to explain all cases of category-specific impairments in noun or verb naming. In other words, the semantic distinction between nouns and verbs is not reducible to a difference in abstractness or imageability.

8.2.2   Visual and sensorimotor features

A different variation on the theme of the SFT maintains that nouns and verbs differ primarily not in the proportion of functional or nonperceptual information with which they are associated, but in the kind of sensory information by which they are prototypically defined. Nouns are characteristically names of concrete objects, with semantic representations that include primarily visual sensory information; verbs, on the other hand, typically denote actions, with semantic representations more heavily invested in motor schemata.

In the literature on this subject, this line of reasoning has been closely linked to specific claims about the organization of cortical systems for processing motor and visual–perceptual information. Indeed, the originators of the SFT argued that putative verb deficits in aphasic patients are more accurately described as reflecting problems in retrieving action words, while noun deficits are equivalent to problems with object naming (McCarthy & Warrington, 1985). Damasio and Tranel (1993), replicating an observation made earlier by Miceli *et al.* (1984) (and concurrently by Daniele *et al.*, 1994), reported that patients with verb production deficits tend to have lesions in the left prefrontal cortex, while noun production deficits tend to co-occur with damage to the left middle temporal cortex. They proposed that these areas represent "convergence zones" – in other words, the termini of cortical processing streams for spatial–motor (dorsal) and visual–sensory (ventral) information.

Likewise, Pulvermüller and colleagues (Pulvermüller, 1999; Pulvermüller, Lutzenberger, & Preissl, 1999) have argued that the semantic representations of nouns and verbs are distributed over the cerebral cortex in a pattern closely related to the processing of visual and sensorimotor information. This association is supposed to hold true at even the finest grain of cortical function; for example, they have shown that the recognition of verbs denoting actions of the mouth, hand, and leg produces evoked potentials in the corresponding regions of motor cortex. Interestingly, Neininger and Pulvermüller (2003) have also reported that patients with damage in the *right* premotor and temporal–occipital cortices can also be shown to have subtle deficits in the recognition of verbs and nouns, respectively. They interpret these findings as evidence that semantic representations include even visual and sensorimotor areas outside the language system as it has traditionally been conceived.[1]

Either the model of Damasio and Tranel (1993) or that of Pulvermüller and colleagues (Pulvermüller, 1999; Pulvermüller, Lutzenberger, & Preissl, 1999) — we will call them collectively the "visual/sensorimotor theory" (VST) — would account for some cases of deficits in naming and comprehension of nouns in patients with fluent primary progressive aphasia or semantic dementia (Hillis, Oh, & Ken, 2004), who have disproportionate atrophy in anterior and inferior/middle temporal cortex (Gorno-Tempini *et al.*, 2004). The VST would also neatly account for the disproportionate impairment of verb naming and comprehension in patients with motor neuron disease—dementia—aphasia syndrome, whose prominent pathology is in the posterior frontal cortex (Bak *et al.*, 2001). Indeed, as we shall see, it is difficult to find cases for which the VST is an explicitly deficient explanation.

At first glance, the VST, like the ESFT and related hypotheses, seems vulnerable to counter-evidence from patients with modality-specific deficits. It is improbable that damage to parts of the brain housing stores of visual information, for example, should affect production of nouns in only one modality of output. The hypothesis can be "rescued," however, by assuming that the lesions in these cases affect not areas of the brain important for storing semantic information, but connections between those areas and areas that store written and oral word forms.

A particular strength of the visual/sensorimotor approaches is that they make specific anatomic predictions about the disposition of the areas that would have to be disconnected. In the version proposed by Pulvermüller and colleagues (Pulvermüller, 1999; Pulvermüller, Lutzenberger, & Preissl, 1999), for example, a putative deficit in written verb production could be explained by postulating a disruption in the relay of information from motor and premotor areas bilaterally to parts of the perisylvian language network important for written output.[2]

---

[1] We should note that in the study by Neininger and Pulvermüller (2003), the patients with right temporo-occipital lesions, who were impaired in the rapid recognition of highly visual nouns, did not have comparable difficulty with nouns that had both visual and motor associations. Nor were the patients with right frontal lesions impaired with bimodal nouns. These findings already suggest that right-hemisphere "semantic" regions might not be crucial for lexical retrieval.

[2] The same argument can be advanced for concreteness-based variants of the SFT (Rapp & Caramazza, 1998), provided that there are differences in the anatomical distribution of cortical areas that represent concrete and abstract (or thematic) semantic knowledge. Unfortunately, it is not readily apparent where in the brain such areas might be found, notwithstanding several attempts to localize them (Perani *et al.*, 1999). In the case of the ESFT, based as it is on a protean notion of "imageability," it is not clear *what* could be disconnected to produce the specific deficits that have been observed in patients (Shapiro & Caramazza, 2001).

In a similar vein, Tranel *et al.* (2001) showed that action naming deficits most commonly result from lesions in the left frontal operculum, including the underlying white matter and insula; especially severe deficits in action naming additionally involved lesions in prefrontal and premotor regions, along with the left mesial occipital cortex and the paraventricular white matter underlying posterior perisylvian gyri. The authors proposed that the frontal opercular areas are involved in implementing action word production, while the latter areas are involved in mediating retrieval, a function that includes access to conceptual semantic information.

This kind of model supplies a plausible interpretation not only for stable modality specific deficits (which, in the cases described thus far, have tended to occur in the setting of large perisylvian infarctions) and worsening modality-specific verb deficits observed in some cases of nonfluent primary progressive aphasia, but also for observations of transient deficits in the setting of acute stroke. Hillis *et al.* (2003) showed that, in two patients, hypoperfusion of the left posterior inferior frontal and precentral gyri was associated with a selective impairment in writing verbs. When blood flow was restored to these areas, written verb naming recovered completely.

What about cases in which the noun–verb dissociation is sensitive not to the modality of production, but to the difference between production and comprehension? It turns out that some patients with primary progressive aphasia are selectively impaired at naming verbs (compared to nouns), but have spared comprehension of verbs (Hillis *et al.*, 2004). One could apply the logic of disconnection here as well, on the assumption that, again, different brain areas are assigned to the processing of input and output word forms.

Here, too, the VST and similar hypotheses coincide agreeably with widely accepted axioms about the anatomy of the brain. In a recent study of 56 patients with primary progressive aphasia, the pattern of impaired verb naming with intact verb comprehension was strongly associated with motor speech deficits (dysarthria or apraxia; Hillis, Heidler, Ken, & Newhart, 2006). Perhaps this association reflects a close spatial relationship between neural systems important for speech production and those important for representing the semantics (or phonological representations) of verbs, such that damage to the former frequently impinges on afferent connections from the latter. This could certainly be true if, for instance, the representation of verb semantics or verb phonological representations and the motor control of speech both relied on networks within the left posterior frontal cortex. Conversely, in the same study, impaired naming and comprehension of nouns relative to verbs was observed only in patients without motor speech deficits. This observation is consistent with the hypothesis that the representation of noun meaning depends on brain areas distant (and cleanly separable) from motor speech centers, like the left medial and ventral temporal lobe.

There are some cases of selective deficits in noun and verb naming, however, for which even a disconnection account based on the SFT fails to provide an adequate explanation. In these cases, the impairment in producing nouns or verbs is demonstrably unrelated to the specific semantic representations of these words. Instead, these patients seem to have difficulty accessing and utilizing the grammatical properties of nouns or verbs, which govern the use of words in the context of phrases and sentences.

The first case so described was that of patient JR, an English-speaking patient with an extensive left-hemisphere lesion affecting the inferior frontal and parietal lobes, who was able to produce verbs with at a high rate of accuracy in picture naming, repetition, and sentence completion tasks, but was impaired in producing nouns in the same contexts (Shapiro, Shelton, & Caramazza, 2000). JR's difficulty with nouns was not correlated with imageability or concreteness in the way predicted by the ESFT. Moreover, JR was able to use meaningless pseudo-words, such as *wug*, as verbs (*he wugs*) but not as nouns (*these are wugs*).

The mirror deficit — difficulty with verbs and pseudo-verbs, but not nouns or pseudo-nouns, independent of concreteness — has been observed in an English-speaking patient RC (Shapiro & Caramazza, 2003a) and in an Italian-speaking patient MR (Laiacona & Caramazza, 2004), both with lesions extending superiorly along the convexity of the frontal lobe. For all of these three patients, impairments in producing words of one category seem to be delimited not by those words' semantic content, but by their grammatical context. The fact that these patients' difficulties extend to confrontation naming implies that every instance of lexical production involves access to grammatical features, and possibly even the construction of a minimal syntactic frame for a noun or verb phrase.

What is more, there is evidence to suggest that grammatical knowledge can be distinguished from conceptual knowledge in comprehension as well as in production. Kemmerer (2000) has reported a double dissociation between perceptual knowledge about verbs, on the one hand, and knowledge about their grammatical properties on the other. In a test that required access to fairly subtle features of verb meaning that were grammatically irrelevant (for example, the distinction between *pour* and *sprinkle*), two patients performed well, but a third (2011SS) performed poorly. In contrast, patient 2011SS performed well, but the other two performed poorly, on judging the grammaticality of sentences incorporating the same verbs.

8.3   Nouns, verbs, objects, and actions

At this point it is reasonable to object that our argument against the SFT and similar proposals merely kicks the can down the road, since it leaves a number of important observations unaccounted for. In contrast to patients such as JR, MR, and RC, there are also several patients who present with relatively selective deficits in noun or verb naming, but entirely spared grammatical processing for words of both categories. For example, an English-speaking patient HG was worse at naming verbs than naming nouns, but showed no impairment in producing morphologically inflected forms of either nouns or verbs (Shapiro & Caramazza, 2003a); Italian-speaking patient EA showed the reverse pattern of impairment (Laiacona & Caramazza, 2004).

We should note that the ESFT is also inadequate to account for the deficits in these patients, since their deficits in noun and verb naming do not appear to be sensitive to dimensions such as imageability or concreteness. Whether the VST fares better is at present somewhat ambiguous; generally speaking, these patients' access to visual and sensorimotor semantic knowledge has not rigorously been tested.

One pretheoretical problem with this class of hypotheses is that while they do offer some interesting insights into the way in which knowledge about objects and actions is accessed in the brain, they speak less to the distinction between nouns and verbs as such. On the one hand, it is uncontroversial that prototypical nouns refer to concrete objects, while prototypical verbs refer to actions. On the other hand, this correlation is by no means exclusive; some nouns refer to actions or abstractions, while verbs can refer to states, processes, or relations. Patients such as JR, MR, and RC demonstrate that true grammatical category-specific impairments extend to nonprototypical category members, including even pseudo-words with no stored semantic representation.

To date, most studies of cortical distribution of word naming have focused explicitly on the action–object distinction, rather than on the noun–verb distinction. In the paper by Tranel et al. (2001), which mapped regions of lesion overlap between patients with action naming impairments, the authors proposed that the areas they identified as "mediational" structures − including the prefrontal/premotor region and left mesial occipital cortex − are related to processing conceptual properties of actions. A later study by the same group specifically assessed nonverbal retrieval of knowledge about actions, and found that lesions in patients with deficits in these tasks overlapped most consistently in the left premotor and prefrontal cortex, the left parietal region, and white matter tracts underlying the left posterior middle temporal lobe (Tranel et al., 2004). The authors point out that these regions are thought to be linked to systems for processing movements of the body, motions of objects, spatial relationships, and so forth.[3]

If this is true, however, it is reasonable to assume that they are important for the semantic representation of *all* action words, including nouns that refer to actions, and therefore that they play no role in the neuroanatomical distinction between nouns and verbs. At any rate, this seems to be true for primary sensorimotor areas, which are thought by some to form part of the conceptual network underlying the representation of actions and objects (Pulvermüller, 1999). In a study using paired-pulse transcranial magnetic stimulation, Oliveri *et al.* (2004) showed that activation in the hand region of left motor cortex increases more when subjects produce both nouns and verbs related to actions (i.e. verbs referring to hand movements and nouns that name manipulable objects) than when they produce words of either category that are not related to actions.

8.3.1 A "semantic core" approach

So far, then, we have argued that not all impairments in naming nouns or verbs are explicable in terms of imageability or concreteness, and probably not all can be explained by appeal to distinctions between the semantic properties of actions and objects. Some of these "true" grammatical category impairments seem to result from problems in deploying syntactic features such as morphological inflection, but others do not. The question, then, remains: how does the brain identify individual words as nouns or verbs?

One possibility is that the categories "noun" and "verb" are anchored by semantic properties that are not directly related to perceptual information, and are sufficiently broadly defined to admit exemplars of varying degrees of abstractness, imageability, specificity, and so on. O'Grady (1997) has proposed that these kinds of properties, or semantic "cores," are critical for the acquisition and organization of the category-based grammar of human language. The criterial feature for nouns, on this view, is reference to an entity that can be individuated (or atomized, as it were). For verbs, the crucial property is reference to an event.

Some evidence consistent with the idea that the categorization of words as nouns or verbs depends on a "core" semantic structure comes from a recent study

---

[3] Interestingly, a functional magnetic resonance imaging (fMRI) study by Kable *et al.* (2002) showed that a conceptual matching task with action words and pictures activated part of the lateral occipitotemporal cortex thought to be important for motion processing, but not the prefrontal, occipital, or parietal regions identified by Tranel *et al.* (2001) or (2004). However, this may be attributable in large part to the specific materials included in this study. For example, the "action" picture matching task relied heavily on perceived trajectories of motion (e.g. judging that a line of waddling geese is more similar to a moving locomotive than to a loaf of bread being sliced by a knife). By contrast, Tranel *et al.* (2004) measured conceptual knowledge about actions using tests that probed more than one kind of attribute (e.g. which action makes the loudest sound?).

using event-related functional magnetic resonance imaging (fMRI) with English-speaking subjects. Subjects in this study produced real words and pseudo-words in the context of short phrases, a paradigm much like that used with patients JR and RC. The analysis identified regions that were commonly activated by the production of real words of different semantic types (abstract or concrete), morphological types (regular or irregular inflection), and pseudo-words used in a noun or verb context. It was found that verbs — including pseudo-verbs — produced activation in parts of the left prefrontal cortex and left posterior parietal cortex; by contrast, nouns produced activation in the left fusiform gyrus (Shapiro, Moo, & Caramazza, 2006).

Although this study was designed to identify brain regions responsible for the grammatical processing of nouns and verbs, it seems unlikely, a priori, that the observed areas of activation are in fact crucial for inflectional morphology. A more plausible hypothesis is that they represent core semantic properties of nouns and verbs, and are engaged whenever the language production system is called upon to classify a word as a member of one category or the other. A positron emission tomography (PET) study with a similar design, conducted in German, also found that the production of real verbs and pseudo-verbs commonly activated the left prefrontal cortex; production of nouns and pseudo-nouns activated the left fusiform gyrus, along with the right superior temporal cortex (Shapiro *et al.*, 2005).

The situation of these putative core areas near other areas thought to be important for conceptual knowledge about objects (ventrolateral occipitotemporal cortex) and actions (prefrontal and parietal cortex) may reflect the close ontogenetic relationship between nouns and verbs, on the one hand, and objects and actions on the other (Caramazza, 1994).

REFERENCES

Bak, T. H., *et al.* (2001). Selective impairment of verb processing associated with pathological changes in Brodmann areas 44 and 45 in the motor neurone disease—dementia—aphasia syndrome. *Brain*, **124**(Pt. 1): 103—20.

Berndt, R. S., Haendiges, A. N., and Burton, M. W. (2002). Grammatical class and imageability in aphasic word production: their effects are independent. *Journal of Neurolinguistics*, **15**(3—5): 353—71.

Bird, H., Howard, D., and Franklin, S. (2000). Why is a verb like an inanimate object? Grammatical category and semantic category deficits. *Brain & Language*, **72**(3): 246—309.

Caramazza, A. (1994). Parallels and divergences in the acquisition and dissolution of language. *Philosophical Transactions of the Royal Society of London, Series B*, **346**(1315): 121—7.

Caramazza, A. and Hillis, A. E. (1991). Lexical organization of nouns and verbs in the brain. *Nature*, **349**: 788−90.

Caramazza, A. and Mahon, B. Z. (2003). The organization of conceptual knowledge: the evidence from category-specific semantic deficits. *Trends in Cognitive Science*, **7**(8): 354−61.

Damasio, A. R. and Tranel, D. (1993). Nouns and verbs are retrieved with differently distributed neural systems. *Proceedings of the National Academy of Sciences*, USA, **90**(11): 4957−60.

Daniele, A., *et al.* (1994). Evidence for a possible neuroanatomical basis for lexical processing of nouns and verbs. *Neuropsychologia*, **32**(11): 1325−41.

Gorno-Tempini, M. L., *et al.* (2004). Cognition and anatomy in three variants of primary progressive aphasia. *Annals of Neurology*, **55**(3): 335−46.

Hillis, A. E., *et al.* (2003). Neural regions essential for writing verbs. *Nature Neuroscience*, **6**(1): 19−20.

Hillis, A. E., Oh, S., and Ken, L. (2004). Deterioration of naming nouns versus verbs in primary progressive aphasia. *Annals of Neurology*, **55**: 268−75.

Hillis, A. E., Tuffiash, E., and Caramazza, A. (2002). Modality-specific deterioration in naming verbs in nonfluent primary progressive aphasia. *Journal of Cognitive Neuroscience*, **14**(7): 1099−108.

Hillis, A. E., Heidler-Gary, J., Newhart, M., Chang, S., Ken, L., Bak, T. (2006). Naming and comprehension in primary progressive aphasia: the influence of grammatical word class. *Aphasiology*, **20**, 246−56.

Kable, J. W., Lease-Spellmeyer, J., and Chatterjee, A. (2002). Neural substrates of action event knowledge. *Journal of Cognitive Neuroscience*, **14**(5): 795−805.

Kemmerer, D. (2000). Grammatically relevant and grammatically irrelevant features of verb meaning can be independently impaired. *Aphasiology*, **14**: 997−1020.

Laiacona, M. and Caramazza, A. (2004). The noun/verb dissociation in language production: Varieties of causes. *Cognitive Neuropsychology*, **21**: 103−24.

Luzzatti, C., *et al.* (2002). Verb−noun double dissociation in aphasic lexical impairments: the role of word frequency and imageability. *Brain & Language*, **81**(1−3): 432−44.

Marshall, J., Chiat, S., and Robson, J. (1996). Calling a salad a federation: an investigation of semantic jargon. Part 2: Verbs. *Journal of Neurolinguistics*, **9**(4): 251−60.

Marshall, J., Pring, T., and Chiat, S. (1996). Calling a salad a federation: an investigation of semantic jargon. Part 1: Nouns. *Journal of Neurolinguistics*, **9**(4): 237−50.

McCarthy, R. A. and Warrington, E. K. (1985). Category specificity in an agrammatic patient: the relative impairment of verb retrieval and comprehension. *Neuropsychologia*, **23**(6): 709−27.

Miceli, G., *et al.* (1984). On the basis for the agrammatic's difficulty in producing main verbs. *Cortex*, **20**(2): 207−20.

Neininger, B. and Pulvermüller, F. (2003). Word-category specific deficits after lesions in the right hemisphere. *Neuropsychologia*, **41**(1): 53−70.

O'Grady, W. (1997). *Syntactic Development*. Chicago: University of Chicago Press.

Oliveri, M., Finocchiaro, C., Shapiro, K., Gangitano, M., Caramazza, A., and Pascual-Leone, A. (2004). All talk and no action: a transcranial magnetic stimulation study of motor cortex activation during speech production. *Journal of Cognitive Neuroscience*, **16**(3): 374−81.

Perani, D., Cappa, S. F., Schnur, T., Tettamanti, M., Collina, S., Rosa, M. M., and Fazio, F. (1999). The neural correlates of verb and noun processing. A PET study. *Brain,* **122**(Pt. 12): 2337–44.

Pulvermüller, F. (1999). Words in the brain's language. *Behavioral and Brain Sciences,* **22**(2): 253–79.

Pulvermüller, F., Lutzenberger, W., and Preissl, H. (1999). Nouns and verbs in the intact brain: evidence from event-related potentials and high-frequency cortical responses. *Cerebral Cortex,* **9**(5): 497–506.

Rapp, B. and Caramazza, A. (1998). A case of selective difficulty in writing verbs. *Neurocase,* **4**: 127–39.

Rapp, B. and Caramazza, A. (2003). Selective difficulties with spoken nouns and written verbs: a single case study. *Journal of Neurolinguistics,* **15**(3–5): 373–402.

Shapiro, K. and Caramazza, A. (2001). Sometimes a noun is just a noun: comments on Bird, Howard, and Franklin (2000). *Brain & Language,* **76**(2): 202–12.

Shapiro, K. and Caramazza, A. (2003a). Grammatical processing of nouns and verbs in left frontal cortex? *Neuropsychologia,* **41**(9): 1189–98.

Shapiro, K. and Caramazza, A. (2003b). Looming a loom: evidence for independent access to grammatical and phonological properties in verb retrieval. *Journal of Neurolinguistics,* **16**(2–3): 85–111.

Shapiro, K., Shelton, J., and Caramazza, A. (2000). Grammatical class in lexical production and morphological processing: evidence from a case of fluent aphasia. *Cognitive Neuropsychology,* **17**: 665–82.

Shapiro, K. A., Moo, L. R., and Caramazza, A. (2006). Cortical signatures of noun and verb production. *Proceedings of the National Academy of Sciences USA,* **103**(5): 1644–9.

Shapiro, K. A., *et al.* (2005). Dissociating neural correlates for nouns and verbs. *NeuroImage,* **24**: 1058–67.

Tranel, D., *et al.* (2001). A neural basis for the retrieval of words for actions. *Cognitive Neuropsychology,* **18**(7): 655–74.

Tranel, D., *et al.* (2004). Neural correlates of conceptual knowledge for actions. *Cognitive Neuropsychology,* **20**(3–6): 409–32.

Warrington, E. K. and Shallice, T. (1984). Category specific semantic impairments. *Brain,* **107**(3): 829–54.

Warrington, E. K. and McCarthy, R. A. (1983). Category specific access dysphasia. *Brain,* **106**(4): 859–78.

Warrington, E. K. and McCarthy, R. A. (1987). Categories of knowledge. Further fractionations and an attempted integration. *Brain,* **110**(5): 1273–96.

Part V

Critical Role of Subcortical Nuclei in Semantic Functions

9

Role of the basal ganglia in language and semantics: supporting cast

Bruce Crosson[1,2], Michelle Benjamin[1,2] and Ilana Levy[2]

[1]Malcolm Randall VA Medical Center
[2]University of Florida

The role of the basal ganglia in language and semantics has been debated since Broadbent (1872), Wernicke (1874), Kussmaul (1877) and Marie (1906) first addressed the topic. Interest was resurrected in the late 1950s and 1960s when the pallidotomies were conducted for relief of Parkinson's disease. After dominant pallidotomy, some patients demonstrated aphasia (Svennilson *et al.*, 1960). Further, stimulation of the dominant globus pallidus during operative procedures interrupted ongoing language (Hermann *et al.*, 1966), and stimulation of the dominant caudate head produced phrases and short sentences not relevant to the ongoing situation (Van Buren, 1963, 1966; Van Buren *et al.*, 1966). Interest peaked in the late 1970s and 1980s, as use of computerized tomography (CT) scans demonstrated basal ganglia infarcts and hemorrhages in the dominant hemisphere that were accompanied by aphasia (Brunner *et al.*, 1982; Cappa *et al.*, 1983; Damasio *et al.*, 1982; Fisher, 1979; Hier *et al.*, 1977; Knopman *et al.*, 1984; Murdoch *et al.*, 1989; Wallesch, 1985, to mention a few).

Much has happened since the latter studies to clarify the role of the basal ganglia in language and semantics. Now, it can be definitively stated that the basal ganglia are not directly involved in primary language or semantic functions. Yet it is becoming equally clear that the basal ganglia play a pervasive, but subtle role in cognitive processing that cuts across a number of functions. Most probably, this role lies within the realm of intention and attention, involving the enhancement of selected actions and cognitions and the suppression of competing action programs and cognitions. The impact on cognition is to sharpen the focus of cognitive activity by enhancing the signal-to-noise ratio in cognitive processing, thereby increasing speed, efficiency, and accuracy of processing. Thus the impact of basal ganglia injury and disease on linguistic and semantic processes is more subtle than the symptoms of aphasia or agnosia. Nonetheless, patients with

This work was supported by Department of Veterans Affairs Rehabilitation Research and Development Service grant # B3470S Research Career Scientist Award to Bruce Crosson.

basal ganglia damage or disease have consistently demonstrated impairment on tests of executive language functions and in semantic priming paradigms. After describing basal ganglia organization and addressing the evidence that the basal ganglia are not involved in basic linguistic and semantic functions, the bulk of this chapter endeavors to develop a conceptual framework for understanding how the basal ganglia impact semantic and related language functions. The goal is to establish a framework from which hypotheses can be developed and tested.

9.1   The basal ganglia impact cortical activity through closed circuits

The basal ganglia are a series of nuclei lying deep within the cerebral hemispheres. They consist of the striatum, the globus pallidus, and the subthalamic nucleus. The striatum can be subdivided into the neostriatum, which consists of the caudate nucleus and putamen, and the archistriatum, which consists of the nucleus accumbens and olfactory tubercle. The globus pallidus can be subdivided into its medial and lateral segments. A ventral pallidum also is connected to the archistriatum. Basic description and illustration of the structure and location of the basal ganglia is not within the scope of this chapter; the reader can consult any good neuroanatomy text for these details.

However, the material in this chapter will rely upon an understanding of how the basal ganglia are organized into circuits that influence cortical functioning (Alexander *et al.*, 1986; Middleton & Strick, 2000). Any basal ganglia circuit begins in a specific cortical region that ultimately is also the target of the closed loops that comprise the circuit. Mostly, these circuits originate in frontal cortical regions, including: primary motor cortex, ventral premotor cortex, dorsal premotor cortex, supplementary motor area (SMA), pre-supplementary motor area (pre-SMA), anterior cingulate cortex, dorsal lateral prefrontal cortex, and orbital frontal cortex (Akkal *et al.*, 2002; Alexander *et al.*, 1986; Inase *et al.*, 1999; Strick *et al.*, 1995). It has been suggested that Broca's area also has a unique loop (Ullman, 2004). Recent evidence further indicates that temporal and parietal loops may exist (Middleton & Strick, 2000).

Furthermore, each basal ganglia circuit can be decomposed into three separate loops. Figure 9.1 illustrates the three loops within pre-SMA circuit; similar loops exist for other basal ganglia circuits. The three loops are as follows: (1) In the "direct" loop, the cortical focus of the circuit projects to its striatal component using glutamate, an excitatory neurotransmitter. The striatal component then projects to the medial pallidal component of the circuit using gamma amino butyric acid (GABA), an inhibitory neurotransmitter. The medial pallidal

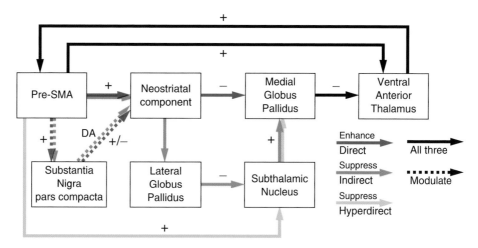

Figure 9.1.   Pre-SMA–basal ganglia circuit. The three loops within the pre-SMA–basal ganglia circuit and their connections are represented in this diagram. The direct loop is involved in enhancing behavior, and its connections are indicated by red arrows. The indirect loop is involved in suppressing behavior, and its connections are indicated by blue arrows. The hyperdirect loop is also involved in suppression, and its connections are indicated in green. Black arrows indicate connections involved in all three loops. Broken arrows indicate modulatory pathways.

component projects to a specific thalamic nuclear target using GABA, and the thalamic component of the loop projects back to the cortex using glutamate as a neurotransmitter (Alexander *et al.*, 1986). Activity in the direct loop is thought to enhance selected actions and cognitions (Gerfen, 1992; Mink, 1996; Penney & Young, 1986). (2) In the "indirect" loop, again, the cortical focus projects to the striatal component of the loop using glutamate. However, in this loop, the striatal component projects to a lateral pallidal component using its GABAergic projections. The lateral pallidal component in turn projects to the segment of the subthalamic nucleus subserving its circuit using GABA as a neurotransmitter. The subthalamic nucleus component projects to the circuit's medial pallidal component using glutamate as its neurotransmitter. Subsequently, the medial pallidal component uses GABAergic projects to influence the thalamic component of the loop, which in turn projects back to the cortical target from which the loop originated using glutamate as a neurotransmitter (Gerfen, 1992; Nambu *et al.*, 2002; Penney & Young, 1986). Activity in the indirect loop is thought to suppress actions or cognitions that compete with selected actions and cognitions. (3) More recently, a "hyperdirect" loop has been described (e.g. Nambu *et al.*, 2000, 2002). In this loop, the cortical component projects directly to its subthalamic nucleus component using glutamatergic projections. The subthalamic nucleus component, in turn, projects to its medial pallidal component also using glutamate as a neurotransmitter. The medial pallidal component projects to the thalamic component of the circuit using GABA, and the thalamic component projects to the cortex using glutamate as a neurotransmitter. Action in the hyperdirect loop is thought to have a suppressing effect on actions and cognitions.

There is good evidence that the impact of the glutamate and GABA in these three loops can be interpreted in a straightforward manner. Specifically, if the neurotransmitter is excitatory its action will increase the output of the target structure, and if it is inhibitory it will suppress output of the target structure. Further, enhancement of corticothalamic activity will tend to trigger actions which the loop influences, while decreased corticothalamic activity will result in suppression of the actions which the loop impacts (Gerfen, 1992; Mink, 1996; Mitchell et al., 1989; Penney & Young, 1986). In contrast, the actions of dopamine within basal ganglia circuitry are less straightforward than the actions of glutamate and GABA. The substantia nigra pars compacta sends dopaminergic projections to the striatal component of the circuitry. Dopamine appears to have both tonic and phasic influences on striatal neurons. The direct loop is modulated primarily by D1 receptors. Stimulation of these receptors seems to have an excitatory influence on the output of the striatal projection neurons in the direct loop (Gerfen, 1992). The indirect loop is modulated primarily by D2 receptors (ibid.). Although D2 receptor activity seems to have an inhibitory influence on striatal output neurons, it also decreases basal activity in cholinergic interneurons. The influence of cholinergic activity on striatal output is still poorly understood (Maurice et al., 2004; O'Donnell, 2003). We shall return to the topic of dopaminergic modulation of basal ganglia circuitry later, as the model of basal ganglia functions is developed.

9.2 The basal ganglia are not directly involved in core language and semantic functions

First, however, we should briefly discuss the evidence that the basal ganglia are not directly involved in language and semantic processing. Nadeau and Crosson (1997) examined cases of left striatocapsular infarction in the literature at the time. Striatocapsular infarcts have a very characteristic distribution affecting the head of the caudate nucleus, the anterior limb of the internal capsule, the putamen, and sometimes the globus pallidus. With such a characteristic lesion distribution, it should be relatively easy to describe an aphasia syndrome if the basal ganglia are involved in language. However, no such syndrome emerged. Patients sometimes had fluent output, and sometimes had nonfluent output. Sometimes, they had impairment of comprehension, and sometimes not. Repetition of words and phrases also showed variable impairment, and so on. An examination of acute cerebral blood flow studies of such cases indicated that when language symptoms occurred, cortical hypoperfusion was present and that the location of such hypoperfusion was consistent with language symptoms.

Indeed, the work of Weiller *et al.* (1993) gave much insight into the nature of these infarcts. Striatocapsular infarcts are most commonly caused by blockage of the initial segment of the middle cerebral artery, before the lenticulostriate arteries emerge to irrigate the caudate head, putamen, and anterior limb of the internal capsule, but they also can be caused by blockage of the internal carotid artery. In these cases, end-to-end anastomosies connecting major arterial territories keep the cortex from infarcting. Yet these anastomosies vary in their patency, and cortical areas that do not show cystic infarction may be hypoperfused or even have ischemic neuronal dropout. Patients with early recanalization of the blocked artery and good anastomotic circulation tend not to demonstrate aphasia with dominant basal ganglia lesions. However, when anastomotic circulation is not adequate to provide for normal cortical perfusion and recanalization does not occur until relatively late in recovery, aphasia is seen in dominant striatocapsular infarction.

Recently, Hillis *et al.* (2002) performed the definitive study on this phenomenon. Using perfusion and diffusion weighted magnetic resonance imaging (MRI), they demonstrated that aphasia occurs acutely in dominant basal ganglia infarction only when the cortex is inadequately perfused. Thus the evidence leaves little room for argument. The basal ganglia do not appear to participate in core language or semantic functions. Otherwise, basal ganglia lesion alone would be sufficient to cause aphasia. Nonetheless, it has become equally clear that the basal ganglia do provide an intention and attention infrastructure for language and other cognitive functions. To better understand how the basal ganglia support language and semantics, we must discuss recent concepts of basal ganglia function.

9.3   The basal ganglia participate in intention

At the most general level of discussion, the basal ganglia can be best understood through their role in intention and attention. Heilman *et al.* (2003) have divided attention into two basic systems: attention proper and intention. Attention is the readiness to process incoming information and the ability to select for further processing one source of information from among several competing sources. The inferior parietal lobe, posterior cingulate gyrus, and thalamus all play roles in the regulation of information processing. Intention is the ability to select for execution one action among multiple, competing actions, and to initiate the selected action. Intention systems involve medial frontal cortex (SMA, pre-SMA, rostral cingulate zone), lateral frontal structures, and basal ganglia loops. Because intention is related to action, it is intimately associated with the frontal lobes, the part of the brain dealing with the planning and execution of actions. Fuster (2003) refers to intention as "executive attention," but it is basically the same concept. He further noted that the investigation of intention in the available literature has been sparse and inadequate.

Thus the basal ganglia can be seen as involved in intention. This conceptualization is consistent with their predominant relationship with the frontal lobes. Although intention and attention have been discussed separately, they are intimately associated. Because the actions we choose to perform affect the items to which we attend, intention guides attention as we execute actions. For example, when we intend to pour a cup of coffee, we must attend to the location of the cup. Otherwise the desired results are not achieved and a mess is created.

9.4   The basal ganglia enhance selected actions and suppress competing action programs

Since the 1980s there has been some agreement that the impact of the basal ganglia on movement can best be understood not as initiating movement per se, but as influencing movement in a more subtle fashion. The basal ganglia are thought to facilitate movement by enhancing selected movements and suppressing competing movements (Mink, 1996; Penney & Young, 1986). This concept can be applied both to action in general, and more specifically to cognitive activities. In other words, the basal ganglia are thought to facilitate cognitive activities through facilitating selected cognitive activities while at the same time suppressing competing ones.

This concept can be best understood through example. Suppose that a subject is asked to generate the name of a single bird. From among the vast number of birds one could name, the name of a single bird must be selected for production. Many factors may influence what bird is selected. Perhaps the bird that one most commonly sees will have the highest level of activation in the semantic system, making it the most likely to be selected. Or perhaps some recent experience has left a more rarely encountered bird at a higher level of activation than other members of the category. According to current concepts, the basal ganglia will enhance the tendency to say the name of the selected bird, while the tendency to say the name of other birds will be suppressed. This mechanism reduces the possibility of confusion as the selected action, saying "eagle," is performed. Figure 9.2 represents this example. The selected item "eagle" in the center white circle is

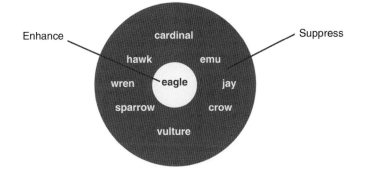

Figure 9.2.   Category member generation. When a subject is asked to generate a member of the category "birds", the selected word (inner white circle) will be enhanced while words representing other birds will be suppressed (outer dark gray circle). This process results in an enhanced signal-to-noise ratio, which will increase the accuracy and efficiency of the system.

enhanced, while at the same time other competing items such as "crow," "cardinal," "hawk," "emu," "jay," "wren," "sparrow," and "vulture" in the outer gray circle are suppressed. The result is an increased signal-to-noise ratio in favor of the selected item, increasing the speed and accuracy of response.

9.5   The basal ganglia are involved in retrieval of lexical items during word generation

This model can be used to understand how the basal ganglia participate in word generation. Crosson *et al.* (2003) recently used fMRI to determine how frontal, basal ganglia, and thalamic structures were engaged by three facets of language generation: the lexical vs. nonlexical status of the items generated, the semantic vs. phonological information used in language generation, and the fast vs. slow rate of generation. During fMRI, 21 neurologically normal subjects performed four tasks: generation of nonsense syllables given beginning and ending consonant blends, generation of words given a rhyming word, generation of words given a semantic category at a fast rate (matched to the rate of nonsense syllable generation), and generation of words given a semantic category at a slow rate (matched to the rate of generating of rhyming words). Tasks were presented in a block format; i.e. the initial stimulus was given and subjects generated as many words or syllables as they could during the remainder of the 17.4 s blocks. Word or syllable generation was alternated with 17.4 s periods of rest during which subjects focused on a fixation cross. Activity of the basal ganglia in both hemispheres was associated with the generation of words without respect to whether a semantic cue (category) or a phonological cue (rhyming word) was used to generate words. No basal ganglia activity in either hemisphere was found during nonsense syllable generation. Thus, because the focus of this chapter is basal ganglia functions, we will concentrate our discussion on the lexical vs. non-lexical component of this experiment.

Components of a left pre-SMA—dorsal caudate nucleus—ventral anterior thalamic loop were active during word generation from rhyming or category cues but not during nonsense syllable generation. Figure 9.3 shows activity in this loop during slow category member generation; activity was similar during fast category member generation and during generation of words from rhyming cues. Thus this basal ganglia loop supports both the semantic and phonological generation tasks. Because structures of this loop are not active during nonsense syllable generation, we conclude that this loop is involved in retrieving words from pre-existing lexical stores. The discussion above suggests that the role of the basal ganglia in lexical retrieval most likely was to enhance words selected for generation and to suppress those not selected for generation.

While this left-hemisphere loop was active only in lexical generation tasks, frontal activity was evident in all tasks, depending upon the nature of the cue used for generation. For semantically based generation tasks (fast and slow category member generation) activity was most robust along the left inferior frontal sulcus

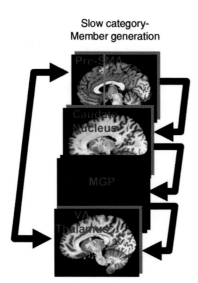

Figure 9.3.   Activation in the pre-SMA—basal ganglia loop during word generation. Whether generating category members or words to a rhyming cue, the pre-SMA loop becomes active. Activity (red and yellow) was elicited in pre-SMA, the dorsal caudate nucleus, and the ventral anterior thalamus. These panels show activity during slow category-member generation.

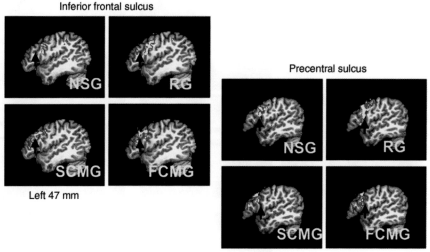

Figure 9.4.   Left lateral frontal activity during word generation. Activity along the inferior frontal sulcus (arrows in left panels) is most robust during semantic tasks. Activity in the precentral sulcus (arrows in right panels) is most robust during phonological tasks NSG = nonsense syllable generation; RG = rhyme generation; SCMG = slow category member generation; FCMG = fast category member generation.

(Figure 9.4). However, for phonologically based generation tasks, activity was most robust in left premotor cortex.

The picture in the right hemisphere was substantially different (Figure 9.5). There was relatively diffuse activity in the right caudate nucleus and putamen that also occurred during word generation tasks but not during nonsense syllable generation. No right frontal activity was present during the word generation tasks, with the exception of a small area of cortex at the juncture of the insula and the frontal operculum. Given the notable lack of right frontal activity, we suggest that the right basal ganglia activity served to suppress right frontal activity, preventing right frontal structures from interfering with language production. This interpretation is consistent with the concept that the basal ganglia suppress unselected activity to facilitate performance of the selected activity.

9.6   Enhancement and suppression are temporally scaled in the basal ganglia

While we noted above that the effects of the glutamatergic and GABAergic activity between structures of the basal ganglia circuitry can be interpreted in a relatively straightforward fashion, dopaminergic actions in the striatum are not

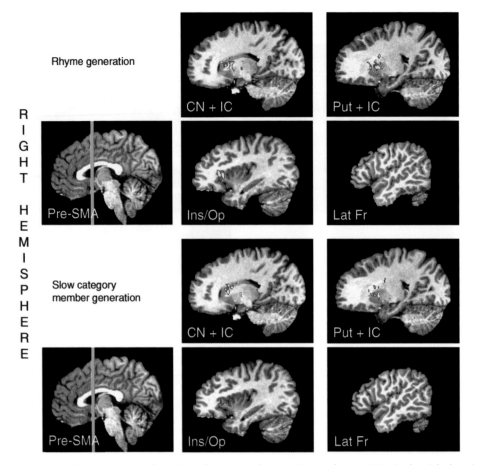

Figure 9.5.   Right basal ganglia activity during word generation. Robust activity in the right basal ganglia (caudate nucleus and putamen) occurs during word generation. At the same time, very little right frontal activity occurs.

so straightforward. Parkinson's disease, a state of dopamine depletion in the striatum, has long been used as a model of basal ganglia dysfunction. However, it will be necessary to understand dopaminergic activity in the striatum to truly understand the mechanisms of Parkinson's disease. Activity of D1 receptors has been fairly well described and can be useful in understanding activity of the direct loop because those receptors tend to populate the striatal neurons that project to the direct loop (Gerfen, 1992; Penney & Young, 1986). Striatal spiny output neurons reside in two states (Figure 9.6): a hyperpolarized state sometimes referred to as the down state, and a less polarized state sometimes referred to as the up state. Action potentials occur only in the up state. Spiny output neurons spontaneously cycle between relatively brief periods in the up state and longer periods of quiescence in the down state, with cycles averaging about a second

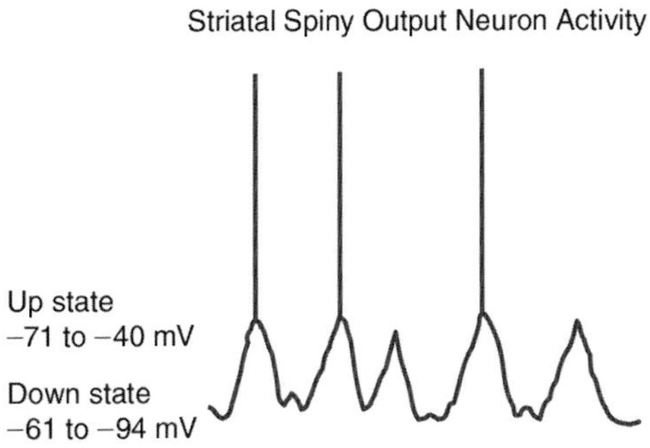

Striatal Spiny Output Neuron Activity

Up state
−71 to −40 mV

Down state
−61 to −94 mV

Figure 9.6.   Representation of striatal spiny neuron output. Long periods of quiescence in the down (hyperpolarized) state are punctuated by relatively brief periods in the up state. Axonal action potentials only occur in the up state. This pattern not only occurs spontaneously, it also is associated with activity of the organism.

in length. These states are also seen during various behaviors of the organism and are believed to play an important role in the phasic influences of the striatum. Excitatory glutamatergic connections from the cortex are known to synapse sparsely on a relatively large number of striatal spiny output neurons. In the down state, excitatory inputs from a few passing fibers can be inactivated by internal mechanisms in striatal spiny neurons. Thus it takes coordinated activity by a relatively large number of cortical inputs to change the neuron from the down to the up state, where action potentials are possible. D1 receptor activity is believed to make transitions to the up state easier as well as to lengthen the period during which the neuron stays in the up state. Dopamine antagonists are known to reduce the duration of the up state evoked by stimulation, but they do not prevent transition to the up state. When D1 receptor activity is reduced, it takes a greater amount of excitatory input to striatal spiny neurons to transition from the down to the up state or to prolong the up state (O'Donnell, 2003; West & Grace, 2002; Wilson & Kawaguchi, 1996). These facts suggest one possible mechanism of action for striatal neurons in the direct loop that are affected by D1 receptors. They may facilitate selected actions or cognitions through prolonging the activity supporting them.

As previously noted, activity of D2 receptors in the indirect loop is not well understood, and we will not belabor the topic further here. However, there is evidence relevant to temporal scaling in the indirect loop that we must address. Nambu *et al.* (2000) electrically stimulated primary motor cortex, and then recorded activity down stream in the medial pallidal segment. Starting at about 8 ms after the stimulation, a wave of excitatory input hit the medial globus pallidus. The origin of this activity was thought to be the hyperdirect loop. Exciting the medial globus pallidus will increase its inhibition of the thalamus that, in turn, will dampen thalamocortical activity. Thus this wave of excitation to the medial pallidum is thought to have a suppressing effect on actions and cognitions. The purpose of this initial wave of suppression may be to reset the basal ganglia circuitry in preparation for changing to a new activity (Nambu *et al.*, 2002). Subsequently, at about 21 ms post stimulation, a wave of inhibitory activity arrives at the medial globus pallidus. The origin of this activity appears to be the direct loop. The net effect of this activity is to free thalamocortical projections from pallidal inhibition, thereby enhancing thalamocortical activity. Finally, at about 30 ms post cortical stimulation, a second wave of excitation hits the medial globus pallidus. Both the hyperdirect and the indirect loops are thought to influence the second wave of excitation. The net effect of the excitation, again, is to suppress thalamocortical activity by increasing pallidal inhibition of its thalamic target.

Nambu *et al.* (2002) conjectured as to the function of this suppress–enhance–suppress sequence. We will translate their concepts to the realm of cognition as follows. Keep in mind that thalamocortical transmission is thought to enhance cognitive processes represented in their cortical targets while an absence of thalamocortical input is thought to have the impact of suppressing the represented cognitive processes. In developing a conceptual framework, it will be helpful to expand upon the word generation example in Figure 9.2. Figure 9.7 represents the sequence of suppression and enhancement we just discussed. In the inner and outer circles, the darker the gray, the greater the state of relative suppression, and the lighter gray and white represent relative states of enhancement. Suppose that the task now is to produce the names of as many birds as possible in a given period of time. Let us further suppose that the subject produces the word "eagle" as the first response. The first diagram (upper left, time −1) represents the state of the system at this time with "eagle" enhanced and all other responses suppressed. The subject's job now is to produce a different name of a bird. The second diagram (time 0) represents the first wave of suppression. Its purpose is to reset the system in preparation for producing a new response, a different bird name than on the previous response. The primary impact of this first wave of suppression is to suppress the previous response ("eagle") to the point where it can be replaced with a different bird name. At time +1, the new response, "crow," has replaced the previous response as the selected response, the wave of enhancement hits, and all available bird names are enhanced to some degree. Since all responses are enhanced, the signal-to-noise ratio is not yet optimal for facilitating the new response. Finally, the second wave of suppression hits. The purpose of this second wave is to suppress all but the most strongly enhanced of the potential responses, thereby yielding the optimal signal-to-noise ratio resulting in facilitation of the new response, "crow." Once this

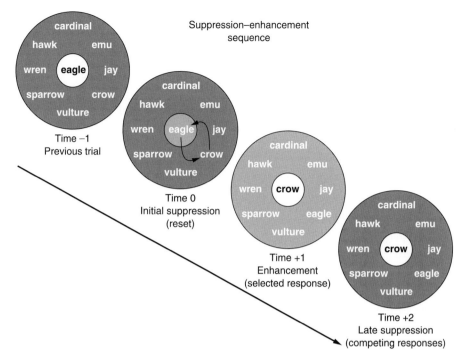

Figure 9.7. Suppression-enhancement-suppression cycle during word generation. The subject must generate all the bird names that they can. Time −1 represents a previous trial in which "eagle" was spoken. At time 0, the first wave of suppression resets the system and "crow" replaces "eagle" as the selected word. At time +1, the wave of enhancement enhances all category members to some degree. At time +2, a second wave of suppression suppresses all but the most highly activated word "crow", thereby enhancing the signal-to-noise ratio and improving the efficiency of the word production system.

response has been given, the system resets itself to begin a new cycle of suppression−enhancement−suppression. While this example has been developed in the realm of intention (i.e. it is focused on competing actions for category member generation), the principles can be applied to intentionally guided attention during semantic priming, as we shall see shortly.

A final point regarding the cycle of suppression and enhancement should be made. The time scale described by Nambu *et al.* (2000) cannot be directly applied to our discussion for two reasons. First, exogenous electrical stimulation is not the manner in which the motor cortex usually influences the basal ganglia and may have distorted the temporal characteristics of the suppress−enhance−suppress sequence. Second, we are interested in cognitive applications, which are fairly far up stream from the motor cortex and, therefore, should evince a longer time course between stimulation and response. Nonetheless, the sequence of suppress−enhance−suppress can provide a template useful in exploring semantic priming paradigms thought to involve suppression. Replication of a similar sequence during priming could be useful in identifying cognitive processes influenced by the hyperdirect and indirect loops.

9.7 Semantic priming studies illustrate the role of the basal ganglia in intentionally guided attention

Since 2000 a number of semantic priming studies have been done with basal ganglia lesion and Parkinson's disease. Parkinson's disease is a movement disorder caused primarily by deterioration of nigrostriatal pathways that supply dopaminergic input to the striatum. Many semantic priming studies have used a lexical decision paradigm for semantic priming. In the simplest of such paradigms, two sets of letter strings are presented in rapid succession. The first string is known as the prime, and it is almost always a real word. The second string is called the target, and sometimes is a real word and sometimes a nonword letter string. In the version of the task most frequently used with basal ganglia lesion and disease, the subject pushes a button as rapidly as they can when the target is a real word and refrains from pressing the button when the target is a nonword letter string. When the target is a real word and the prime and target are semantically related (e.g. bark—dog), normal subjects usually respond more quickly to the target than when the prime and the target words have no semantic relationship (e.g. river—dog). There are many versions of semantic priming tasks. In some, the major effects appear to be related to enhancement of the ability to respond to the target, but other versions are more sensitive to suppression. It is this variable sensitivity to enhancement and suppression of cognitive activity that makes semantic priming useful in understanding how Parkinson's disease and basal ganglia lesion affect cognitive processes.

Semantic priming paradigms are probably best understood as an interface between intention and intentionally guided attention. In these paradigms, the primes act as cues that either speed up (enhance) or slow down (suppress) reaction times to targets. In other words, attending to the information in the cue allows the subject to analyze and respond to the target more quickly when the cue and the target are semantically related. Attention to the cue is a product of the intention to engage in the task and impacts the ability to respond.

However, this facet of the task does not mean that the relationship between the prime and the target is always subject to deliberation by the subject. Indeed, one frequent interpretation of short stimulus—onset asynchronies (usually 100 to 200 ms) is that such short intervals do not allow time for top—down (i.e. controlled) processing. Only the longer intervals (often of a second or more) are subject to conscious deliberations regarding the prime and its potential value in the task (i.e. controlled processing). While this conceptualization has a great deal of validity, we will take a different approach to interpreting temporal phenomena in semantic priming. Our analysis of the literature leads us to believe that temporal phenomena are the product of the physiological properties of the systems that produce them and that the limitations and capabilities of the physiological systems will be reflected in the cognitive processing that arises from these systems. If we can successfully map the properties of cognitive processing onto the physiological processes of the system, we will gain a greater under-standing of the cognitive processes and their limitations. Shortly, we will discuss two semantic priming studies that map particularly well onto known physiological processes.

9.8   The participation of the basal ganglia in semantic priming and word generation can be most parsimoniously explained by connections at the lexical level of processing

Before discussing these semantic priming studies, however, one digression regarding the nature of lexical–semantic processing is apropos. Recent models of lexical–semantic processing agree that separate lexical and semantic levels contribute to word processing. However, the structure of these levels of processing and how they interact has been the topic of considerable debate, which is not likely to end any time soon (Levelt, 1999). Although two models have dominated much of the discussion (i.e. Dell *et al.*, 1998; Levelt, 2001), it is the work of Balota and Paul (1996) that has provided the most parsimonious explanation of semantic priming effects. These investigators showed that the effects of semantic priming actually can be accounted for by connections within the lexical level of processing, unless the paradigm in question involves overt semantic processing (e.g. making an overt semantic judgment about an item, such as whether it represents an animate or inanimate object). The semantic priming paradigms we discuss below do not involve explicit semantic processing. Apparently, the lexical items acquire connections (i.e. associations) with each other due to the fact that semantically related items are likely to be mentioned together. This observation suggests that the lexical level of processing acquires some degree of semantic knowledge by virtue of these connections. Indeed, some evidence suggests semantic processing can be modality specific to verbal and visual modalities (e.g. Hart & Gordon, 1992). Resolution of this debate about lexical–semantic processing is beyond the scope of this chapter. However, given Balota and Paul's (1996) evidence and the parsimonious character of their assumptions as applied to the current discussion, we model processes in semantic priming at a single level of processing, the lexical level. The model for word generation that we discussed above also has made this assumption, which is consistent with the fact that the basal ganglia in both hemispheres respond to the lexical rather than the semantic properties of production tasks (Crosson *et al.*, 2003).

9.9 Modulation of the direct loop by D1 activity can be used to understand enhancement during semantic priming

As noted above, some semantic priming paradigms seem to reflect more the enhancement side of the equation and some seem to reflect more the suppression side of the equation. We begin our discussion of semantic priming with an example of priming thought to rely more heavily on the enhancement than the suppression properties of basal ganglia functions, the triplet paradigm of lexical ambiguity priming. In lexical ambiguity priming, a word with two or more meanings is used as a prime. For example, the word "bank" can represent a place where money is kept or the land beside a river. In the triplet paradigm, three words are presented: a contextual cue, the prime, and the target. The target sometimes is a real word and sometimes is a nonword letter string. In the version that has been used with basal ganglia lesion and disease, the subject pushes a button as quickly as possible when the target is a real word and withholds responding when the target is a nonword letter string. There are four conditions in the triplet priming paradigm that are based on the semantic relationships between the contextual cue, prime, and target words. In the concordant condition, the contextual cue has a meaning that is consistent with the semantic relationship between the prime and the target (e.g. teller–bank–money). In the discordant condition, the contextual cue has a meaning that is related to the prime, but inconsistent with the semantic relationship between the prime and the target (e.g. river–bank–money). In the neutral condition, the contextual cue has no semantic relationship to the prime, but the prime and the target are semantically related (e.g. dog–bank–money). Finally, in the unrelated condition, both the contextual cue and the target are unrelated to the prime (e.g. dog–rain–money). The concordant, neutral, and discordant conditions are compared to the unrelated condition. If reaction times in the former conditions are significantly faster than in the latter condition, semantic priming is said to occur. In normal subjects at short interstimulus intervals (ISIs), priming is greatest in the concordant condition, intermediate in size in the neutral condition, and smallest in the discordant condition. In other words, a concordant contextual cue can be thought of as strengthening the relationship between the prime and the target, and a discordant contextual cue can be thought of as weakening the relationship during the presentation of the triplet.

Copland (2000) gave this triplet priming paradigm to Parkinson's disease patients, to patients with dominant-hemisphere non-thalamic subcortical lesions, to patients with dominant-hemisphere cortical lesions, and to neurologically normal controls, using a short ISI (100 ms) and a long ISI (1250 ms) At the short ISI, the performance of all the patient groups was for the most part similar to that of the controls. At the long ISI, the controls lost the priming effect for the discordant condition but otherwise performed similarly to their performance at the short delay. At the long ISI, the cortical lesion patients continued to prime in all conditions but lost the differences between the priming conditions; in other words the contextual cues seemed to have no impact. The nonthalamic subcortical lesion patients, whose lesions included the basal ganglia or surrounding white matter, lost all priming effects at the long ISI. This finding was consistent with the fact that destruction of striatal neurons (or the impact on their output down stream from the striatum) would result in a loss of enhancement at the longer ISI through destruction of the direct loop. At the longer ISI, Parkinson's disease patients showed priming only during the concordant condition. This finding is consistent with the description of the influence of D1 receptor activity on the enhance circuitry. Specifically, the loss of D1 receptor stimulation appears to result in an inability to enhance responding for all but the strongest stimulus, the condition with the concordant contextual cue.

To summarize, let us return to the direct loop and the D1 receptor system. At the outset, it is important to note that the basal ganglia appear to influence priming primarily at the long ISIs, but have only subtle impact at the short ISIs. The direct loop is thought to participate in enhancement of selected cognitions during intentionally guided attention. Thus destruction of structures or pathways of the direct loop should lead to an inability to perform their enhancement functions. This is exactly what happened at the long ISI with subcortical lesion in Copland's (2000) study. As discussed above, D1 receptor activity in the striatum appears to make transitions from the down to the up state easier and to prolong duration of the up state. Loss of D1 receptor activity (as in Parkinson's disease) does not prevent transitions to the up state; it simply makes the transitions harder to achieve and decreases the amount of time in the up state. Thus it takes very strong excitatory stimulation by incoming fibers from the cortex to cause a shift to and to prolong the up state. These facts are consistent with Copland's (2000) finding that only the strongest (concordant) condition produced semantic priming in Parkinson's disease patients at the long ISI. Thus it can be concluded that the direct loop of the basal ganglia functions primarily to prolong cortically generated activity, which would make that activity accessible to modification during controlled processing. Finally, the fact that basal ganglia lesion or disease has very little impact on activity at the short ISIs suggests that these paradigms are not sensitive to striatal disturbance at short ISIs.

9.10 Suppression during semantic priming may be implemented by the hyperdirect and indirect loops

Now we will turn to a different lexical ambiguity priming paradigm, one that appears to be more sensitive to suppression processes. In this paradigm, only the prime and the target are presented, and the subject again must press a button when the target is recognized as a real word and withhold responding to nonword letter strings. The ambiguous prime has two meanings, one of which can be considered dominant, i.e. more frequently used (e.g. bank—money) and the other of which can be considered subordinate, i.e. less frequently used (e.g. bank—river). The precise mechanisms for this type of priming are controversial. For the sake of the current discussion, the relatively simple diagram in Figure 9.8 will suffice as a model. The center white circle represents words connected with the dominant meaning of bank (a place where money is kept). By virtue of their connection

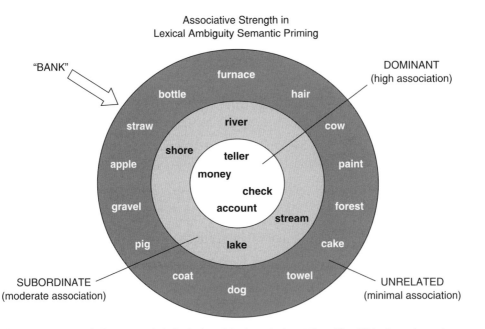

Figure 9.8.   Associative strength in lexical ambiguity priming. When "bank" is the prime, the strongest associations are to words connoting the dominant meaning. Associations to words connoting the subordinate meaning are more modest, and associations to unrelated words are minimal.

with the more commonly used meaning of bank, these words will have the strongest association with the lexical item of bank. In the next circle out from the center (light gray) are words connected with the subordinate meaning of bank (land on the side of a river). These words have a moderately strong association with the word bank through their connection with its subordinate meaning. That is, the strength of association of these words with bank is weaker than for words connected to the dominant meaning, but it is stronger than for words with minimal association to bank. The words in the outer, dark gray circle are unrelated to bank, and therefore have minimal association with the word. When no contextual cues are present, there is a tendency to gravitate toward (i.e. attend to) the dominant meaning because words associated with this meaning will have a greater strength of association to the word bank. Under these circumstances, there is evidence that the subordinate meaning is actively suppressed at longer ISIs in priming paradigms.

However, for ultra-short stimulus onset asynchronies (SOAs), Simpson and Burgess (1981) also found an absence of priming for the subordinate meaning while the dominant meaning was primed. At their 16 ms SOA, dominant but not subordinate meanings were primed. At intermediate SOAs (100 to 500 ms), both the dominant and subordinate meanings were primed, but at their longer SOA (700 ms), only the dominant meaning was again primed. While these data have been interpreted in various ways, there is a striking resemblance in the suppression–enhancement–suppression sequence for the subordinate meaning to the suppression–enhancement–suppression sequence of basal ganglia activity described by Nambu *et al.* (2000, 2002). This raises the question of how patients with Parkinson's disease or patients with lesions of the basal ganglia would respond to this paradigm.

Copland (2003) did perform the relevant experiment, only he did not use the ultra-short ISI. The priming paradigm was administered to Parkinson's disease patients, patients with nonthalamic subcortical lesions, patients with cortical lesions, and neurologically normal controls at an intermediate ISI (200 ms) and a long ISI (1250 ms). At the intermediate ISI, all subjects primed both the dominant and subordinate meanings. At the long ISI, normal controls and cortical lesion patients primed only the dominant and not the subordinate meaning. However, both the Parkinson's disease patients and nonthalamic subcortical lesion patients showed priming of both the dominant and subordinate meanings at the long SOA. In other words, the patients with basal ganglia impairment showed a failure to suppress the subordinate meaning at the long SOA.

These findings raise two interesting questions. The first is why Parkinson's disease and subcortical lesion patients show the same pattern of failure to suppress the subordinate meaning at the long ISI. The failure to suppress of the lesion patients can easily be explained by the fact that the suppression as well as the enhancement circuitry has been destroyed. However, in the Parkinson's disease patients, there is a loss of dopaminergic modulation via the activity of D2 receptors. D2 receptors are known to have an inhibitory influence on striatal spiny output neurons projecting into the indirect loop. Removal of this inhibitory influence should enhance activity within the indirect loop, and the corresponding expectation is that suppression of cognitive activity should be increased. Nonetheless, as explained above, the ultimate actions of the D2 receptor system within the striatum are poorly understood, and we conclude that the cognitive data at this time are more likely to give us insight into how the circuitry works than is our incomplete understanding of the D2 system in the striatum. The second question is how Parkinson's disease patients would respond to the ultra-short SOA in this priming paradigm. Based upon the assumption that ultra-short suppression is a function of the hyperdirect loop, which by passes the primary site of impairment in Parkinson's disease (i.e. the striatum), one might predict that suppression will be intact at the ultra-short interval, but this remains to be seen.

To summarize, for this lexical ambiguity paradigm in which no contextual cues are given, priming appears to be sensitive to the suppression function of the basal ganglia. Indeed, one early study of the paradigm demonstrates the suppression—enhancement—suppression sequence that might be predicted from the physiology of the system (Nambu *et al.*, 2000). Both nonthalamic subcortical lesion and Parkinson's disease patients demonstrate a failure to suppress the subordinate meaning at the long ISI. Once again, it is at the long ISI when the effects of basal ganglia dysfunction are seen. However, we must be cautious in our interpretation because the ultra-short interval has yet to be assessed in these patient populations.

9.11 Further research is needed to refine this model

Before a few concluding remarks, we will briefly recap the highlights of the model described herein. The basal ganglia are not directly involved in semantic functions but influence them through the realms of intention and intentionally guided attention. They facilitate action and cognitive processing by enhancing selected actions and cognitions while at the same time suppressing competing action plans and unattended cognitions. This facilitates selected actions and processing of attended cognitions by increasing the signal-to-noise ratio, resulting in increased speed, efficiency, and precision of action and cognition processing.

This facilitation occurs primarily in the late stages of realizing actions or cognitive processing and has the effect of making the actions and cognitions more available to controlled, top–down processing and modification.

Actions and cognitions are enhanced through the direct loop of the basal ganglia. Enhancement is modulated by D1 receptor activity, which has the effect of facilitating and prolonging the enhancement. In contrast, suppression is accomplished through the hyperdirect and indirect loops. An early wave of suppression has the effect of resetting basal ganglia systems to a relatively neutral state so that new actions or cognitions can be facilitated. This first wave is a product of activity in the hyperdirect loop. After a brief period in which widespread enhancement dominates basal ganglia circuitry, a second wave of suppression occurs. This second wave suppresses all but the most strongly activated actions or cognitions. It is the product of the indirect and hyperdirect loops. The action of the indirect loop is modulated by D2 receptor activity, but the net impact of this receptor system on behavior is poorly understood. The fact that both patients with basal ganglia lesions and patients with Parkinson's disease fail to suppress subordinate meanings in lexical ambiguity semantic priming at long SOAs suggests that the loss of dopaminergic modulation will result in the loss of the late suppression component of the suppress–enhance–suppress sequence. This finding is incompatible with a simple interpretation of the inhibitory effects of D2 activity on striatal spiny output neurons and, therefore, suggests that the incomplete knowledge about D2 modulation of the indirect loop is currently inadequate to clearly translate the physiological phenomena into predictions about actions and cognitions.

Semantic priming studies hold great promise for continuing to unravel the impact of basal ganglia functions on semantics. For example, studies already have been conducted addressing the impact of administering of L-dopa on semantic priming in neurologically normal subjects (e.g. Angwin *et al.*, 2004; Kischka *et al.*, 1996). We have not attempted to interpret these studies. What is needed to do so is a clear understanding both of how the specific priming paradigms entail enhancement and suppression of cognition and of how increased dopamine availability impacts D1 and D2 receptor systems in normal subjects. Such knowledge should lead to clear predictions of priming results. Functional MRI studies also will be helpful in further delineating the role of the basal ganglia in semantics. However, one caveat regarding fMRI should be mentioned. In our experience (Crosson *et al.*, 2003) basal ganglia activity is difficult to image. We have found consistent activity in basal ganglia loops only with relatively large numbers of subjects (18 or greater) and with a large number of activity blocks. Thus there are obstacles to the use of priming and fMRI studies to study the basal ganglia. Yet these obstacles seem to be surmountable, and it appears we will continue to develop our knowledge about how the basal ganglia influence action and cognition by using these techniques.

Another agenda is to expand the disease models that are studied. For example, in Huntington's disease there is a loss of striatal output neurons. Therefore, it would be pertinent to compare the performance of Huntington's disease patients to the performance of patients with other basal ganglia dysfunctions on the various tasks we have discussed. Additionally, there is a significant loss of dopaminergic activity during normal aging (Bäckman & Farde, 2005). It would be of interest to determine how this decrease affects cognition in aging.

To conclude, it is clear that more research will lead to a greater understanding of how basal ganglia functions influence semantic and other cognitive functions. This research should lead to the refinement of the current model, or possibly even rejection of it. This understanding is important for a variety of reasons. It will help us to manage or even mitigate the cognitive deficits that occur in Parkinson's disease, in lesions of the basal ganglia, or in other basal ganglia dysfunctions. Further, there is evidence that the degree of intactness of the basal ganglia influences how language is lateralized after dominant-hemisphere strokes that cause aphasia. For example, it appears that in chronic aphasia, language production lateralizes to the left frontal lobe when the basal ganglia are intact, but not when the basal ganglia are damaged (Crosson *et al.*, 2005; Kim *et al.*, 2002). This knowledge may have implications for rehabilitation. Put simply, continuing research on how the basal ganglia influence semantic processing and other cognitive activity could have an important impact on a variety of patients and, therefore, should have a high priority on our research agenda.

REFERENCES

Akkal, D., Dum, R. P., and Strick, P. L. (2002). Cerebellar and basal ganglia inputs to the pre-supplementary area (Pre-SMA). *Society for Neuroscience Abstract Viewer/Itinerary Planner*, Online, Program No. 462.14.

Alexander, C. E., DeLong, M. R., and Strick, P. L. (1986). Parallel organization of functionally segregated circuits linking the basal ganglia and cortex. *Annual Review of Neuroscience*, **9**: 357–81.

Angwin, A. J., Chenery, H. J., Copland, D. A., Arnott, W. L., *et al.* (2004). Dopamine and semantic activation: an investigation of masked direct and indirect priming. *Journal of the International Neuropsychological Society*, **10**: 15–25.

Bäckman, L. and Farde, L. (2005). The role of dopamine systems in cognitive aging. In R. Cabeza, L. Nyberg, and D. Park (eds.), *Cognitive Neuroscience of Aging: Linking Cognitive and Cerebral Aging*. New York: Oxford University Press, pp. 58–84.

Balota, D. A. and Paul, S. T. (1996). Summation of activation: Evidence from multiple primes that converge and diverge within semantic memory. *Journal of Experimental Psychology: Learning, Memory, and Cognition*, **22**: 827–45.

Broadbent, W. H. (1872). On the cerebral mechanisms of speech and thought; in *Proceedings of the Royal Medicinal and Chirurgical Society of London*, pp. 25–9. (Cited by Wallesch and Papagno, 1988.)

Brunner, R. J., Kornhuber, H. H., Seemuller, E., Suger, G., and Wallesch, C.-W. (1982). Basal ganglia participation in language pathology. *Brain and Language*, **16**: 281–99.

Cappa, S. F., Cavallotti, G., Guidotti, M., Papagno, C., and Vignolo, L. (1983). Subcortical aphasia: two clinical–CT scan correlation studies. *Cortex*, **19**: 227–41.

Copland, D. A. (2000). *A Real-Time Examination of Lexical Ambiguity Resolution Following Lesions of the Dominant Nonthalamic Subcortex*. Doctoral Dissertation: University of Queensland, Brisbane, Australia.

Copland, D. A. (2003). Basal ganglia and semantic engagement. *Journal of the International Neuropsychological Society*, **9**: 1041–52.

Copland, D. A., Chenery, H. J., and Murdoch, B. E. (2000a). Persistent deficits in complex language function following dominant nonthalamic subcortical lesions. *Journal of Medical Speech–Language Pathology*, **8**: 1–15.

Copland, D. A., Chenery, H. J., and Murdoch, B. E. (2000b). Processing lexical ambiguities in word triplets. *Neuropsychology*, **14**: 370–90.

Crosson, B., Bacon Moore, A., Gopinath, K., White, K. D., *et al.* (2005). Role of the right and left hemispheres in recovery of function during treatment of intention in aphasia. *Journal of Cognitive Neuroscience*, **17**: 392–406.

Crosson, B., Benefield, H., Cato, M. A., Sadek, J. R., Moore, A. B., *et al.* (2003). Left and right basal ganglia and frontal activity during language generation: Contributions to lexical, semantic, and phonological processes. *Journal of the International Neuropsychological Society*, **9**: 1061–77.

Damasio, A. R., Damasio, H., Rizzo, M., Varney, N., and Gersh, F. (1982). Aphasia with nonhemorrhagic lesions in the basal ganglia and internal capsule. *Archives of Neurology*, **39**: 15–20.

Dell, G. S., Schwartz, M. F., Martin, N., Saffran, E. M., and Gagnon, D. A. (1997). Lexical access in aphasic and nonaphasic speakers. *Psychological Review*, **104**: 801–38.

Demonet, J.-F. (1987). *Les Aphasies Sous-corticales: Etude Linguistique, radiologique et hemodynamique de 31 observations*. Thèse Pour le Doctorat D'Etat en Medicine, Université Paul Sabatier-Toulouse III, Facultés de Medecine.

Fisher, C. M. (1979). Capsular infarcts: the underlying vascular lesions. *Archives of Neurology*, **36**: 65–73.

Fuster, J. M. (2003). *Cortex and Mind: Unifying Cognition*. New York: Oxford University Press.

Gerfen, C. (1992). The neostriatal mosaic: multiple levels of compartmental organization in the basal ganglia. *Annual Review of Neuroscience*, **15**: 285–320.

Hart, J. and Gordon, B. (1992). Neural subsystems for object knowledge. *Nature*, **359**: 60–4.

Heilman, K. M., Watson, R. T., and Valenstein, E. (2003). Neglect and related disorders. In K. M. Heilman and E. Valenstein (eds.), *Clinical Neuropsychology*, 4th edn. New York: Oxford University Press, pp. 296–346.

Hermann, K., Turner, J. W., Gillingham, F. J., and Gaze, R. M. (1966). The effects of destructive lesions and stimulation of the basal gangalia on speech mechanisms. *Confinia Neurologica*, **27**: 107–207.

Hier, D. B., Davis, K. R., Richardson, E. P., Jr., and Mohr, J. P. (1977). Hypertensive putaminal hemorrhage. *Annals of Neurology*, **1**: 152–9.

Hillis, A. E., Wityk, R. J., Barker, P. B., Beauchamp, N. J., *et al.* (2002). Subcortical aphasia and neglect in acute stroke: the role of cortical hypoperfusion. *Brain*, **125**: 1094–104.

Inase, M., Tokuno, H., Nambu, A., Akazawa, T., and Takada, M. (1999). Corticostriatal and corticosubthalamic input zones from the presupplementary motor area in the macaque monkey: comparison with the input zones from the supplementary motor area. *Brain Research*, **833**: 191–201.

Kim, Y.-H., Ko, M.-H., Parrish, T. B., and Kim, H.-G. (2002). Reorganization of cortical language areas in patients with aphasia: a functional MRI study. *Yonsei Medical Journal*, **43**: 441–5.

Kischka, J., Kammer, T. H., Maier, S., Weisbrod, M., *et al.* (1996). Dopaminergic modulation of semantic network activation. *Neuropsychologia*, **23**: 1107–13.

Knopman, D. S., Selnes, O. A., Niccum, N., and Rubens, A. B. (1984). Recovery of naming in aphasia: Relationship to fluency, comprehension, and CT findings. *Neurology*, **34**: 1461–70.

Kussmaul, A. (1877). *Die Storungen der Sprache*. Leipzig: Vogel. (Cited by Wallesch & Papagno, 1988.)

Levelt, W. J. M. (2001). Spoken word production: a theory of lexical access. *Proceedings of the National Academy of Sciences*, **98**: 13464–71.

Levelt, W. J. M. (1999). Models of word production. *Trends in Cognitive Science*, **3**: 223–32.

Marie, P. (1906). Revision de la question de l'aphasie: Que faut-il penser des aphasies sous-courticales (aphasies pures)? *La Semaine Medicale*, 42. October (Cited by Démonet, 1987.)

Maurice, N., Mercer, J., Chan, C. S., Hernandez-Lopez, S., *et al.* (2004). D2 dopamine receptor-mediated modulation of voltage dependent Na+ channels reduces autonomous activity in striatal cholinergic interneurons. *Journal of Neuroscience*, **24**: 10289–301.

Middleton, F. A. and Strick, P. L. (2000). Basal ganglia and cerebellar loops: motor and cognitive circuits. *Brain Research Review*, **31**: 236–50.

Mink, J. W. (1996). The basal ganglia. *Progress in Neurobiology*, **50**: 381–425.

Mitchell, I. J., Jackson, A., Sambrook, M. A., and Crossman, A. R. (1989). The role of the subthalamic nucleus in experimental chorea. *Brain*, **112**: 1533–48.

Murdoch, B. E., Chenery, H. J., and Kennedy, M. (1989). Aphemia associated with bilateral striato-capsular lesions subsequent to cerebral anoxia. *Brain Injury*, **3**: 41–9

Nadeau, S. E. and Crosson, B. (1997). Subcortical aphasia. *Brain and Language*, **58**: 355–402.

Nambu, A., Tokuno, H., Hamada, I., Kita, H., *et al.* (2000). Excitatory cortical inputs to pallidal neurons via the subthalamic nucleus in the monkey. *Journal of Neurophysiology*, **84**: 289–300.

Nambu, A., Tokuno, H., and Takada, M. (2002). Functional significance of the cortico-subthalamo-pallidal "hyperdirect" pathway. *Neuroscience Research*, **43**: 111–17.

Penney, J. B. and Young, A. B. (1986). Striatal inhomogeneities and basal ganglia function. *Movement Disorders*, **1**: 3–16.

O'Donnell, P. (2003). Dopamine gating of forebrain neural ensembles. *The European Journal of Neuroscience*, **17**: 429–35.

Simpson, G. and Burgess, C. (1985). Activation and selection processes in the recognition of ambiguous words. *Journal of Experimental Psychology, Human Perception, and Performance*, **11**: 28–39.

Strick, P. L., Dum, R., and Picard, N. (1995). Macro-organization of the circuits connecting the basal ganglia with the cortical motor areas. In J. C. Houk, J. L. Davis, and D. G. Beiser (eds.), *Models of Information Processing in the Basal Ganglia*. Cambridge, MA: MIT Press, pp. 117–30.

Svinnilson, E., Torvik, A., Lowe, R., and Leksell, L. (1960). Treatment of Parkinsonism by stereotactic thermolesions in the pallidal region. *Acta Psychiatrica et Neurologica Scandinavia*, **35**: 358–77.

Ullman, M. T. (2004). Contributions of memory circuits to language: the declarative/procedural model. *Cognition*, **92**: 231–70.

Van Buren, J. M. (1963). Confusion and disturbance of speech from stimulation in the vicinity of the head of the caudate nucleus. *Journal of Neurosurgery*, **20**: 148–57.

Van Buren, J. M. (1966). Evidence regarding a more precise localization of the frontal-caudate arrest response in man. *Journal of Neurosurgery*, **24**: 416–17.

Van Buren, J. M., Li, C. L., and Ojemann, G. A. (1966). The fronto-striatal arrest response in man. *Electroencephalography and Clinical Neurophysiology*, **21**: 114–30.

Wallesch, C.-W. (1985). Two syndromes of aphasia occurring with ischemic lesions involving the left basal ganglia. *Brain and Language*, **25**: 357–61.

Wallesch, C.-W. and Pagagno, C. (1988). Subcortical aphasia. In F. C. Rose, R. Whurr, and M. A. Wyke (eds.), *Aphasia*. London: Whurr Publishers, pp. 256–87.

Weiller, C., Willmes, K., Reiche, W., Thron, A., *et al.* (1993). The case of aphasia or neglect after striatocapsular infarction. *Brain*, **116**: 1509–25.

Wernicke, C. (1874). *Der Aphasische Symptomencomplex*. Breslau: Cohn & Weigert. (Cited by Wallesch & Papagno, 1988.)

West, A. R. and Grace, A. A. (2002). Opposite influences of endogenous dopamine D1 and D2 receptor activation on activity states and electrophysiological properties of striatal neurons: studies combining In Vivo intracellular recordings and reverse microdialysis. *Journal of Neuroscience*, **22**: 294–304.

Wilson, C. J. and Kawaguchi, Y. (1996). The origins of two-state spontaneous membrane potential fluctuations of neostriatal spiny neurons. *Journal of Neuroscience*, **16**: 2397–410.

Part VI

Conceptual Models of Semantics

10

Process and content in semantic memory

Phyllis Koenig and Murray Grossman

University of Pennsylvania School of Medicine

To identify something is to group it with like objects called by the same name; that is, to place it in a category. This process begins in our earliest days of acquiring language: the toddler who learns that his spherical rubber toy is a "ball" will spontaneously use that same word for striped beach balls and fuzzy tennis balls. Categorization allows us to make assumptions about an object at hand based on experience with related ones; without this capacity we would be first-time visitors to our own planet with every new experience, unable to understand our surroundings. Hence categorization is essential to the organization of semantic memory, that is, our long-term representation of meaningful non-episodic information.

How does categorization take place? Semantic content knowledge (e.g. appearance, specific features, and functions) and ability to process that knowledge (e.g. select appropriate features and make comparisons) are both necessary. Consider this scenario: someone describes a 45-year-old female traffic cop who strictly disciplines her grandchild as "not what one usually thinks of as a grandmother." Presumably the speaker is referring to characteristics commonly associated with grandmothers, e.g. being elderly, sedentary, sweet-natured, and eager to spoil their grandchildren. Of course, the speaker also knows that what qualifies someone as a grandmother is being a mother of a parent, age, appearance, and lifestyle notwithstanding. This scenario illustrates two primary categorization processes: similarity-based and rule-based (Smith *et al.*, 1998). Similarity-based categorization is relatively quick, automatic, and perceptually based, involving global comparison with an established category representation such as a proto-type or representative exemplars (Medin, Goldstone, & Gentner, 1993; Medin & Schaffer, 1978; Smith & Medin, 1981; Ashby, Alfonso-Reese, Turken, & Waldron,

This work was supported in part by National Institutes of Health (AG17586, AG15116, NS44266) and the Charles A. Dana Foundation. We express our deep appreciation to the patients and their families for allowing us conduct this research.

1998). Since most of our classification judgments are instantaneous and seemingly effortless, similarity-based categorization is presumably our default process, employed most of the time. Unlike the "atypical grandmother" example, our accrued world knowledge of typicality generally leads to correct classifications: small flying animals are usually BIRDS (we use capitals to indicate a superordinate category), legless broad-tailed aquatic creatures are usually FISH. In contrast, rule-based categorization assumes that certain features have special diagnostic status, while other features, no matter how salient, are irrelevant or even misleading (Smith, Langston, & Nisbett, 1992). This is the process we would employ for exceptional examples such as the young traffic-cop grandmother, or in classifying bats and dolphins as MAMMALS rather than as BIRDS and FISH. We probably also use this process when, as novices in some field, we attempt to classify unfamiliar things before we have accumulated enough experience with the category to support a prototypical representation (Johansen & Palmeri, 2002). Hence rule-based categorization is relatively effortful, and requires executive resources such as selective attention, working memory, and inhibitory control to assess and evaluate appropriate features.

Theories of semantic memory have tended to focus on knowledge content. Semantic memory impairments in patients with neurodegenerative diseases, manifested in difficulties naming, recognizing, or describing objects, are well documented. Many investigators have observed apparent category-specific impairments, such as deficits limited to manufactured objects (e.g. tools) while spared for natural kinds (e.g. animals) or vice versa (Cappa *et al.*, 1998; Chertkow & Bub, 1990; Garrard *et al.*, 1998, 2001; Gonnerman *et al.*, 1997; Montanes *et al.*, 1995; Moss & Tyler, 2000; Silveri *et al.*, 1991; Warrington, 1975). Although such observations have sometimes proven inconsistent or amenable to alternative explanations, they have given rise to a rich body of hypotheses whose common thread is a focus on content-related distinctions among categories. For example, the "sensory–motor" hypothesis posits that features are stored in modality-specific brain regions (Warrington & Shallice, 1994; Farah & McClelland, 1991). In this view, categories of knowledge are distinguished by the predominance of features of a particular modality, such as visual features for ANIMALS and motor features for TOOLS. For instance, our feature knowledge of giraffes, by which we differentiate them from other ANIMALS, includes their long neck, long legs, and spotted hide, while our knowledge of hammers, by which we differentiate them from other TOOLS, includes their use for pounding in nails. From this perspective, a category-specific deficit should reflect damage to brain regions (e.g. visual cortex) in which most feature knowledge for that category (e.g. ANIMALS) is stored. The "distributed" hypothesis, in contrast, posits that feature representation is scattered throughout the cortex (Gonnerman *et al.*, 1997; Moss & Tyler, 2000). Category-specific deficits arise because categories differ in the extent of feature overlap among members; redundancy of feature representation allows for compensation of lost knowledge about one member by retained knowledge about another. For instance, ANIMALS share many features, such as heads, legs, and tails: lost knowledge about a feature such as *tail* of a horse can thus be "filled in" by retained knowledge about exemplars of the category, such as cows and mules, that share this feature. TOOLS, in contrast, tend to have unique features: lost knowledge about a saw's blade cannot be compensated for by retained knowledge about hammers and chisels. Hence minimal cortical damage should disproportionately impair semantic memory for categories with fewer shared features, and categories with many shared features should become increasingly affected as damage spreads and formerly redundant knowledge becomes degraded. While these two hypotheses differ in their predictions of which location-specific brain damage will result in a particular category-specific deficit, they share emphases on feature-type distinctions among categories and where that feature knowledge is stored. A third hypothesis, the "evolutionary" view, does not address cortical location of represented knowledge, but like the first two hypotheses, focuses on stored knowledge: according to this view, knowledge of natural kinds has a privileged status resulting from our evolutionary history in the natural world in which successful identification of predators and food was essential to survival (Caramazza, 1998). Thus this hypothesis posits that category-specific deficits reflect inherently separate representations of categories for artifacts and for natural kinds.

We believe that knowledge content is only part of the story, and that processes such as categorization also play a role in semantic memory. These processes serve to integrate feature knowledge into coherent concepts. Thus a patient with semantic memory impairment who misclassifies a carrot as a FRUIT could be doing so for several reasons: the patient could have lost content knowledge about carrots, and hence not be able to make a similarity-based comparison between carrots and some general representation of FRUITS or of VEGETABLES. Alternatively, the patient could have retained the knowledge that carrots are *long, crunchy, sweet, orange, roots*, and so on, but be unable to apply rules such as *edible roots are VEGETABLES* or *FRUIT must have seeds*. In turn, this apparent rule-based deficit could reflect loss of knowledge of a particular feature's diagnosticity (i.e. that being a *root* determines a carrot's status as a VEGETABLE rather than a FRUIT), or it could reflect deficits in the rule-based process itself, i.e. in the executive resources needed to ignore the fruit-like feature *sweet* and select the appropriate feature *root*.

Neurologically healthy individuals, including the elderly, are able to appropriately use similarity- or rule-based categorization, both in daily functioning (as in correctly classifying the atypical grandmother) and in controlled studies (Allen & Brooks, 1991; Grossman *et al.*, 2003; Patalano, Smith, Jonides, & Koeppe, 2001; Rips, 1989; Smith & Sloman, 1994; Sloman & Rips, 1998). For instance, one study asked participants to place a brief verbal description of an object (e.g. "a round object three inches in diameter") in one of two probe categories (e.g. pizzas or quarters). Only one of the categories could vary along the provided dimension (e.g. a pizza can vary in size, but a quarter cannot), qualifying it as the category of the described object, and the value mentioned in the object description was intermediate between the fixed size of one category and the typical size of the other. During one condition, categorization took place under instructions emphasizing the overall similarity of the described object to a category; during a second condition, participants categorized the object description under instructions emphasizing rule-based categorization. Healthy elderly participants successfully used rule-based processing in deciding the probe category to which the item must belong (e.g. pizza), and were appropriately flexible in using similarity-based processing in choosing the category to which the item was most similar. In contrast, neurologically impaired patients with frontotemporal dementia (FTD) or with Alzheimer's disease (AD) were only able to make similarity-based categorization judgments (Grossman *et al.*, 2003). Their rule-based categorization was significantly impaired.

We assessed whether this rule-based categorization deficit was due to loss of feature knowledge by biasing categorization judgments with the addition of a phrase that was applicable to either category, e.g. "a round object three inches in diameter *found in arcades*," but was more strongly associated with the fixed-dimension category (e.g. quarter). Patients and healthy elderly participants were both influenced by the added phrase; that is, they increased their likelihood of choosing the fixed-dimension category regardless of instruction condition. Hence the patients, as well as the healthy seniors, demonstrated knowledge of semantic features associated with the categories. However, the patients remained limited to similarity-based categorization, while the healthy participants could again use either process. These findings are consistent with a processing-based deficit in these patient groups. Moreover, since these patients are known to have difficulty on measures of executive functioning such as working memory, selective attention, and planning (Kramer *et al.*, 2003; LaFleche & Albert, 1995; Libon *et al.*, 2007; Patterson *et al.*, 1996; Perry & Hodges, 1999), these observations support the view that rule-based categorization intimately depends on executive resources.

This task was also administered to young healthy participants while regional brain activity was monitored with functional magnetic resonance imaging (fMRI), a technique that has rapidly advanced our understanding of the neural basis of semantic memory in the past decade. While in the bore of the magnet, participants were monitored during similarity-based categorization and rule-based categorization, using the identical materials described above (Grossman *et al.*, 2002). We found activation of temporal−parietal cortex and dorsolateral prefrontal cortex during both rule-based categorization and similarity-based categorization, suggesting that these brain regions are critical to categorization. The temporal−parietal area is a multimodal association region that has reciprocal projections with sensory-specific association cortices, and seems particularly well suited to the process of integrating features into a coherent concept. A direct contrast of these categorization conditions, moreover, showed significantly greater activation of dorsolateral prefrontal cortex during rule-based categorization. As many studies associate this prefrontal brain region with the executive resources we implicate in rule-based categorization, these findings are quite consistent with our process-and-content model of categorization.

We turn now to some work investigating semantic knowledge and semantic categorization processes in greater detail. This study involved teaching a novel semantic category to three groups of neurologically impaired patients using rule-based and similarity-based processes. In the "pizza-versus-quarter" study referred to above, the use of familiar probe categories could not definitively isolate the cause of the patients' difficulties with rule-based categorization. Patients' responses were compatible with a processing-based inability to apply rules; however, although we monitored patients' sensitivity to feature knowledge during the task and assessed feature knowledge in a post-test study, we could not fully rule out a loss of essential content knowledge about quarters and pizzas, including a loss of the diagnostic value associated with particular features. Indeed, even if knowledge of these features is preserved, there may be unequal exposure frequency or familiarity with these categories. One way to manage issues and potential confounds related to knowledge of familiar categories is to examine semantic categorization of a meaningful but novel category. In our protocol, the requisite feature knowledge is available to the patient, including the diagnostic status of individual features, so that categorization does not depend on previously held knowledge that may have become degraded (Koenig *et al.*, 2006). In addition, unlike the meaningless dot patterns, geometric shapes, consonant letter strings, and schematized figures used in many categorization studies (e.g. Knowlton & Squire, 1996; Reber *et al.*, 1998; Allen & Brooks, 1991; Medin *et al.*, 1984), the novel category was intended to capture some of the characteristics of categories spontaneously formed over the course of ordinary life. Specifically, we created a set of realistically illustrated, biologically plausible animals with variable features. Furthermore, in forming the category around a prototype, we designated membership based on presence of features that were empirically determined to contribute particularly strongly to subjective assessments of inter-item resemblance. Hence, while the category was novel, it was psychologically coherent rather than arbitrary, and presumably at least somewhat reflective of "real-life" experience.

Our stimuli were a set of 64 novel animals representing all possible combinations of six features, each having two values, e.g. a long or a short snout, or a straight or a curly tail. We chose one animal at random as the prototype, and constructed a category based on the four features that had been previously established as contributing most to perceived resemblance among items. The remaining two features varied randomly and were irrelevant to category membership, thus capturing some of the complexity and "noise" of naturally formed categories. Animals with at least three of the four prototypical features were designated as members; low-distortion items were those animals with exactly two of those features, and high-distortion items had no more than one. (Examples are shown in Figure 10.1.) Training pairs were created by forming 40 unique combinations of eight members and eight high-distortion items, and these pairs were presented in sequence via computer. There were two training conditions, Similarity and Rule. Participants were taught about an animal called a *crutter* in both conditions, but in different ways: for similarity-based training, the training pairs were accompanied by the prototype, presented as an example of a *crutter* (see Figure 10.2, top), and participants were asked to select which animal in each pair was likewise a *crutter* based on its overall resemblance to the example. For rule-based training, the training pairs were accompanied by captioned outline drawings of the four relevant features (see Figure 10.2, bottom). Participants were told that an animal called a *crutter* must have at least three of these features, and they were asked to select which animal in each pair was a *crutter* based on its adherence to the at-least-three-features rule. Feedback was provided by the experimenter for each trial. Testing was identical following both training conditions: participants saw the entire set of 64 animals in sequence, that is, the full array of members, low-distortion, and high-distortion items, and judged whether each was or was not a *crutter*, in accordance with how they had been trained. No feedback was given. To ensure that patients' responses reflected the categorization processes of interest rather than episodic memory, participants were provided with a "reminder" card at test, showing the prototype following similarity-based training, or the four relevant features following rule-based training. This standard technique for testing amnesic patients has been shown to reveal patterns of performance that would otherwise be masked by floor effects resulting from episodic memory impairment

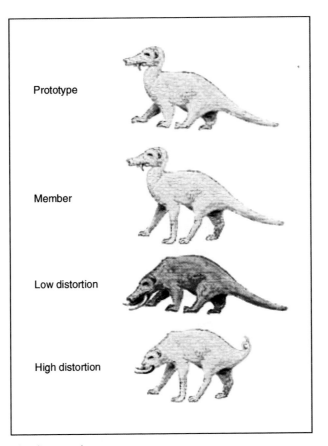

Figure 10.1. Stimulus samples.

(Oscar-Berman & Samuels, 1977). Patients participated in both conditions at least six weeks apart, in order to avoid influence of one categorization condition over the other; healthy individuals participated in one condition only.

Our measure of performance was frequency of endorsement at test for each of the three types of stimulus items; that is, how often members, low-distortion items, and high-distortion items were deemed *crutters*. Consider what a hypothetical "perfect learner" would do: following similarity-based training, the perfect learner would endorse items in accordance with their general resemblance to the prototype. Thus members would be endorsed most of the time and high-distortion items would usually be rejected. However, low-distortion items would be equivocal, as they resemble high-distortion items as much as they resemble the prototype; consequently, endorsing them as *crutters* would be a "judgment call." Hence the perfect learner would endorse them about half the time. In short, the perfect learner's endorsement patterns for similarity-based categorization would

Similarity-based training

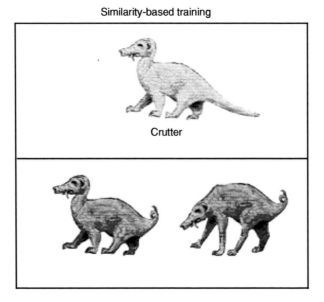

Crutter

Rule-based training

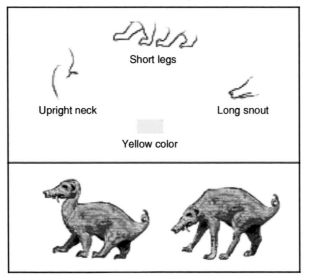

Short legs

Upright neck   Long snout

Yellow color

Figure 10.2. Training trial displays.

be graded in accordance with each item's overall resemblance to the prototype, and an item's overall resemblance would reflect the extent to which the item contained prototypical features. In contrast, rule-based categorization requires that only members be endorsed as such. Thus the perfect learner would endorse *all* members, and reject *all* other items, resulting in a sharply bounded or categorical endorsement pattern. The crucial distinction between rule-based and similarity-based categorization, then, would lie in the judgments of low-distortion items: they would receive chance endorsements by similarity-based criteria, but would be rejected by rule-based criteria.

Among the neurologically impaired participants were 17 patients with probable Alzheimer's disease (AD) and six patients with semantic dementia (SD), one of the phenotypes associated with FTD. Patients were mildly to moderately impaired; demographic information and Mini Mental State Examination (MMSE) scores (Folstein *et al.*) are summarized in Table 10.1. While the hallmark of AD is episodic memory loss, semantic memory impairment is also common, and has been observed in 30–50 percent of patients with AD (Grossman *et al.*, 1996, submitted). In addition, difficulties with executive resources have been demonstrated in AD (LaFleche & Albert, 1995; Libon *et al.*, 2007; Patterson *et al.*, 1996; Perry & Hodges *et al.*, 1999), suggesting that individuals with this disease should have particular difficulty with rule-based processes, consistent with the results in the familiar-category study mentioned above (Grossman *et al.*, 2003). SD, in contrast, is characterized by semantic rather than episodic memory loss, clinically manifested in deficits of single word comprehension, object comprehension, and naming (Lambon Ralph *et al.*, 2001; Libon *et al.*, 2007; Rogers *et al.*, 2004). To the extent that these patients' semantic impairment reflects lost content rather than impaired processing, rule-based categorization should be preserved, particularly as participants are provided with the feature knowledge associated with *crutters*.

We identified AD patients with impaired semantic memory for familiar objects and words using the Semantic Category Decision task (Grossman *et al.*, 1996). This involves judging the category membership status of pictures and printed words for two probe categories, VEGETABLES and CARPENTER'S TOOLS. For each probe category, half of the test items are category members (e.g. *celery* is a kind of VEGETABLE). The remaining half

Table 10.1. Mean (standard deviation) participant demographics

Group	Sex	Age (yrs)	Education (yrs)	MMSE (max = 30)
Healthy elderly	13f, 7m	68.2 (6.2)	15.1 (2.5)	29.1 (1.2)
SD	2f, 4m	61.0 (6.3)	15.8 (3.4)	23.0 (4.9)
AD	9f, 8m	73.6 (7.0)	14.9 (3.5)	21.6 (3.3)

Note: Education level was equivalent among groups, $F(2,39) = 0.16$, ns. Patient groups differed in age, $t(21) = 3.88$, $p < 0.001$, reflecting the typically later onset of AD relative to SD. Patient MMSE scores did not differ, $t(21) = 0.75$, ns.

includes nonmember foils. Half of these foils are semantically *unrelated* (e.g. for the category VEGETABLE, unrelated foils include kinds of TOOLS and FURNITURE like *lamp*), and half are semantically *related* (e.g. for the category VEGETABLE, kinds of FRUIT like *banana*). For the CARPENTER'S TOOL category, the unrelated foils are exemplars of FRUITS and VEGETABLES, and the related foils are FURNITURE. Patients are shown items blocked by probe category and by presentation modality, and respond "yes" or "no" to the question "*Is this a vegetable?*" for half of the trials and to the question "*Is this a carpenter's tool?*" for the remaining half. Hence task demands are minimal: naming and word generation are not involved, so that difficulty with word retrieval is not a factor. Executive search strategies and self-generated concept production, as in category naming tasks, are not required. In addition, episodic memory is not involved. The performance on the Semantic Category Decision task by patients who participated in the *crutters* study was closely correlated with their performance on the Pyramids & Palm Trees task, a standard assessment of semantic impairment, $r = 0.86$, $p < 0.01$.

Scoring for the Semantic Category Decision task reflected category membership decision accuracy out of the total of 48 stimuli. The six SD patients' mean score was 36.5 (76 percent correct), and scores did not exceed 43. This was significantly impaired relative to the performance of the healthy elderly partic-ipants ($t(14) = 3.60$; $p < 0.01$), whose mean score was 45.1 (94 percent correct). We divided the AD patients into two groups: the eight "semantically impaired" AD patients' scores matched those of the SD patients, that is, they also did not exceed 43, with a mean of 39.1 (81 percent correct) that is statistically equivalent to SD patients ($t(12) = 0.92$; ns) and differed significantly from controls ($t(15) = 5.45$; p < 0.01). The nine "semantically normal" AD patients all scored above 43, with a higher mean of 46.2 (96 percent correct). This did not differ from control subjects ($t(17) = 1.72$; ns).

We did not expect any of our participants — even the neurologically healthy ones — to be perfect learners. Rather, we looked for approximations of the process-specific patterns, and adopted two criteria: first, the endorsement patterns for the two conditions must be characteristically distinct (as captured in an analysis of variance (ANOVA) showing an interaction between process-specific training and stimulus endorsement scores). Second, following rule-based training, the differences between endorsement of members and low-distortion items must exceed the difference between low-distortion and high-distortion items. This captures the rule-based categorical process of endorsing members while rejecting both low- and high-distortion items. Figure 10.3 shows the test results. All participant groups demonstrated successful similarity-based categorization to an equivalent degree; that is, judgment profiles were graded, and an ANOVA showed

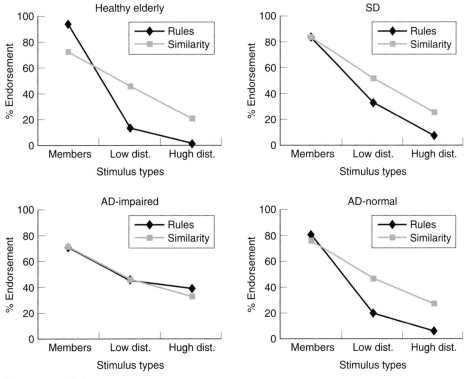

Figure 10.3. Endorsements at test.

no overall differences among participant groups $(F(3,28) = 0.51$, ns) nor any group by stimulus type interaction $(F(6,56) = 1.09$, ns). However, there were distinctions following rule-based training: the healthy seniors showed a pattern of judgments characteristic of rule-based categorization with the requisite interaction, $F(2,36) = 31.5$, $p = 0.001$. The AD-normal patients subgroup and the SD patients both demonstrated some success at rule-based categorization, $F(2,28) = 4.95$, $p = 0.01$ and $F(2,16) = 3.15$, $p = 0.07$, respectively. However, the subgroup of AD patients with a semantic memory impairment performed no differently than they had following similarity-based training. That is, the AD-impaired subjects alone were completely unable to categorize the novel animal stimuli in a manner consistent with rule-based processing. The SD patients and the AD-normal patients thus demonstrated comparable success at rule-based categorization, despite the differences in their semantic memory and despite SD patients' difficulties with categorization demonstrated in two tasks involving familiar objects, i.e. the Semantic Category Decision task and the "pizza versus quarter" study.

SD patients and the subgroup of AD patients who were not semantically impaired were both able to categorize the novel animal stimuli by applying rules.

The AD patients in the subgroup who were semantically impaired at a level comparable to the SD patients, in contrast, were unable to categorize by rules. However, both the SD patients and the semantically impaired AD patients had difficulties categorizing the related foils on the Semantic Category Decision task; that is, they tended to endorse *bananas* as VEGETABLES and *lamps* as TOOLS, but never endorsed *lamps* as VEGETABLES or *bananas* as TOOLS. We posit that judging related foils, but not related foils, requires rule-based processing, as the judgment involves selecting appropriate features to distinguish the related foils from the probe category, whose members they resemble but to which they do not belong. Furthermore, we have posited that rule-based processing deficits reflect executive resource-related difficulties with the rule-based process. The results of the novel animal study suggest that the semantically impaired AD patients are deficient in applying rules to what they know, while the SD patients have degraded content knowledge for known objects, since their rule-based categorization ability is as least partially intact. We find support for these conclusions in other observations concerning these patient populations: SD patients can be retaught formerly familiar objects (Graham *et al.*, 1999), although the information is not retained over the long run. Presenting novel objects and providing explicit criteria for categorizing them seems comparable to reteaching degraded content knowledge for familiar objects. When content knowledge is available in SD, the processes that act on it thus seem to still be available. AD patients, by comparison, are known to have executive resource deficits. In assessing our entire group of AD patients with standard clinical tests of executive functions such as working memory, planning/switching, attention, and inhibitory control, we found significant correlations between success on those assessments and success at categorizing novel *crutters* by rules (ranging from $r = 0.56$ to $r = 0.79$, $p < 0.05$). However, no such correlation was found with episodic memory, the hallmark deficit of AD ($r = 0.08$; ns). Moreover, AD patients' success at the Semantic Category Decision task correlated highly with their success at categorizing *crutters* by rules ($r = 0.84$; $p < 0.01$), but not with categorizing them by similarity-based judgments ($r = 0.01$; ns) (Koenig *et al.* 2007). Hence, even when content information and the nature of the rules were readily available, AD patients who demonstrated impaired categorization of familiar objects were unable to muster the resources necessary to attend to, evaluate, and keep track of the requisite features for using rules to identify a *crutter*.

This interpretation of semantic memory functioning in SD and AD is consistent with the pattern of cortical activation seen in an fMRI study using these novel animal materials in healthy young adults (Koenig *et al.*, 2005). Subjects participated in either similarity-based or rule-based training, followed by a test period, while in the scanner. At test, activation during similarity-based processing was seen in temporal-parietal cortex, the region playing a critical role in the integration of feature knowledge represented in sensory association cortex. We also observed activation in anterior prefrontal cortex and posterior cingulate, areas important for the successful recall of previously encountered knowledge such as the *crutter* stimuli used during the training period. By comparison, rule-based categorization at test showed activation of cortical regions that support executive resources such as anterior cingulate, inferior frontal, and parietal cortices.

The novel animal categorization task was designed to separate content from process and to relate the findings to semantic memory. We have concluded from our *crutters* study that there is a processing deficit in AD patients stemming from their impaired executive resources, and a deficit in SD due to degradation of previously acquired knowledge. However, there is a finer grain of content knowledge that the study leaves unaddressed. A patient with intact feature knowledge but who cannot correctly classify a *carrot* as a VEGETABLE may be unable to use rules to selectively attend to the appropriate feature *edible root* from among the other salient features of color, texture, and shape. An alternate explanation is that the patient could have retained knowledge of the features and could be potentially able to attend to a particular one, but could have lost the knowledge associated with a feature that indicates its diagnosticity. That is, the patient no longer knows that *edible root* is diagnostic of the category VEGETABLE, and that *orange color* is not. Since the *crutter* study clearly specified which features were diagnostic, the nature of content knowledge loss in SD was not addressed.

Another study from our lab suggests that it is feature diagnosticity, rather than general feature knowledge, that is degraded in SD — at least in the relatively early stages of the disease represented by the patients who participated in these studies. This study was modeled after a classic investigation into concept development in children by Susan Carey (1999). It involves inductive reasoning about the presence of features in various things, both living and nonliving, that represent a continuum of decreasing resemblance to *human beings*. Participants are told that *human beings* have some particular biological property, e.g. a *methylmalonic enzyme*, and are then asked whether each of the other items likewise contains that property. The other living items, in order of decreasing resemblance to *humans*, include stimuli such as *cat*, *squirrel*, and *spider*; the manufactured items include *robot*, *doll*, and *bicycle*. Neurologically healthy adults and AD patients seem to base their decisions about the presence of the newly taught property on two factors: the target item's resemblance to humans, and the target item's category membership status as living or man-made. Thus both AD patient and healthy control groups think that a *cat* is somewhat more likely than a *squirrel* to have a *methylmalonic enzyme*, and a *squirrel* is somewhat more likely to have it than a *spider*. They also think that a *robot* is somewhat more likely to have the property than a *doll*, and a *doll* is somewhat more likely to have the property than a *bicycle*. However, they will think that a *spider* is *much* more likely to have a *methylmalonic enzyme* than a *robot* is. That is, the AD patients and healthy seniors recognize the categorical break between living and manufactured things, even within the context of a continuum, and they do not assume that a property of humans and animals is present in man-made objects. In contrast, SD patients seem to base their decisions exclusively on the target item's resemblance to *humans*. That is, their judgments about the presence of the property appear to mirror the continuum of resemblance to *humans*, but their decisions do not reflect the categorical distinction between living and nonliving things.

We posit that the systematically graded responses by the SD patients reflect their having retained enough content knowledge about the target objects to make inter-item comparisons. Such knowledge retention is also consistent with their accuracy in classifying unrelated foils in the Semantic Category Decision task. For instance, SD patients may know that a *cat*, like a *human*, has a head, and that a *squirrel*, like a *cat*, has four legs, and that a *robot*, like a *squirrel*, moves about. They may also know that *humans*, *cats*, and *squirrels* breathe, unlike *robots* — but they may have lost the knowledge that marks *breathing* as a crucial feature that distinguishes living things like *humans*, *cats*, and *squirrels* from *robots* and the other manufactured objects. AD patients, whose deficits are due to a processing limitation rather than degraded semantic content, seem to have retained both feature knowledge and knowledge of the diagnostic status of these features.

We have characterized most inquiries into semantic memory as content-focused. In particular, such work apparently seeks to explain category-specific deficits through appeals to the distinguishing nature of a category's features, and hypothesizes that each separate set of features is stored in a partially distinct portion of the brain. The "sensory–motor" hypothesis and the "distributed" hypothesis specifically contrast feature representations for natural kinds and manufactured objects. Our results are not mutually exclusive of these hypotheses. However, *crutters* are distinguishable only by a subset of visual features, and the descriptions in the familiar-category study could involve only a limited set of objects, so we could not systematically investigate the role of specific feature knowledge posited by the "sensory–motor" hypothesis. Because we created the *crutter* stimuli to have a set number of features and a set range of feature overlap, we may have violated characteristics of real-world feature distributions that contribute to the "distributed" hypothesis. Our study is even somewhat compatible with the "evolutionary" hypothesis: in establishing the relative contributions of our novel animals' six variable features to judged inter-item resemblance, we found that *heads* were overwhelmingly more salient than *tails*. That is, all of our participating judges were more likely to evaluate two animals with identical heads as highly similar than two animals with identical tails, even though the objective distinctions between tail shapes were greater than the distinctions between head shapes. In addition, when asked to specify the animals' most noticeable feature, viewers generally indicated the color, even though color contributed only weakly to resemblance assessments. These discrepancies suggest that perceptual salience was not the overriding factor in categorizing our novel stimuli; that is, *crutters* constitute a conceptual category, rather than a purely perceptual one. We speculate that the *crutters'* convincingly animal-like appearance caused viewers, including neurologically impaired patients, to regard them as they would actual animals. A tendency to attend to heads more than tails could be hard-wired, reflecting the special status of our mental representations of the natural world.

Rather than contradicting existing theories about semantic memory, our findings summarized above suggest that those theories may not account for the whole story. Processing matters, and it may be that category-specific deficits arise because different categories are more or less conducive to particular categorization processes, which can be selectively compromised. Additionally, knowledge of the diagnostic status of features, as well as executive resources, appears to be a necessary component of rule-based processing: if TOOLS are identified by critical features, then perhaps whether one identifies a *drill* by knowledge of its hole-boring function or by visual representation of its characteristic spiraled bit is less important than knowing which features are critical, be they visual, functional, or motor. And, once known, features must be appropriately integrated to form coherent concepts. Thus content and process have interactive roles in semantic memory.

REFERENCES

Allen, S. W. and Brooks, L. R. (1991). Specializing the operation of an explicit rule. *Journal of Experimental Psychology: General*, **120**: 3—17.

Ashby, F. G., Alfonso-Reese, L. A., Turken, U., and Waldron, E. M. (1998). A neuropsychological theory of multiple systems in category learning. *Psychological Review*, **105**: 442—81.

Cappa, S. F., Binetti, G., Pezzini, A., Padovani, A., Rozzini, L., and Trabucchi, M. (1998). Object and action naming in Alzheimer's disease and Fronto-temporal dementia. *Neurology*, **50**: 351—5.

Caramazza, A. (1998). The interpretation of semantic category-specific deficits: what do they reveal about the organization of conceptual knowledge in the brain? *Neurocase*, **4**: 265—72.

Carey, S. (1999) Sources of conceptual change. In E. K. Scholnick (ed.), *Conceptual Development: Piaget's Legacy*, Mahwah, NJ: Lawrence Erlbaum, pp. 293—325.

Chertkow, H. and Bub, D. N. (1990). Semantic memory loss in dementia of the Alzheimer's type: what do the various measures measure? *Brain*, **113**: 397–417.

Farah, M. J. and McClelland, J. L. (1991). A computational model of semantic impairment: modality specificity and emergent category specificity. *Journal of Experimental Psychology: General*, **120**: 339–57.

Folstein, M. F., Folstein, S. F., and McHugh, P. R. (1975). "Mini Mental State." A practical method for grading the cognitive state of patients for the clinician. *Journal of Psychiatric Research*, **12**: 189–98.

Garrard, P., Lambon Ralph, M. A., Watson, P. C., Powis, J., Patterson, K., and Hodges, J. R. (2001). Longitudinal profiles of semantic impairment for living and nonliving concepts in dementia of the Alzheimer's type. *Journal of Cognitive Neuroscience*, **13**: 892–909.

Garrard, P., Patterson, K., Watson, P. C., and Hodges, J. R. (1998). Category specific semantic loss in dementia of Alzheimer's type: functional–anatomic correlations from cross-sectional analyses. *Brain*, **121**: 633–46.

Gonnerman, L. M., Andersen, E. S., Devlin, J. T., Kempler, D., and Seidenberg, M. S. (1997). Double dissociation of semantic categories in Alzheimer's disease. *Brain and Language*, **57**: 254–79.

Graham, K. S., Patterson, K., Pratt, K. H., and Hodges, J. R. (1999). Relearning and subsequent forgetting of semantic category exemplars in a case of semantic dementia. *Neuropsychology*, **13**: 359–80.

Grossman, M., D'Esposito, M., Hughes, E., Onishi, K., Biassou, N., White-Devine, T., and Robinson, K. M. (1996). Language comprehension difficulty in Alzheimer's disease, vascular dementia, and fronto-temporal degeneration. *Neurology*, **47**: 183–9.

Grossman, M., Smith, E. E., Koenig, P., Glosser, G., Rhee, J., and Dennis, K. (2003). Categorization of object descriptions in Alzheimer's disease and frontotemporal dementia: limitation in rule-based processing. *Cognitive, Affective, and Behavioral Neuroscience*, **3**(2): 120–32.

Johansen, M. K. and Palmeri, T. J. (2002). Are there representational shifts during category learning? *Cognitive Psychology*, **45**: 482–553.

Knowlton, B. J. and Squire, L. R. (1996). Artificial grammar learning depends on implicit acquisition of both abstract and exemplar-specific information. *Journal of Experimental Psychology: Leaning, Memory, and Cognition*, **22**: 169–81.

Koenig, P., Smith, E. E., Glosser, G., DeVita, C., Moore, P., McMillan, C., Gee, J., and Grossman, G. (2005). The neural basis for novel semantic categorization. *NeuroImage*, **24**: 369–83.

Koenig, P., Smith, E. E., and Grossman, G. (2006). Semantic categorisation of novel objects in frontotemporal dementia. *Cognitive Neuropsychology*. **23**: 541–62.

Koenig, P., Smith, E. E., Moore, P., Glosser, G., and Grossman, M. (2007). Categorization of novel animals by patients with Alzheimer's disease and corticobasal degeneration. *Neuropsychology*.

Kramer, J. H., Jurik, J., and Sha, S. J. (2003). Distinctive neuropsychological patterns of frontotemporal dementia, semantic dementia, and Alzheimer's Disease. *Cognitive and Behavioral Neurology*, **16**: 211–18.

LaFleche, D. and Albert, M. S. (1995). Executive function deficits in mild Alzheimer's disease. *Neuropsychology*, **9**: 313–20.

Lambon-Ralph, M. A., McClelland, J. L., Patterson, K., Galton, C. J., and Hodges, J. R. (2001). No right to speak? The relationship between object naming and semantic impairment: neuropsychological evidence and a computational model. *Journal of Cognitive Neuroscience*, **13**: 341–66.

Libon, D. J., Xie, S. X., Moore, P., Farmer, J., Antani, S., McCawley, G., Cross, K., and Grossman, M. (2007). Patterns of neuropsychological impairment in frontotemporal dementia: A factor analytic study.

Medin, D. L., Altom, M. W., and Murphy, T. D. (1984). Given versus induced category representations: Use of prototype and exemplar information in classification. *Journal of Experimental psychology: Learning, Memory, and Cognition*, **1013**: 333–52.

Medin, D. L., Goldstone, R. L., and Gentner, D. (1993). Respects for similarity. *Psychological Review*, **100**: 254–78.

Medin, D. L. and Schaffer, M. M. (1978). A context theory of classification learning. *Psychological Review*, **85**: 207–38.

Montanes, P., Goldblum, M. C., and Boller, F. (1995). The naming impairment of living and nonliving items in Alzheimer's disease. *Journal of the International Neuropsychological Society*, **1**: 39–48.

Moss, H. E. and Tyler, L. K. (2000). A progressive category-specific deficit for non-living things. *Neuropsychologia*, **38**: 60–82.

Oscar-Berman, M. and Samuels, I. (1977). Stimulus preference and memory factors in Korsakoff's syndrome. *Neuropsychologia*, **15**(1): 99–106.

Patalano, A., Smith, E. E., Jonides, J., and Koeppe, R. (2001). PET evidence for multiple strategies of categorization. *Cognitive, Affective, and Behavioral Neuroscience*, **1**: 360–70.

Patterson, M. B., Mack, J. L., Geldmacher, D. S., and Whitehouse, P. J. (1996). Executive functions and Alzheimer's disease: problems and prospects. *European Journal of Neurology*, **3**: 5–15.

Perry, R. J. and Hodges, J. R. (1999). Attention and executive deficits in Alzheimer's disease: a critical review. *Brain*, **122**: 383–404.

Reber, P. J., Stark, C. E. L., and Squire, L. R. (1998). Cortical areas supporting category learning identified using functional MRI. *Proceedings of the National Academy of Sciences*, **95**: 747–50.

Rips, L. J. (1989). Similarity, typicality, and categorization. In S. Vosniadou and A. Ortony (eds.), *Similarity and analogical reasoning*. Cambridge: Cambridge University Press, pp. 21–59.

Rogers, T. T., Lambon Ralph, M. A., Garrard, P., Bozeat, S., McClelland, J. L., Hodges, J. R., and Patterson, K. (2004). Structure and deterioration of semantic memory: a neuropsychological and computational investigation. *Psychological Review*, **111**: 205–35.

Silveri, M. C., Daniele, A., Giustolisi, L., and Gainotti, G. (1991). Dissociation between living and nonliving things in dementia of the Alzheimer type. *Neurology*, **41**: 545–6.

Sloman, S. A. and Rips, L. J. (1998). Similarity as an explanatory construct. *Cognition*, **65**: 87–101.

Smith, E. E. and Medin, D. L. (1981). *Categories and Concepts.* Cambridge, MA: Harvard University Press.

Smith, E. E. and Sloman, S. A. (1994). Similarity- versus rule-based categorization. *Memory and Cognition*, **22**: 377–86.

Smith, E. E., Langston, C., and Nisbett, R. E. (1992). The case for rules in reasoning. *Cognitive Science*, **16**: 1–40.

Smith, E. E., Patalano, A. L., and Jonides, J. (1998). Alternative strategies of categorization. *Cognition*, **65**: 167–96.

Warrington, E. K. (1975). The selective impairment of semantic memory. *Quarterly Journal of Experimental Psychology*, **27**: 635–57.

Warrington, E. K. and Shallice, T. (1984). Category specific semantic impairments. *Brain*, **107**: 829–54.

11

The conceptual structure account: A cognitive model of semantic memory and its neural instantiation

Kirsten I. Taylor[1,2], Helen E. Moss[1], and Lorraine K. Tyler[1]

[1]University of Cambridge, England
[2]University Hospital Basel, Switzerland

The work described in this chapter is motivated by the conviction that a cognitive theory of semantic memory is best suited to investigate the functional and neural bases of the semantic memory system. The advantage of this approach is that detailed hypotheses about the structure and function of the semantic system can be formulated and then tested in behavioral experiments with healthy individuals and neurologically impaired patients. The challenge is then to identify the neural correlates of these experimentally validated cognitive structures and processes, i.e. their neural substrates and mechanisms. The cognitive model provides a detailed framework for this investigation which, when combined with the appropriate functional−neuroanatomical technique, provides the potential to meet this challenge.

The first part of this chapter describes the Conceptual Structure Account (CSA), a cognitive model developed at the Centre for Speech, Language and the Brain. We will present the results of neuropsychological studies with patients and healthy volunteers that have tested the main claims of this model.[1] The CSA has been the driving force in the generation of hypotheses on the neural organization of semantic memory. In the second part of this chapter, we will describe our attempts to investigate the neural instantiation of the CSA using functional imaging techniques. In particular, we will concentrate on our recent research efforts which have combined the hypotheses of the CSA with those of a hierarchical model of object processing in the ventral temporal lobe, developed in nonhuman primates,

---

[1] A discussion of the computational modeling studies investigating the CSA lie beyond the scope of this chapter, and can be found elsewhere (Durrant-Peatfield et al., 1997; Greer et al., 2001; Moss et al., 2002; Randall et al., 2004; Tyler et al., 2000a).

This research was supported by an MRC Programme Grant to LKT. The support of the Roche Research and Olga Mayenfisch Foundations is gratefully acknowledged (KIT).

to guide the fine-grained testing of neural systems involved in semantic memory of objects (Bright *et al.*, 2005; Moss *et al.*, 2005; Tyler *et al.*, 2004).

11.1   The conceptual structure account: a cognitive model of semantic memory

11.1.1   The model

Patients with selective deficits in one specific category of knowledge have stimulated the development of exciting new classes of neural models of semantic memory. The most common form of these category-specific semantic deficits is an impairment for living things (Forde & Humphreys, 1999), a pattern we will focus on in the current text. One class of models that have been proposed to account for this pattern are modular in nature: they postulate that neuroanatomically distinct regions house different categories or domains (i.e. living and nonliving things) of knowledge (e.g. the categories of living animate, living inanimate, conspecifics, and perhaps tools; Caramazza & Shelton, 1998; Caramazza & Mahon, 2003, 2005) or the features that typify living and nonliving things (e.g. visual semantic features central to the representation of living things, functional semantic features for nonliving things; Warrington & McCarthy, 1983, 1987; Warrington & Shallice, 1984; see also Martin & Chao, 2001; Martin *et al.*, 2000, for a more recent characterization of this view). Alternatively, Tranel and colleagues (Tranel *et al.*, 1997) suggested that distinct neural regions do not actually store concept representations belonging to different categories (e.g. persons, animals, and tools), but rather are critical for the concerted retrieval of information belonging to the concepts in different categories. Category-specific semantic deficits for living things are hypothesized to arise when the neural tissue housing e.g. animals (Caramazza & Shelton, 1998), the visual semantic features claimed to be central to the representation of living things (Warrington & McCarthy, 1987), or the region responsible for retrieving features belonging to animals (Tranel *et al.*, 1997) is damaged.

However, two aspects of the qualitative neuropsychological performances of patients with category-specific semantic deficits for living things appear at odds with modular theories and provided the impetus for an alternative account of these deficits. First, patients' performances with concepts from the "spared," nonliving domain are rarely within normal limits; nor do patients lose all information about concepts in the impaired, living domain. Instead, their deficits are graded, with *relatively* more deficient performance with living compared to nonliving things (Moss *et al.*, 2002). This pattern is inconsistent with a modular view that proposes that different domains of knowledge are represented in distinct neural regions. Secondly, the *kind* of conceptual information about living things that is lost is relatively specific: those features of a living thing that distinguish it from other concepts in the category are impaired (e.g. that a tiger *has stripes*), while the information that many living things share (i.e. nondistinctive information) is typically spared (e.g. that a *tiger has four legs, has a tail* and *has eyes*; Moss *et al.*, 1998, see also Hart & Gordon, 1992). This pattern of feature loss is strikingly evident in the drawings of a herpes simplex encephalitis (HSE) patient (SE) who presented with a category-specific semantic impairment for living things (see Figure 11.1). SE's drawings of nonliving things contained both distinctive and nondistinctive features, allowing these objects to be distinguished from one another and identified (Figure 11.1a). His depictions of animals, on the other hand, contained nondistinctive information that typically co-occurs in many animals (e.g. *four legs, has a tail*), but lacked the distinctive features required to uniquely identify each animal (e.g. the hump of a camel; see Figure 11.1b; target concepts in figure footnote; Moss *et al.*, 1997). Since modular theories do not distinguish between these two kinds of features, they are not able to explain how SE's brain damage resulted in the selective impairment of the distinctive features of animals without additional assumptions about the internal organization of separate categories of knowledge.

These two observations — the graded nature of category-specific semantic deficits and the specificity with which certain kinds of features are damaged — were among those central to the development of the Conceptual Structure

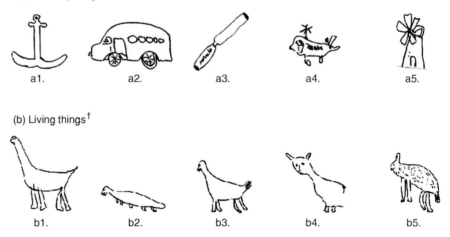

(a) Nonliving things*

a1.   a2.   a3.   a4.   a5.

(b) Living things†

b1.   b2.   b3.   b4.   b5.

*a1. anchor; a2. bus; a3. chisel; a4. helicopter; a5. windmill
†b1. camel; b2. crocodile; b3. duck; b4. penguin; b5. zebra

Figure 11.1. Drawing performance of patient SE.

Account (CSA) of semantic memory (Tyler *et al.*, 2000a; Tyler & Moss, 2001). The basic assumptions in our model are that concepts are instantiated in a distributed connectionist system composed of units representing semantic properties and where the processing of a concept corresponds to overlapping patterns of activation across units representing the concept (Greer *et al.*, 2001; Moss *et al.*, 2002; Tyler & Moss, 2001; Tyler *et al.*, 2000a; see Devlin *et al.*, 1998; Masson, 1995; and McRae *et al.*, 1997, for similar proposals). Thus the CSA differs fundamentally from modular theories of semantic memory in that it contends that categories of knowledge are represented in a distributed network containing the conceptual features of all knowledge categories with no explicit category or domain boundaries. Such distributed systems are ideally suited to account for the neuropsychological findings of graded deficits, i.e. relatively poorer performance of one domain of knowledge over the other, as has been demonstrated by the graceful degradation of computational simulations of these systems (Devlin *et al.*, 1998; Plaut & Shallice, 1993). Moreover, the CSA adopts a set of claims about the nature of features in the distributed system which can explain the selective feature deficit in category-specific semantic impairments for living things. Specifically, the CSA proposes that all features in the distributed system vary in the extent to which they are shared by different concepts (or, alternatively, the degree to which they are distinctive for a particular concept) and the frequency with which they co-occur with other features. These two dimensions, distinctiveness and correlation, respectively, give rise to the internal structure of the semantic system.

SE's animal drawings (see Figure 11.1b) illustrate how some features can be more informative about a concept than others. Those features that are shared by many concepts, e.g. *has ears, has a tail*, are indicative of category membership (animals) but are not helpful in identifying what the specific object is, while other features (e.g. *has a hump*) are distinctive to certain objects and therefore much more informative about the object. Thus features vary in the extent to which they are shared or distinctive, with shared features typically indicating category membership and distinctive features being highly discriminatory and critical for the unique identification of a concept. Distinctive features therefore occupy a special status in object processing (identification, recognition), and appear to be those selectively lost in category-specific semantic deficits for living things.

But how could the semantic system be organized such that brain damage affects only the distinctive (but not shared) features of living (but not nonliving) things? A lower frequency of distinctive relative to shared features may provide part of the answer, as object and object feature familiarity are known to influence the vulnerability of objects to brain damage (Funnell & Sheridan, 1992; Funnell, 1995). However, patients show specific deficits with distinctive, living features compared to distinctive, nonliving features even when feature frequency is controlled for (Moss & Tyler, unpublished observations). The critical factor may not be the frequency of occurrence and associated familiarity, but the frequency of feature *co*-occurrence.

Features also vary in the degree to which they are correlated with, or co-occur with, other features (Cree & McRae, 2003; Devlin *et al.*, 1998; McRae *et al.*, 1997, 1999; Rosch, 1978): we rarely see a creature with eyes but no nose, and we rarely encounter a creature with eyes that cannot see. Thus the feature *has eyes* commonly co-occurs with other object features (*has a nose, can see*), the entire set being co-activated upon each encounter with an object. Within a Hebbian-like framework, this mutual co-activation is thought to strengthen the connections between the features, making highly correlated features more resilient to the effects of brain damage (Devlin *et al.*, 1998; Gonnerman *et al.*, 1997). Conversely, those features that do not typically co-occur (e.g. *has a hump, has a nose*) do not benefit from a strengthened association and are more vulnerable to the effects of brain damage.

Feature distinctiveness and correlation are two dimensions that are hypothesized to structure the semantic space (see Figure 11.2), with the former playing a critical role in object identification and the latter in protecting features from the effects of brain damage. The critical claim of the CSA, and that which differentiates it from similar models (Caramazza *et al.*, 1990; Devlin *et al.*, 1998; McRae *et al.*, 1997), is that distinctiveness and correlation interact with domain, giving rise to qualitatively different internal structures for living and nonliving things. In other words, the CSA claims that the two domains differ with respect to the degree to which their distinctive and shared object features are correlated with the other features of the object. While living things tend to have many shared, highly correlated properties (e.g. *has eyes, has a nose*; see also Humphreys *et al.*, 1988; Keil, 1986; Malt & Smith, 1984), their distinctive properties are weakly correlated with the object's other features (e.g. *has a hump, has a nose*). Nonliving things (e.g. tools), on the other hand, tend to have highly distinctive features that are

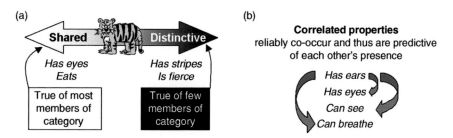

Figure 11.2. Dimensions manifesting the internal structure of concepts.

richly correlated with the other features of the nonliving object, partly as a result of strong form–function mappings (e.g. *has a blade* and *used for cutting*), whereas their shared features are relatively fewer in number and less densely correlated (e.g. *has a blade, has a handle*). Since correlated properties are more resilient to damage in this kind of network, the CSA predicts that the distinctive, but not shared, properties of living things will be particularly vulnerable to damage, while the distinctive features of nonliving things will be relatively spared by damage (see Figure 11.3). Clearly, distinctiveness and correlation are inversely related – highly distinctive properties occurring for only a few concepts tend to be less

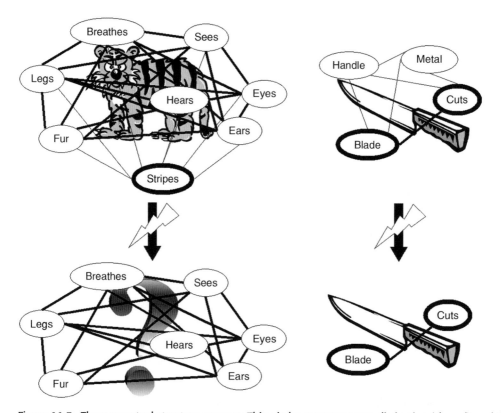

Figure 11.3. The conceptual structure account. Thin circles represent non-distinctive (shared) and thick circles distinctive features. Thin straight lines represent weak and thick lines strong correlations between features. The distinctive features of living things (left panel) are weakly correlated with other features, making them susceptible to damage, while the distinctive features of nonliving things (right panel) are strongly correlated, protecting them from damage. Since distinctive features are relatively more important for the identification of objects, brain damage will more likely result in a category-specific semantic impairment for living things.

correlated since they are infrequent. However, the CSA stresses the *relative*, and not absolute, differences in the degree of correlation between distinctive living and nonliving features. The experimental neuropsychological studies that test these central predictions of the CSA are presented below.

11.1.2   Behavioral evidence

Property generation studies

One way to acquire a model of a feature-based semantic system with which to test the CSA's claims is to ask healthy individuals to provide one. Accordingly, property generation studies instruct healthy participants to list all the features they can think of for specific concepts. The distinctiveness of properties can be estimated as the inverse of the number of concepts for which a property occurs (Devlin *et al.*, 1998). For example, a unique feature such as *has an udder*, which is listed for only one concept, would have a maximal distinctiveness value of 1 (1/1), whereas a shared feature such as *has fur* would have a low distinctiveness value (1/[a high number of concepts]). Features can also be categorized as distinctive or shared by setting an arbitrary cut-off point, e.g. distinctive features are those that occur in two or fewer concepts. The degree to which features co-occur with the other features of a concept can be estimated with Pearson product−moment correlations among feature pairs, as well as the number of feature pairs whose Pearson product−moment correlation exceeds an arbitrarily defined cut-off point (correlated property pairs; e.g. $p < 0.05$). The featural structures of concepts in the two domains can then be statistically compared (Greer *et al.*, 2001; McRae & Cree, 2002; McRae *et al.*, 2005; Randall *et al.*, 2004).

We conducted a property generation study in which 45 healthy participants listed the features of concepts belonging to the living (31 animals, 16 fruits) and nonliving (22 tools, 24 vehicles) domains (as well as 47 filler items; Randall *et al.*, 2004; see also Greer *et al.*, 2001). As illustrated in Table 11.1, living things had larger clusters of correlated features (CPPs; see also Devlin *et al.*, 1998; McRae *et al.*, 1993), but the mean distinctiveness of features was greater in the nonliving than living domain. The shared features of living things were more correlated with other features of living things than the shared features of nonliving things. Critically, however, the distinctive features of nonliving things were significantly more correlated with the other features of nonliving things than the distinctive features of living things. Thus these differences in the distinctiveness and correlation of features in the living and nonliving domains support the CSA's claims, providing a framework with which to explain category-specific semantic deficits for living things: since a high correlation is thought to protect features from the effects of brain damage, the relatively weakly correlated distinctive

Table 11.1. Results of a property generation study (n = 45) of 93 living (animals, fruits; n = 47) and nonliving (tools, vehicles; n = 46) concepts (Randall *et al.*, 2004)

	Living things	Nonliving things	*p*
Number of correlated property pairs (CPPs)[a]	**60**	25	<0.001
Mean distinctiveness[b] of properties	0.33	**0.45**	<0.001
Correlational strength[c] of shared properties	**0.35**	0.32	<0.001
Percentage of distinctive CPPs[d]	16	**30**	<0.001

[a]Defined as any property pair with a significant (*p* < 0.05) Pearson product–moment correlation.
[b]Defined as the inverse of the number of concepts for which a feature was listed.
[c]Defined as the mean correlation between a given feature and all other features of a concept.
[d]Defined as CPPs occurring in two or fewer concepts.

features of living things will be more vulnerable than the relatively more strongly correlated distinctive features of nonliving things. Since distinctive features are more important for the differentiation and identification of specific objects, this loss will pattern as a category-specific semantic deficit for living things.

Naturally, the internal structures of concepts in different categories in the living and nonliving domains are not identical, but vary slightly from the typical pattern described above. For example, vehicles tend to have more properties that are also more highly correlated and on average less distinctive than the properties of tools (but not as highly correlated or shared as the properties of animals). Therefore, the CSA predicts that patients with category-specific semantic impairments for living things will perform worse with vehicles than with tools (but not as poorly as with animals). This pattern has indeed been demonstrated in case studies of patients with category-specific semantic impairments (see Tyler & Moss, 2001). The internal structure of the fruits and vegetable category also deviates from the prototypical structure of living things: they have fewer distinctive properties, and these are even more weakly correlated than those of animals. Of course, the fruits and vegetable and the vehicle categories differ from other categories in their respective domains in many other ways. These differences are examined in detail by Cree & McRae (2003). Thus the CSA predicts that the fruits and vegetable category will be most impaired at any level of damage (Moss *et al.*, 2002). Indeed, an isolated category-specific semantic impairment for fruits and vegetables has been documented (Hart *et al.*, 1985; Sheridan & Humphreys, 1993), and some patients with category-specific semantic deficits for living things perform worse with fruits and vegetables than with animals (Bunn *et al.*, 1998; Laiacona *et al.*, 1997; but see De Renzi & Lucchelli, 1994). These patterns highlight a key premise of the CSA, namely that it is not domain per se, but the nature of the internal structure of the properties of concepts in these domains (and categories) that determine which domain (and category) will be spared and impaired following brain damage.

Neuropsychological patient studies

The CSA generates a number of predictions about the kinds of information and types of processes that will be impaired and spared in patients with category-specific semantic impairments. The most obvious prediction is that category-specific semantic impairments for living things should be more frequent than specific impairments with nonliving things, as indeed appears to be the case (see Forde & Humphreys, 1999; Gainotti, 2000 for overviews). As described above, the CSA proposes that the weak correlation of living things' distinctive features makes them vulnerable to the effects of brain damage, since correlation is thought to strengthen the association between features, a protective effect. A further consequence of this relationship is that as the severity of brain damage increases, more and more strongly correlated features will be lost. At the same time, we know that familiarity protects features from the effects of brain damage (Funnell & Sheridan, 1992; Funnell, 1995), such that, at comparable levels of correlation, more familiar, shared features will have an advantage over less familiar, distinctive features since the former are more frequent. Thus the CSA predicts that the distinctive properties of nonliving things will be affected at more severe levels of brain damage, resulting in an additional semantic impairment for nonliving things (i.e. a global semantic impairment). At the most severe level of brain damage, only the most strongly correlated and familiar features will survive. These features are most likely to be the shared features of living things, as they are greater in number and more highly correlated than the shared features of nonliving things (see Table 11.1). The availability of these shared features of living things will presumably support some conceptual processing of living things, such that the overall pattern of performance will cross over to reflect a category-specific semantic impairment for nonliving things[2] albeit in the context of very poor overall performance (see Figure 11.4a; Moss & Tyler, 2000; Moss et al., 2002; see also Moss et al., 1998).

Thus the CSA predicts that category-specific semantic impairments for nonliving things will be associated with severe damage to the semantic system. It follows that the detection of these patients may be hampered by their severe

---

[2] See Durrant-Peatfield et al. (1997), and Tyler et al. (2000a) for computational modeling support for these claims.

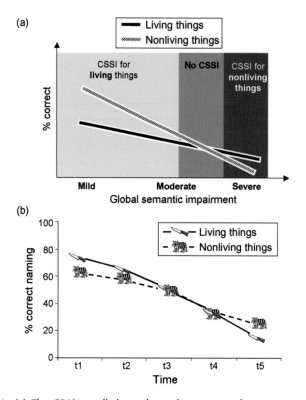

Figure 11.4. (a) The CSA's predictions about the pattern of category-specific semantic impairments at difference degrees of global semantic impairment (see text for details). (b) The longitudinal naming performance of a patient with progressive cerebral atrophy supports the prediction outlined in (a) (Moss & Tyler, 2000, 1997).

conceptual deficits. Published accounts of category-specific semantic impairments for nonliving things provide mixed support for this prediction: while two such patients suffered from severe global dysphasia (Warrington & McCarthy, 1983, 1987), others were mildly impaired (Hillis & Caramazza, 1991; Sacchett & Humphreys, 1992). A more informative approach might be the longitudinal assessment of patients with degenerative diseases affecting the semantic system. One such patient, ES, initially presented with semantic impairments which were either nonspecific or worse for living things, depending on the task. ES was tested biannually for 2.5 years with picture naming, spoken property verification, semantic priming, definition, and naming to description tasks. As predicted by the CSA, ES's performance on all but the naming to description tasks showed an increasing, selective impairment with nonliving compared to living things over time (Moss & Tyler, 1997, 2000; see also Moss *et al.*, 2002). The course of ES's picture naming performance was most striking: an initial disproportionate impairment for living things crossed over to a specific impairment for nonliving things with time (see Figure 11.4b). We documented a similar progressive, nonliving things deficit in a second progressive aphasic patient (AA; Moss *et al.*, 2002). These patterns are consistent with the CSA: at milder levels of damage, the most vulnerable, weakly correlated distinctive properties of living things are affected, resulting in a category-specific semantic deficit for living things. As damage to the semantic system progresses, the more highly correlated, less familiar distinctive features of nonliving things are affected, resulting in an additional impairment with nonliving things, i.e. no category-specific semantic deficit. At the most severe levels of damage, only the most highly correlated and familiar (shared) features are available. Since living things have many more correlated, shared features than nonliving things, performance, while poor on concepts from both domains, will be relatively better with living things; a category-specific semantic impairment for nonliving things emerges. A further implication of this set of claims is that not all patients with progressive neurodegenerative diseases affecting the semantic system will suffer from a category-specific semantic impairment for living things; instead, whether and which specific domain is impaired depends on the level of damage to the semantic system, i.e. what stage of the disease the patient is in (see Figure 11.4a).

Other authors have failed to find the predicted cross-over from a category-specific semantic impairment for living to nonliving things in cross-sectional studies of patients with Alzheimer's disease (Garrard *et al.*, 1998; Zannino *et al.*, 2002). Moreover, category-specific semantic impairments for nonliving things have been reported in patients with relatively mild impairments (Hillis & Caramazza, 1991; Sacchett & Humphreys, 1992). Thus this prediction of the CSA remains controversial. Additional longitudinal studies of patients with category-specific deficits for living things would help to resolve these conflicting findings.

The CSA also predicts that damage to a distributed featural system will result in graded, as opposed to all-or-none, deficits, with relatively greater impairments in the affected compared to the "spared" domain. This prediction was recently tested in a study with seven HSE patients who had varying degrees of category-specific semantic deficits for living things. The patients and a group of demographically matched control participants were tested on three semantic tasks: picture naming (Bunn *et al.*, 1998), word–picture matching and naming to verbal description. Figure 11.5 shows each patient's performance on all tasks and for each domain separately, as well as the ranges of the control participant's scores on each task (collapsed over domain; control participants performed at ceiling on the word–picture matching task). All patients performed poorer with living

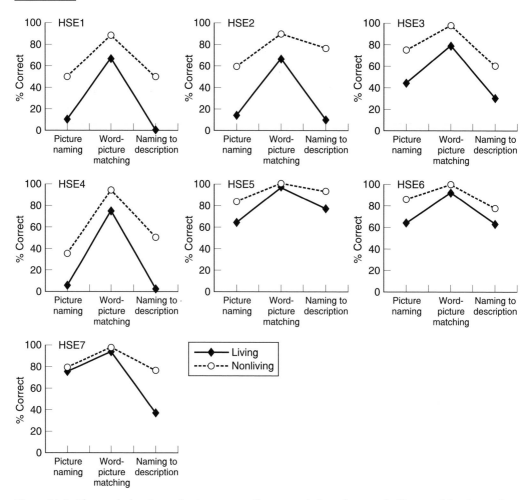

Figure 11.5. The graded nature of category-specific semantic impairments is illustrated by the performances of seven herpes simplex patients presenting with category-specific semantic impairments for living things.

compared to nonliving things. However, their performances with nonliving things were also moderately impaired, falling in most cases well below the range of the control participants' performances (Moss & Tyler, unpublished observations). These performance patterns illustrate the graded nature of deficits typically encountered in patients with "category-specific" semantic impairments, patterns we believe can most parsimoniously be explained by postulating a distributed featural system with no explicit category or domain boundaries (see also, e.g. Basso *et al.*, 1988; Moss *et al.*, 1998; Sartori and Job, 1988; Sartori *et al.*, 1993; Warrington & Shallice, 1984).

At the featural level, the CSA generates hypotheses about the types of features that will be impaired in patients with category-specific semantic deficits for living things. Specifically, the CSA claims that the distinctive, weakly correlated properties of living things will be disadvantaged relative to their shared, strongly correlated properties, and also with respect to the relatively strongly correlated shared and distinctive properties of nonliving things. This set of hypotheses can be directly tested with property verification tasks in which patients judge whether specific (living and nonliving) concepts have specific (shared and distinctive) features. For example, patients are asked: "butterfly — does it have legs?", "ambulance — does it have wheels?" (shared features), or "zebra — does it have black and white stripes?", "drum — is it round and hollow?" (distinctive features; filler and false trials are also included). We administered this task to an HSE patient (RC) with an established category-specific semantic deficit for living things. As predicted by the CSA, RC performed significantly worse with the distinctive features of living things compared to all other feature types (Moss *et al.*, 1998; see also Moss *et al.*, 2002). A specific deficit with the distinctive features of living things can also be demonstrated with other tasks, e.g. sorting concepts with respect to specific semantic properties (Moss *et al.*, 1998), and presumably underlies patients' impairments in e.g. naming and word—picture matching of living things: because such patients lack an appreciation of the distinctive visual features, living things become visually confusable and difficult to discriminate from one another and thus uniquely identify.

Patients with category-specific semantic deficits for living things still retain knowledge of the shared features of concepts in this domain. While not providing information about what the object is, features that are shared by many concepts are indicative of category membership (e.g. many animals *have four legs, have a tail, have eyes*, etc.). Therefore the CSA predicts that patients with category-specific semantic impairments for living things will indeed be able to perform some analyses of living things if the task requires access to category-level, as opposed to concept-level, information. This appears to be the case. For example, RC, although unable to identify individual exemplars of living things, could successfully sort these same exemplars into their appropriate superordinate category (Moss *et al.*, 1998). This interaction of task demands with conceptual structure (and indeed the precedence of task demands over domain per se) is a topic we will discuss in greater detail in the second part of this chapter.

We believe that the studies described above support the CSA's main claims. However, it is critical that the CSA be confirmed in studies with healthy individuals to ensure that the patients' behavioral performances reflected the workings of a merely incomplete but not a pathologically reorganized semantic system. Also, control participants typically provide more reliable measures of online semantic processing (RTs), and thus with the appropriate paradigms, control performances can offer further insights into the workings of the semantic memory system.

Studies with healthy participants

The effects of distinctiveness and correlation on online language comprehension have only recently become the focus of investigation in healthy participants. We will address studies attempting to tap automatic semantic processing, as untimed tasks or paradigms which elicit controlled processing may emphasize cognitive processes taking place outside the semantic system.

McRae and colleagues (1997) were the first to investigate how feature correlation affects online word comprehension with two different priming tasks. In a first priming study with prime and target concept words, similarity in terms of correlated features predicted response times (RTs) to living, but not nonliving concepts (i.e. the higher the correlation, the faster the RTs). McRae *et al.* suggested that the effects of correlation were not apparent with nonliving things because they contain fewer correlated features than living things (see above), and thus a decreased likelihood of observing the effect of correlation. In a second feature verification, priming task, participants were shown prime concepts (e.g. *deer*) followed by target features (e.g. *is hunted*) which were either weakly or strongly correlated with the concept's other features, and verified whether the features were true of the concept or not. Here, correlation strength predicted feature verification RTs to both living and nonliving things. Based on the behavior of an attractor network model designed to simulate these effects, McRae and colleagues suggested that the mutual activation among correlated features results in a faster "rise time" in activation, such that strongly correlated features reach a stable state of activation faster than weakly correlated features. This study has been replicated and extended in a second series of experiments by the same researchers (McRae *et al.*, 1999; see also McRae, 2004).

We recently performed a similar feature verification priming experiment with living and nonliving concepts to test a critical claim of the CSA. Based on the results of McRae *et al.*'s experiments (1997, 1999), we proposed that distinctive properties of living things would be disadvantaged compared to the distinctive properties of nonliving things as only the latter are highly correlated. We therefore hypothesized that the distinctive properties of living things would be activated more slowly than their shared properties, whereas no such effect would be evident for nonliving things. This was indeed what we found in a speeded feature

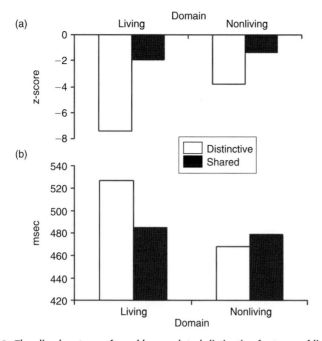

Figure 11.6. The disadvantage of weakly correlated distinctive features of living things as demonstrated by (a) the property verification performance (z-scores, where more negative values indicate increasingly worse performance compared to a control group) of a patient with Herpes Simplex Encephalitis presenting with a category-specific semantic impairment for living things (RC) and (b) the results of a speeded feature verification priming study.

verification task where the emphasis was on early activation of meaningful representations (Randall *et al.*, 2004; see Figure 11.6a). Moreover, no such interaction was evident in an untimed version of the task, suggesting that correlation affects the initial rise time of activation rather than the final level of activation when the network reaches a stable state. Significantly, these findings mirror RC's feature verification performance (described above and shown in Figure 11.6b), strongly suggesting that his deficits indeed reflected an incomplete, but not pathologically reorganized, semantic system, and providing converging evidence for one of the CSA's central claims.

We recently examined the effects of both correlation and distinctiveness of properties on normal, online language processing (Taylor *et al.*, 2004). This study employed a semantic priming paradigm, using a lexical decision task with the prime word denoting a concept (e.g. *elephant*) followed by a target word denoting one of its properties (e.g. *trunk*). We manipulated both the distinctiveness and correlation of the properties using published property norms (McRae *et al.*, in press), which resulted in conditions representing all four combinations (High/Low Distinctiveness × High/Low Correlation). We predicted that highly correlated properties would show greater online priming than weakly correlated properties (McRae *et al.*, 1997; Randall *et al.*, 2004). We also aimed to determine whether highly distinctive properties were likewise facilitated, and whether the effects of correlation and distinctiveness were additive. The multivariate analyses revealed that both increasing distinctiveness and correlation led to greater priming when the opposing variable was low, and that the two variables significantly interacted, such that when both distinctiveness and correlation were high, priming was reduced. This "interference" between the two variables was a surprising result. Exploration of the concept–property pairs in each condition revealed that the High Distinctiveness/High Correlation items had a significantly greater number of features per concept than did items in the other conditions. In a distributed semantic model with bidirectional lexical–semantic connections, word recognition of concepts with many features benefits from greater feedback of activation to the lexical level (Pexman *et al.*, 2003; see also Tyler *et al.*, 2000b). We therefore suggested that the greater feedback activation of the prime word led to an increased inter-lexical competition affecting the activation of the subsequent property target word, negating the advantages associated with the high correlation and distinctiveness of that property. We are currently investigating this and similar hypotheses in a new series of priming studies.

These studies illustrate how complex interactions between distinctiveness and correlation can determine the automatic activation of concept features during online processing. There are now several findings indicating that the number of features associated with a concept may also critically influence how concepts are activated: in the above study (Taylor *et al.*, 2004), the number of features associated with concepts appeared to negate the facilitatory effects of both distinctiveness and correlation on priming of lexical decisions; McRae *et al.* (1997) suggested that their lack of priming of *semantic* decisions[3] for nonliving things was due to their lower number of features, and, as reviewed above, we postulate that patients with severe levels of brain damage will show a category-specific semantic impairment for nonliving things since they have fewer correlated features with which to support the processing of these concepts. Thus this tripartite dimensional structure may provide the basis for emergent category differences in both intact

---

[3] Based on the semantic feedback activation hypothesis (Pexman *et al.*, 2002, 2003), we predict that opposite effects of number of features will be observed in priming tasks of lexical and semantic decisions (i.e. the level at which the target word is processed). The presentation of a prime concept with many features purportedly results in a large activation at the semantic level. This semantic activation feeds back to the orthographic level, i.e. to the orthographic representation of the prime and orthographic representation of semantically associated words. Lexical decisions to the target will be slowed, since semantic feedback activation will have created competition between the prime and target orthographic representations. However, semantic decisions to the target will be facilitated, since activation at the semantic level has co-activated semantically related representations.

and damaged semantic systems. Many more factors are known to influence semantic processing within the normal language system, and clearly the two domains differ with respect to a number of important factors (see, e.g. Cree & McRae, 2003). The objective of the CSA, however, is to determine the minimum number of factors that are both necessary and sufficient to explain category-specific semantic impairments.

11.2   The neural instantiation of the CSA

11.2.1   Category-specific vs. distributed neural systems

The fundamental assumption of the CSA is that semantic knowledge is represented in a distributed, featural system with no explicit category or domain boundaries. The most obvious inference of this assumption is that different categories or domains of knowledge are not represented in neuroanatomically distinct stores, and therefore processing of concepts in these categories or domains will not activate topographically distinct regions in functional imaging experiments. Yet several such studies have reported category- or domain-specific functional activation patterns, and have interpreted these findings as support for a modular organization of semantic knowledge (Cappa *et al.*, 1998; Martin *et al.*, 1996; Moore & Price, 1999; Mummery *et al.*, 1996; Perani *et al.*, 1995). For example, domain-specific activations for living compared to nonliving things have been reported in isolated regions in the right-hemisphere (inferior parietal lobe (Mummery *et al.*, 1996), posterior middle temporal cortex and anterior (Moore & Price, 1999) and anteromedial temporal lobes (Mummery *et al.*, 1996)), extensive left-hemisphere regions (medial occipital gyrus (Damasio *et al.*, 1996), calcarine sulcus (Martin *et al.*, 1996), lingual gyrus (Perani *et al.*, 1995), inferior temporal gyrus (Damasio *et al.*, 1996) including the fusiform (Moore & Price, 1999) gyrus and anterior (Moore & Price, 1999) and anteromedial temporal lobes (Mummery *et al.*, 1996; Phillips *et al.*, 2002)) as well as other visual areas presumably mediating the processing of more complex visual living stimuli (e.g. Martin *et al.*, 1996; Moore & Price, 1999; Perani *et al.*, 1995). A similarly complex set of activations has been associated with the processing of nonliving compared to living things: the right supramarginal gyrus (Martin *et al.*, 1996), and in the left hemisphere, the medial extrastriate (Moore & Price, 1999), the occipitotemporal junction (Moore & Price, 1999; Mummery *et al.*, 1996), inferior temporal gyrus (Damasio *et al.*, 1996) and middle temporal gyrus (MTG; Martin *et al.*, 1996), in particular its posterior portion (Mummery *et al.*, 1996; Damasio *et al.*, 1996), anterior cingulate (Martin *et al.*, 1996) and inferior (Perani *et al.*, 1995) and lateral inferior frontal gyrus (Martin *et al.*, 1996).

Thus different neuroanatomical regions have been associated with the processing of concepts from the two domains across studies. Part of this inconsistency may be due to the different kinds of stimuli used, in particular the modality the stimuli were presented in and their psycholinguistic characteristics (Tyler & Moss, 2001). For example, across a range of tasks, semantic processing of pictures is consistently associated with more occipitotemporal activations, whereas word stimuli activate more anterior temporal regions (Bright *et al.*, 2004). Perhaps more significantly, psycholinguistic stimulus variables such as familiarity, frequency, and imageability have not always been matched across domain. Indeed, our recent event-related functional magnetic resonance imaging (efMRI) study, which controlled for these variables, found that living and nonliving items activated a common left-lateralized network including the left fusiform and superior and middle temporal gyri, with no category- or domain-specific activations (see Figure 11.7; Tyler *et al.*, 2003b). This study was a replication of our previous efMRI (Pilgrim *et al.*, 2002), fMRI and position emission tomography (PET) (Devlin *et al.*, 2000, 2002b; Tyler *et al.*, 2003a) studies which likewise found no domain-specific activations across a range of tasks (e.g. lexical decisions, semantic decisions) and with different stimulus materials (pictures and words; see also Ewbank *et al.*, 2005), supporting the CSA's claim that the conceptual system is distributed, with no neuroanatomic boundaries for different domains of concepts (Tyler & Moss, 2001; Tyler *et al.*, 2003a).

Other investigators have argued that it is not the category or domain membership per se, but the type of semantic property that is the organizing principle of the semantic system (Chao *et al.*, 1999; Martin & Chao, 2001; Martin *et al.*, 2000; Mummery *et al.*, 1996). In an extension of Warrington, McCarthy and Shallice's account (Warrington & McCarthy, 1983; Warrington & Shallice, 1984), Martin and colleagues' sensory–motor model (Martin, 2001; Martin & Chao, 2001; Martin *et al.*, 2000) proposed that an object's sensory and motor attributes are stored in the sensory and motor regions activated when the object was first learned, i.e. near sites responsible for perceiving the object or carrying out the motor actions associated with it. Their claims are supported by the findings of a block-design fMRI study in which participants viewed, matched, and named picture stimuli, and made semantic decisions on written word stimuli from different categories (i.e. animals, tools, houses, and faces; Chao *et al.*, 1999). Regions were identified that were consistently activated by animals and tools across tasks, thus presumably coding for amodal semantic features. Compared with tools, animals commonly activated the lateral fusiform gyrus and the posterior superior temporal sulcus (STS), while tools relative to animals activated

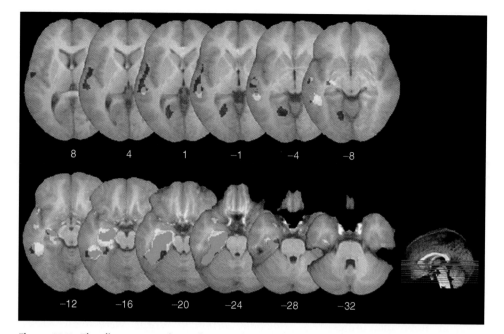

Figure 11.7. The direct comparison of processing animal names (yellow) with tool names (blue) did not result in any regions of significant activation, supporting the CSA's claim that concepts from both the living and nonliving domain are represented in the same, distributed system (sites of overlap represented in green; numbers represent Talairach z-coordinates; red lines represent the level of the sagittal sections; Tyler *et al.*, 2003b). Reprinted from *NeuroImage*, volume 18, Tyler, Stamatakis, Dick, Bright, Fletcher and Moss, "Objects and their actions: evidence for a neurally distributed semantic system", p. 550, copyright 2003, with permission from Elsevier.

the medial fusiform gyrus and posterior MTG. The authors suggested that different regions of the ventral temporal lobe represent object form features related to animals (i.e. lateral fusiform gyrus) and tools (medial fusiform gyrus). They further hypothesized that the posterior STS, which had previously been implicated in the perception of biological motion (Bonda *et al.*, 1996), and the posterior MTG, previously associated with the perception of non-biological object motion (Zeki *et al.*, 1991), stored information about the motion of biological and non-biological concepts, respectively. Thus, according to the sensory–motor model, the processing of animal and tool concepts will automatically activate neural regions storing their amodal object form representations (lateral and medial fusiform, respectively) and amodal object motion information (posterior STS and posterior MTG, respectively; see Martin, 2001; Martin & Chao, 2001; Martin *et al.*, 2000, for overviews).

It remains unclear why the majority of functional imaging studies of animal and tool processing failed to find the associated constellation of activity in the object form and motion regions specified in the sensory–motor model (e.g. Damasio *et al.*, 2004; Devlin *et al.*, 2000, 2002b; Martin *et al.*, 1996; Moore & Price, 1999; Perani *et al.*, 1995; Tyler *et al.*, 2003a). The most robust relationship appears to be between tool processing and activity in the posterior MTG (Devlin *et al.*, 2002a). However, most of the studies reporting this association used verb generation tasks where participants generate the appropriate action upon presentation of a noun concept (Fiez *et al.*, 1996; Martin *et al.*, 1995; Wise *et al.*, 1991), tasks which induce semantic processing of the action word in addition to motion-related information. Thus it is unclear to what extent the reported posterior MTG activity reflected the processing of action words (action verbs) and the motion attributes associated with the noun concept. We attempted to disentangle these two processes in an efMRI study in which participants were presented with nouns representing animals and tools (e.g. *tiger, hammer*) and verbs representing the actions associated with living and nonliving things (e.g. *galloping, drilling*). Words were matched on familiarity, frequency, and letter length, while imageability ratings, which could not be matched across domain, were entered into the analyses as covariates. Participants saw two cue words presented sequentially, followed by a target word to which they made a semantic relatedness decision. Consistent with the sensory–motor model, both object nouns and action verbs activated neural regions in the superior and middle temporal gyri, indicating that object nouns indeed activate the actions associated with them (and/or action verbs automatically activate the object concept with which they are associated). While action words (both for animals and tools) activated the left inferior frontal gyrus more than object words, these effects were attributed to the additional cognitive processes necessary to decode the morphological structures of these regularly inflected verbs (Marslen-Wilson & Tyler, 1997; Tyler *et al.*, 2005). Posterior STS and MTG activity, however, was not specifically associated with animal and tool nouns, respectively; instead, nouns from both object domains activated both regions [please delete carriage returns].

Moreover, animal and tool words did not preferentially activate the lateral and medial fusiform gyrus, respectively. Thus both animal and tool nouns, and the action words associated with them, appear to engage the same distributed network encompassing the left fusiform gyrus and middle/superior temporal lobes purportedly mediating object form and action information, respectively (see Figure 11.8), providing further evidence for a neuroanatomically distributed semantic system (Tyler *et al.*, 2003b).

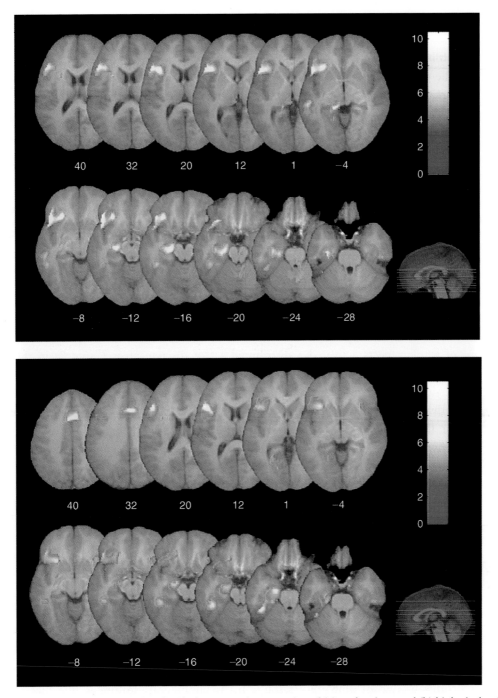

Figure 11.8. Activity associated with the semantic processing of (a) tool actions and (b) biological actions were found in the same distributed system of fusiform, middle and superior temporal gyri (numbers represent Talairach z-coordinates; red lines represent the level of the sagittal sections; Tyler *et al.*, 2003b). Reprinted from *NeuroImage*, vol. 18, Tyler, Stamatakis, Dick, Bright, Fletcher and Moss, "Objects and their actions: evidence for a neurally distributed semantic system", pp. 550–1, copyright 2003, with permission from Elsevier.

11.2.2   A distributed, hierarchical object processing system

The goal of our recent research has been to determine how such a distributed semantic system, and the dimensions purportedly structuring this space (Tyler & Moss, 2001), are instantiated in neural space. Towards this end, we have concentrated on a model system from the animal literature. Research with nonhuman primates suggests that there is a hierarchical, visual object processing system in the ventral occipitotemporal cortex (Ungerleider & Mishkin, 1982; Mishkin *et al.*, 1983). In this feature-based system, more posterior sites process elementary visual features (e.g. line orientation), while more anterior sites operate on the output of these early processes to create increasingly more complex conjunctions of visual features. Visual similarity also appears to be coded in this system, with inferotemporal neurons which respond to similar, moderately complex visual features clustering together in columns perpendicular to the cortical surface (Tanaka, 1993, 1996). Thus visual objects may be represented by the concerted activity of different inferotemporal regions corresponding to columns coding for different stimulus features. Indeed, the presentation of whole objects activated a distributed set of discrete areas ("spots") in the inferotemporal lobes of awake monkeys, while the presentation of simplified versions of these visual objects (i.e. whole objects minus certain visual features) activated only a subset of these areas (Tsunoda *et al.*, 2001; see Haxby *et al.*, 2001, for the human correlate of these findings). Other discrete regions were also activated during the presentation of degraded objects, regions purportedly inhibited during the processing of whole objects (Tsunoda *et al.*, 2001).

Mounting evidence suggests that the perirhinal cortex of the anteromedial temporal lobe represents the endpoint of this hierarchical object processing pathway, integrating the most complex combinations of visual object features (Bussey *et al.*, 2005; Murray & Bussey, 1999; Murray & Richmond, 2001). For example, Buckley, Gaffan, and colleagues found that rhesus monkeys with bilateral perirhinal lesions were impaired on complex object discrimination tasks which required the integration of several stimulus features (e.g. objects degraded with visual masks), but retained the ability to discriminate objects based on simple perceptual features such as color, shape, and size (Buckley *et al.*, 2001; see also Buckley & Gaffan, 1998; Bussey *et al.*, 2003; Eacott *et al.*, 2001). Bussey, Saksida, and colleagues have conceptualized this function of the perirhinal cortex as one of ambiguity resolution. An ambiguous feature is one that is rewarded when it appears together with some, but not other, visual features in a stimulus display. Thus, in order to know which visual stimulus display is meaningful, an animal must integrate the ambiguous visual feature with the other visual features in the display. The demands of visual feature integration increase with the proportion of ambiguous features in a display. As predicted, animals with ablated perirhinal cortices performed increasingly worse as the proportion of ambiguous visual features, i.e. as the complexity of visual feature integration, increased (Bussey *et al.*, 2002; see also Bussey & Saksida, 2002; Bussey *et al.*, 2003).

Theories on how such similarly organized hierarchical object processing pathways could be implemented in the human system have since been forwarded. The conceptual topography theory (CTT; Simmons & Barsalou, 2003), which borrows heavily from Damasio's convergence zone theory (Damasio, 1989a), postulates that each sensory and motor system contains "feature maps" processing the respective elementary sensory object features. These sensory and motor features are bound together into increasing more complex feature conjunctions from early to later regions in a hierarchical system of conceptual "convergence zones" (association areas) in each sensory and motor stream. The CTT differs critically from Damasio's convergence zone hypothesis in that it postulates that groups of bound features can function as stand-alone representations, independent of their sensory and motor feature maps, to support object processing during automatic tasks (e.g. categorization). The perirhinal cortex also plays a key role in the CTT by purportedly performing the most complex conjunction of visual object features.

Thus hierarchical models of object processing in humans (and non-human primates) exhibit two key characteristics. First, objects are represented in a distributed fashion, with several distinct regions in each sensory or motor system coding for the respective sensory and motor features associated with the object. This claim is a neuroanatomical reflection of distributed cognitive theories of semantic memory, such as the CSA, and is supported by our functional imaging studies showing no category- or domain-specific activations (see above). Second, such models hypothesize that increasingly complex combinations of sensory and motor features are coded from early to later regions of each sensory and motor system. This hierarchical organization implies that different regions of the, e.g., ventral occipitotemporal stream will be engaged depending on the complexity of visual analysis required by the task: posterior sites will support simple visual analyses of objects, while more anterior and anteromedial temporal lobe regions will be necessary for complex visual analyses.

Evidence that the human occipitotemporal processing stream may be hierarchically organized has recently emerged from functional imaging studies in humans. Lerner *et al.* (2001) presented healthy participants with intact images of cars and images of the same objects scrambled to different degrees. They postulated that scrambled images would induce activity in regions coding for simple stimulus features, while whole images would engage regions coding more complex feature conjunctions. Consistent with a hierarchical object processing system, these investigators demonstrated that scrambled images predicted activity in more posterior sites (V1, V2, V3, V4/V8) while intact images predicted activity in more anterior regions (lateral occipital sulcus and posterior fusiform gyrus; lateral occipital complex). The hypothesized role of anteromedial structures in complex visual discriminations was confirmed in another series of fMRI studies (Moss *et al.*, 2005; Tyler *et al.*, 2004). In these studies, healthy control participants were presented with two naming tasks. During domain-level naming, participants silently named the domain to which the object belonged, a task which required only a broad visual appraisal of the object, i.e. an appreciation of general visual featural differences, such as curvature. The second task was to actually name the specific object (basic-level naming; e.g. *tiger*). This task required a much more detailed visual analysis of the object to distinguish it from other, visually similar objects (e.g. lion). Critically, the same picture stimuli were employed in both naming tasks. If the ventral temporal stream is organized by stimulus category, then the presentation of objects from one category should result in a circumscribed pattern of activation, irrespective of the task. However, if the system is organized in a hierarchical fashion, then the activation associated with the same stimulus will differ depending on the task demands (i.e. depending on whether a simple or complex visual analysis is required). Consistent with this latter hypothesis, domain-level naming resulted in posterior occipital and ventral temporal activations, while basic-level naming additionally activated the anteromedial temporal lobe including the perirhinal cortex (Tyler *et al.*, 2004; see also Moss *et al.*, 2005; see Figure 11.9). Similar, task-dependent blood-oxygen-level-dependent (BOLD) effects have since been reported in the fusiform gyrus (Raposo *et al.*, 2004; Rogers *et al.*, 2005), and the critical role of the anteromedial temporal lobe, including perirhinal cortex, in complex visual discriminations has been confirmed in several studies with brain-lesioned patients (Barense *et al.*, 2005; Lee *et al.*, 2005; Moss *et al.*, 2005; Tyler *et al.*, 2004). Taken together, these findings provide preliminary support for a distributed, hierarchical visual object processing system in the human ventral occipitotemporal lobe, similar to the nonhuman primate system, which codes for increasingly complex conjunctions of visual features from posterior to anterior and anteromedial regions. The dependency of activation patterns on task may provide an additional explanation of why domain-specific activation patterns have been so variable across studies (see above).

We have recently focused on investigating how the internal structure of concepts – their feature correlation and distinctiveness – relates to the hierarchical object processing system of the ventral temporal lobe. As described in the first part of this chapter, living things tend to have many shared, highly correlated properties, and fewer weakly correlated distinctive properties.

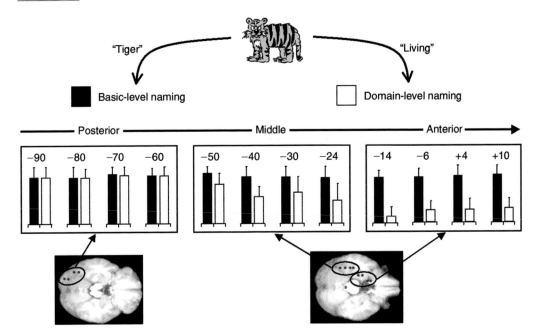

Figure 11.9. Consistent with the predictions of hierarchical object processing models, signal change plots revealed that activity associated with domain-level naming requiring coarse visual analyses was restricted to more posterior occipitotemporal sites, while basic-level naming of the same object stimuli requiring more complex visual discriminations was associated with both posterior occipitotemporal and anteromedial temporal lobe activation (Tyler *et al.*, 2004). (The approximate loci of the signal change plots are indicated on sagittal (top) and axial (bottom) slices of a normalized T1-weighted scan; MNI coordinates are reported.)

Comparatively, nonliving things have more distinctive features that are also more highly correlated with the concept's other features. The greater proportion of shared to distinctive (visual and nonvisual) features for living things renders these concepts more similar to one another. In terms of visual features, they are more visually confusable. We therefore predicted that the basic-level naming of living compared to nonliving things would rely on anteromedial temporal structures supporting complex visual discriminations, i.e. the perirhinal cortex, to a greater extent than the basic-level naming of nonliving things. This prediction was supported by the results of an efMRI study with matched sets of living and nonliving pictures (animals and vehicles, and fruits/vegetables and tools). As shown in Figure 11.10, basic-level naming of animals compared to vehicles, and of fruits and vegetables compared to tools, resulted in anteromedial temporal lobe activity including the entorhinal and perirhinal cortices at a reduced threshold (Moss *et al.*, 2005).

Activity associated with the basic-level naming of living compared to nonliving things reported by Moss and colleagues was centered in the entorhinal cortex (BAs 28, 34), medial to the perirhinal cortex (see Figure 11.10), raising the question of whether the perirhinal or entorhinal cortex is the critical structure for the complex visual discriminations for objects. Several lines of evidence from the animal literature indicate that these structures indeed play different roles in object processing, with perirhinal cortex primarily responsible for the integration of object-related feature information. First, the macaque perirhinal cortex receives the majority of inputs from unimodal sensory regions representing unisensory object features, i.e. the anterior ventral temporal lobe (visual information), the STG (auditory information), and the insular cortex (somatosensory information), and a smaller number of inputs from polymodal association regions (orbitofrontal cortex, dorsal STS, cingulate cortex and the parahippocampal cortex). The entorhinal cortex, on the other hand, receives the majority of its inputs from polymodal association areas (orbitofrontal, parainsular, cingulate, retrosplenial, perirhinal, and parahippocampal cortices and the dorsal STS), with only unimodal olfactory information being sent directly here (olfactory bulb, piriform cortex). Moreover, its inputs are not segregated, such that, e.g. polymodal visual information reaches potentially every region of the entorhinal cortex. Second, both regions are characterized by a network of intrinsic associative connections, indicating that the information each receives is integrated in the respective structure. Third, intraregional connections are feed-forward (ascending projections), typical of hierarchical processing systems. Lavenex and Amaral (2000) employed these characteristics to conceptualize this system as a "hierarchy of connectivity". Taken together, these data indicate that information reaching the

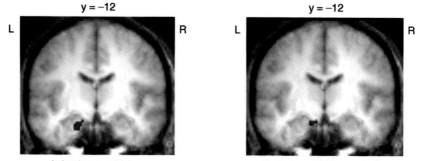

Animals vs. vehicles   Fruits/vegetables vs. tools

Figure 11.10. Anteromedial temporal lobe activity associated with the basic-level naming of matched sets of living compared to nonliving things (numbers refer to Talairach y-coordinates of the associated coronal slices; Moss et al., 2005).

perirhinal cortex, i.e. primarily unimodal object feature information, is both necessary and *sufficient* for the representation of objects, i.e. semantic memories of objects (Murray *et al.*, 2000; Simmons & Barsalou, 2003). Information received by the entorhinal cortex is more highly integrated, suggesting that it binds other, associative or contextual information with the object representation, providing both necessary and sufficient conditions for the formation of episodic memories, consistent with the human lesion literature (Squire *et al.*, 2004). Unfortunately it is not possible for human functional imaging to stop the perirhinal cortex from feeding the information it processes forward to the entorhinal cortex so that the independent contribution of the perirhinal cortex to object processing can be assessed, and we do not know whether participants based their basic-level naming on semantic object representations (e.g. *it has four legs and stripes, growls, and is furry to the touch – it's a tiger*) or episodic memories (e.g. *I saw something like that on TV last night – it's a tiger*). However, the afferent, intrinsic, and intraregional connectivity within the anteromedial temporal lobe strongly suggests that the perirhinal cortex is primarily responsible for processing object-related featural information necessary to represent these meaningful objects in memory.

The convergence of sensory inputs in the perirhinal cortex (Suzuki & Amaral, 1994) indicates that it integrates not only complex visual, but also information across modalities to form multimodal object representations (Murray *et al.*, 1998, Simmons & Barsalou, 2003). Although animal ablation studies have confirmed the role of the perirhinal region in cross-modal flavor–visual (Parker & Gaffan, 1998) and tactile–visual (Murray *et al.*, 1998) association learning, homologous evidence for the human perirhinal cortex is lacking. We recently conducted an efMRI to determine whether human perirhinal cortex is likewise involved in the cross-modal integration of object features (Taylor *et al.*, 2006). Participants were presented with pictures of objects paired with environmental sounds or auditory words (cross-modal conditions) and with two parts of a sound and two parts of a picture (unimodal auditory and visual conditions, respectively). Half of the stimulus pairs in each condition were congruent (i.e. meaningfully related, e.g. a picture of a cat and the sounds *meow*) and half incongruent (i.e. not meaningfully related, e.g. a picture of an elephant and the sound *woof*), and within each congruency condition, half of the stimuli represented living and half nonliving things. We reasoned that since living things have many more shared features than nonliving things, cross-modal integration of living things would place greater demands on the complex feature integration processes supported by the perirhinal cortex. The contrast of cross-modal compared to unimodal integration resulted in two clusters of activation, one centered in the posterior STS/MTG consistent with previous reports (Beauchamp *et al.*, 2004a, 2004b).

Significantly, cross-modal compared to unimodal integration also activated the perirhinal cortex in the group analysis, a finding that was confirmed in individual subjects (see Figure 11.11). Moreover, only perirhinal cortex, but not posterior STS/MTG, activity was modulated by the semantic factors: responses here were greater for living compared to nonliving things, as predicted, and for incongruent compared to congruent stimuli. The behavioral performance patterns of two HSE patients with lesions including the perirhinal cortex, but not two patients whose brain damage primarily involved the left inferior frontal gyrus and whose perirhinal cortices were spared, mirrored these efMRI findings.

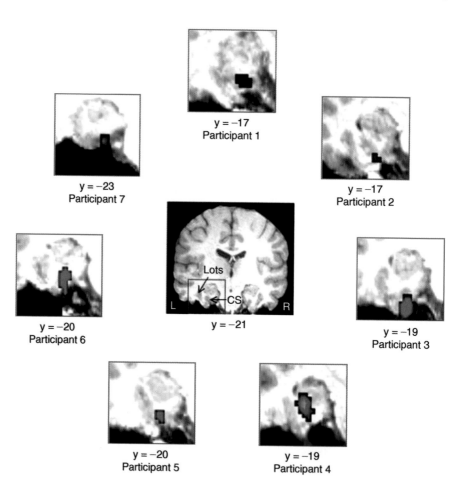

Figure 11.11. The center coronal slice shows the positions of the lateral occipitotemporal sulcus (LOTS) and collateral sulcus (CS). The red box signifies the area shown in the surrounding slices, which show perirhinal cortex activity in single subjects during the crossmodal compared to unimodal integration of audiovisual object features (Taylor *et al.*, unpublished data).

These results extend findings from non-human primates into the human domain by providing converging evidence that human perirhinal cortex is critically involved in binding cross-modal object features into meaningful, multimodal object representations.

Unimodal and multimodal feature binding in the perirhinal cortex may be accomplished by via feedback connections to posterior unimodal sites. The results of a single-unit recording study by Higuchi and Miyashita (1996) provided evidence for this hypothesis. Monkeys underwent anterior commissurotomy to interrupt interhemispheric communication between the anterior inferotemporal lobes, and were then taught to associate different pairs of visual fractal pattern stimuli with one another (e.g. S–S′). After this learning phase, some inferotemporal neurons evidenced "pair-coding" properties (Sakai & Miyashita, 1991), that is, they responded as strongly to S as to S′ when these stimuli were presented in isolation. Higuchi and Miyashita then unilaterally ablated the rhinal sulci of these animals, after which the animals relearned the old stimulus set and were taught a new stimulus set. Inferotemporal lobe neurons in the lesioned hemisphere were again recorded. Remarkably, these neurons no longer exhibited pair-coding properties, neither for the pre-operatively nor the post-operatively learned stimulus pairs, although they responded normally to individual visual stimuli. These findings strongly support the hypothesis that the rhinal sulcus is responsible for the pair-coding properties of posterior inferotemporal lobe neurons, presumably via feedback connections, thus binding these features together. The involvement of the perirhinal cortex in multimodal feature integration (Murray *et al.*, 1998; Taylor *et al.*, 2006) suggests that its role extends beyond one of maintaining purely intramodal visual associations (Higuchi & Miyashita, 1996) to that of a "master binder", integrating not only visual, but the polymodal inputs it receives (Suzuki & Amaral, 1994) into multimodal stimulus associations underlying object representations.

11.3   Future directions

The investigation of the neuroanatomical bases of semantic memory is in its infancy. We have endeavored to contribute to this exciting venture by first developing a cognitive model of semantic memory, the CSA, and then by attempting to identify the neural correlates of the cognitive structures and processes it describes. The results of our work to date suggest that a distributed semantic system, and the combined effects of feature correlation and distinctiveness, can be instantiated in a neural theory of hierarchical object processing in which increasingly complex conjunctions of sensory features are processed from early to late sites, with perirhinal cortex of the anteromedial temporal lobe supporting complex, polymodal feature conjunctions. The emphasis of our current work is on understanding how the effects of feature correlation, distinctiveness, and number of features each influence processing in the hierarchical object processing system. For example, Simmons and Barsalou (2003) suggested that the proximity of clumps of conjunctive neurons coding for category features increases as the similarity of the represented category exemplars increases (the "variable dispersion principle"), i.e. with increasing proportion of shared features. Are these effects demonstrable with high-resolution efMRI imaging? Moreover, Sigala and Logothetis (2002) demonstrated that with training, neurons in the monkey inferotemporal lobe became tuned to the distinguishing features of visual objects. Do human inferotemporal neurons evidence similar tunings for distinguishing features, a subset of distinctive features?

A great number of other intriguing questions await scientific inquiry. Can the seemingly contradictory functional imaging findings in support of modular and distributed semantic systems be reconciled by postulating task-induced processing demands, or is it necessary to postulate that the distributed, hierarchical object processing system contains columns of neurons coding visually similar feature combinations, as in the macaque inferotemporal lobe (Tanaka, 1993, 1996) (does it?)? Is reactivation of feature maps ("reenactment") necessary for conceptual processing, as Damasio (1989b) hypothesizes and preliminary findings from a functional imaging study of semantic dementia patients seem to suggest (Mummery *et al.*, 1999)? Or (/and?) does reactivation of feature maps depend on the automaticity of the processes involved in the task, as Simmons and Barsalou postulate (Simmons & Barsalou, 2003)? How does imagery influence ventral occipitotemporal activation? How can verbs, abstract nouns, and encyclopedic concepts be integrated in these models? We look forward to the results of the studies that will investigate these and other similarly exciting questions about the neuroanatomical bases of our conceptual system.

REFERENCES

Barense, M. D., Bussey, T. J., Lee, A. C. H., Rogers, T. T., Hodges, J. R., Saksida, L. M., Murray, E. A., and Graham, K. S. (2005). Feature ambiguity influences performance on novel object discriminations in patients with damage to perirhinal cortex. *Cognitive Neuroscience Society — 2005 Annual Meeting Program*, p. 129.

Basso, A., Captiani, E., and Laiacona, M. (1988). Progressive language impairment without dementia: a case with isolated category specific semantic impairment. *Journal of Neurology, Neurosurgery & Psychiatry*, **51**: 1201–7.

Beauchamp, M. S., Argall, B. D., Bodurka, J., Duyn, J. H., and Martin, A. (2004a). Unraveling multisensory integration: patchy organization within human STS multisensory cortex. *Nature Neuroscience*, **7**: 1190−2.

Beauchamp, M. S., Lee, K. E., Argall, B. D., and Martin, A. (2004b). Integration of auditory and visual information about objects in superior temporal sulcus. *Neuron*, **41**: 809−23.

Bonda, E., Petrides, M., Ostry, D., and Evans, A. (1996). Specific involvement of human parietal systems and the amygdala in the perception of biological motion. *Journal of Neuroscience*, **16**: 3737−44.

Bright, P., Moss, H., and Tyler, L. K. (2004). Unitary versus multiple semantics: PET studies of word and picture processing. *Brain and Language*, **89**: 417−32.

Bright, P., Moss, H. E., Stamatakis, E. A., and Tyler, L. K. (2005). The anatomy of object processing: The role of anteromedial temporal cortex. *Quarterly Journal of Experimental Psychology*, **58B**: 361−77.

Buckley, M. J. and Gaffan, D. (1998). Perirhinal cortex ablation impairs visual object identification. *Journal of Neuroscience*, **18**: 2268−75.

Buckley, M. J., Booth, M. C. A., Rolls, E. T., and Gaffan, D. (2001). Selective perceptual impairments after perirhinal cortex ablation. *Journal of Neuroscience*, **21**: 9824−36.

Bunn, E. M., Tyler, L. K., and Moss, H. E. (1998). Category-specific semantic deficits: the role of familiarity and property type reexamined. *Neuropsychology*, **12**: 367−79.

Bussey, T. J. and Saksida, L. M. (2002). The organization of visual object representations: a connectionist model of effects of lesions in perirhinal cortex. *European Journal of Neuroscience*, **15**: 355−64.

Bussey, T. J., Saksida, L. M., and Murray, E. A. (2002). Perirhinal cortex resolves feature ambiguity in complex visual discriminations. *European Journal of Neuroscience*, **15**: 365−74.

Bussey, T. J., Saksida, L. M., and Murray, E. A. (2003). Impairments in visual discrimination after perirhinal cortex lesions: testing ''declarative'' vs. ''perceptual−mnemonic'' views of perirhinal cortex function. *European Journal of Neuroscience*, **17**: 649−60.

Bussey, T. J., Saksida, L. M., and Murray, E. A. (2005). The perceptual−mnemonic/feature conjunction model of perirhinal cortex function. *The Quarterly Journal of Experimental Psychology*, **58B**: 269−82.

Cappa, S. F., Perani, D., Schnur, T., Tettamanti, M., and Fazio, F. (1998). The effects of semantic category and knowledge on lexical−semantic access: a PET study. *NeuroImage*, **8**: 350−9.

Caramazza, A., Hillis, A. E., Rapp, B. C., and Romani, C. (1990). The multiple semantics hypothesis: multiple confusions? *Cognitive Neuropsychology*, **7**: 161−89.

Caramazza, A. and Mahon, B. Z. (2003). The organization of conceptual knowledge: the evidence from category-specific semantic deficits. *Trends on Cognitive Sciences*, **7**: 325−74.

Caramazza, A. and Mahon, B. Z. (2005). The organisation of conceptual knowledge in the brain: the future's past and some future directions. *Cognitive Neuropsychology*, **22**: 1−25.

Caramazza, A. and Shelton, J. R. (1998). Domain-specific knowledge systems in the brain: the animate−inanimate distinction. *Journal of Cognitive Neuroscience*, **10**: 1−34.

Chao, L. L., Haxby, J. V., and Martin, A. (1999). Attribute-based neural substrates in temporal cortex for perceiving and knowing about objects. *Nature Neuroscience*, **2**: 913−19.

Cree, G. S. and McRae, K. (2003). Analyzing the factors underlying the structure and computation of the meaning of Chipmunk, Cherry, Chisel, Cheese, and Cello (and many other such concrete nouns). *Journal of Experimental Psychology: General*, 132: 162–201.

Damasio, A. R. (1989a). The brain binds entities and events by multiregional activation from convergence zones. *Neural Computation*, 1: 123–32.

Damasio, A. R. (1989b). Time-locked multiregional retroactivation: a systems-level proposal for the neural substrates of recall and recognition. *Cognition*, 33: 25–62.

Damasio, H., Grabowski, T. J., Tranel, D., Hichwa, R. D., and Damasio, A. R. (1996). A neural basis for lexical retrieval. *Nature*, 380: 499–505.

Damasio, H., Tranel, D., Grabowski, T., Adolphs, R., and Damasio, A. (2004). Neural systems behind word and concept retrieval. *Cognition*, 92: 179–229.

De Renzi, E. and Lucchelli, F. (1994). Are semantic systems separately represented in the brain? The case of living category impairment. *Cortex*, 30: 3–25.

Devlin, J. T., Gonnerman, L. M., Andersen, E. S., and Seidenberg, M. S. (1998). Category-specific semantic deficits in focal and widespread brain damage: a computational account. *Journal of Cognitive Neuroscience*, 10: 77–94.

Devlin, J. T., Russell, R. P., Davis, M. H., Price, C. J., Wilson, J., Moss, H. E., Matthews, P. M., and Tyler, L. K. (2000). Susceptibility-induced loss of signal: comparing PET and fMRI on semantic task. *NeuroImage*, 11: 589–600.

Devlin, J. T., Moore, C. J., Mummery, C. J., Gorno-Tempini, M. L., Phillips, J. A., Noppeney, U., Frackowiak, R. S. J., Friston, K. J., and Price, C. J. (2002a). Anatomic constraints on cognitive theories of category specificity. *NeuroImage*, 15: 675–85.

Devlin, J. T., Russell, R. P., Davis, M. H., Price, C. J., Moss, H. E., Fadili, M. J., and Tyler, L. K. (2002b). Is there an anatomical basis for category-specificity? Semantic memory studies in PET and fMRI. *Neuropsychologia*, 40: 54–75.

Durrant-Peatfield, M., Tyler, L. K., Moss, H. E., and Levy, J. (1997). The distinctiveness of form and function in category structure: a connectionist model. In M. G. Shafto and P. Langley (eds.), *Proceedings of the Nineteenth Annual Conference of the Cognitive Science Society*. Mahwah, NJ: Erlbaum, pp. 193–8.

Eacott, M. J., Machin, P. E., and Gaffan, E. A. (2001). Elemental and configural visual discrimination learning following lesions to perirhinal cortex in the rat. *Behavioural Brain Research*, 124: 55–70.

Ewbank, M. P., Schluppeck, D., and Andrews, T. J. (2005). fMR-adaptation reveals a distributed representation of inanimate objects and places in human visual cortex. *NeuroImage*, 28: 268–79.

Fiez, J. A., Raichle, M. E., Balota, D., Tallal, P., and Peterson, S. E. (1996). PET activation of posterior temporal regions during passive auditory word presentation and verb generation. *Cerebral Cortex*, 6: 1–10.

Forde, E. M. E. and Humphreys, G. W. (1999). Category-specific recognition impairments: a review of important case studies and influential theories. *Aphasiology*, 13: 169–93.

Funnell, E. (1995). Objects and properties: a study of the breakdown of semantic memory. *Memory*, 3: 497–581.

Funnell, E. and Sheridan, J. (1992). Categories of knowledge: unfamiliar aspects of living and non-living things. *Cognitive Neuropsychology*, **9**: 135–53.

Gainotti, G. (2000). What the locus of brain lesion tells us about the nature of the cognitive defect underlying category-specific disorders: a review. *Cortex*, **36**: 539–59.

Garrard, P., Patterson, K., Watson, P.C., and Hodges, J.R. (1998). Category specific semantic loss in dementia of Alzheimer's type: functional–anatomical correlations from cross-sectional analyses. *Brain*, **121**: 633–46.

Gonnerman, L.M., Andersen, E.S., Devlin, J.T., Kempler, D., and Seidenberg, M.S. (1997). Double dissociation of semantic categories in Alzheimer's disease. *Brain and Language*, **57**: 254–79.

Greer, M., van Casteren, M., McClellan, S., Moss, H.E., Rodd, J., Rogers, T., and Tyler, L.K. (2001). The emergence of semantic categories from distributed featural representations. In J.D. Moore and K. Stenning (eds.), *Proceedings of the 23rd Annual Conference of the Cognitive Science Society*. London: Lawrence Erlbaum Associates, pp. 358–63.

Hart, J. and Gordon, B. (1992). Neural subsystems for object knowledge. *Nature*, **359**: 60–4.

Hart, J., Berndt, R.S., and Caramazza, A. (1985). Category-specific naming deficit following cerebral infarction. *Nature*, **316**: 439–40.

Haxby, J.V., Gobbini, M.I., Furey, M.L., Ishai, A., Schuten, J.L., and Pietrini, P. (2001). Distributed and overlapping representations of faces and objects in ventral temporal cortex. *Science*, **293**: 2425–30.

Higuchi, S. and Miyashita, Y. (1996). Formation of mnemonic neuronal responses to visual paired associates in inferotemporal cortex is impaired by perirhinal and entorhinal lesions. *Proceedings of the National Academy of Sciences USA*, **93**: pp. 739–43.

Hillis, A.E. and Caramazza, A. (1991). Category-specific naming and comprehension impairment: A double dissocation. *Brain*, **114**: 2081–94.

Humphreys, G.W., Riddoch, M.J., and Quinlan, P. (1988). Cascade processes in picture identification. *Cognitive Neuropsychology*, **5**: 67–103.

Keil, F. (1986). The acquisition of natural kinds and artifact terms. In W. Demoupoulous and A. Marras (eds.), *Language Learning and Concept Acquisition: Foundational Issues*, Norwood, NJ: Ablex, 133–53.

Laiacona, M., Capitani, E., and Barbarotto, R. (1997). Semantic category dissocations: a longitudinal study of two cases. *Cortex*, **33**: 441–61.

Lavenex, P. and Amaral, D.G. (2000). Hippocampal–neocortical interaction: a hierarchy of associativity. *Hippocampus*, **10**: 420–30.

Lee, A.C., Bussey, T.J., Murray, E.A., Saksida, L.M., Epstein, R.A., Kapur, N., Hodges, J.R., and Graham, K.S. (2005). Perceptual deficits in amnesia: challenging the medial temporal lobe "mnemonic" view. *Neuropsychologia*, **43**: 1–11.

Lerner, Y., Hendler, T., Ben-Bashat, D., Harel, M., and Malach, R. (2001). A hierarchical axis of object processing stages in the human visual cortex. *Cerebral Cortex*, **11**: 287–97.

Malt, B.C. and Smith, E. (1984). Correlated properties in natural categories. *Journal of Verbal Learning and Verbal Behaviour*, **23**: 250–69.

Marslen-Wilson, W. D. and Tyler, L. K. (1997). Dissociating types of mental computation. *Nature*, **387**: 592–4.

Martin, A. (2001). Functional neuroimaging of semantic memory. In R. Cabeza and A. Kingstone (eds.), *Handbook of Functional Neuroimaging of Cognition*. Cambridge, MA: MIT Press, pp. 153–86.

Martin, A. and Chao, L. L. (2001). Semantic memory and the brain: structure and processes. *Current Opinion in Neurobiology*, **11**: 194–201.

Martin, A., Haxby, J. V., Lalonde, F. M., Wiggs, C. L., and Ungerleider, L. G. (1995). Discrete cortical regions associated with knowledge of color and knowledge of action. *Science*, **379**: 649–52.

Martin, A., Ungerleider, L. G., and Haxby, J. V. (2000). Category-specificity and the brain: the sensory-motor model of semantic representations of objects. In M. S. Gazzaniga (ed.), *The Cognitive Neurosciences*. Cambridge, MA: MIT Press, pp. 1023–36.

Martin, Q., Wiggs, C. L., Ungerleider, L. G., and Haxby, J. V. (1996). Neural correlates of category-specific knowledge. *Nature*, **379**: 649–52.

Masson, M. (1995). A distributed memory model of semantic priming. *Journal of Experimental Psychology Learning, Memory, and Cognition*, **21**: 3–23.

McRae (2004). Semantic memory: Some insights from feature-based connectionist attractor networks. In B. H. Ross (ed.), *Psychology of Learning and Motivation*, vol. 45. Amsterdam: Elsevier, pp. 41–86.

McRae, K. and Cree, G. S. (2002). Factors underlying category-specific semantic deficits. In E. M. E. Forde and G. Humphreys (eds.), *Category-specificity in Mind and Brain*. East Sussex: Psychology Press, pp. 211–50.

McRae, K., Cree, G. S., Seidenberg, M. S., and McNorgan, C. (2005). Semantic feature production norms for a large set of living and nonliving things. *Behavior Research Methods, Instruments, & Computers*, **37**: 547–59.

McRae, K., Cree, G. S., Westmacott, R., and de Sa, V. R. (1999). Further evidence for feature correlations in semantic memory. *Canadian Journal of Experimental Psychology*, **53**: 360–73.

McRae, K., de Sa, V., and Seidenberg, M. S. (1993). Semantic priming and the structure of semantic memory. *Journal of Clinical and Experimental Neuropsychology*, **15**: 385–6.

McRae, K., de Sa, V. R., and Seidenberg, M. S. (1997). On the nature and scope of featural representations of word meaning. *Journal of Experimental Psychology: General*, **126**: 99–130.

Mishkin, M., Ungerleider, L. G., and Macko, K. A. (1983). Object vision and spatial vision: two cortical pathways. *Trends in Neurosciences*, **6**: 414–17.

Moore, C. J. and Price, C. J. (1999). A functional neuroimaging study of the variables that generate category-specific object processing differences. *Brain*, **122**: 943–62.

Moss, H. E., Rodd, J. M., Stamatakis, E. A., Bright, P., and Tyler, L. K. (2005). Anteromedial temporal cortex supports fine-grained differentiation among objects. *Cerebral Cortex*, **15**: 616–27.

Moss, H. E. and Tyler, L. K. (1997). A category-specific impairment for non-living things in a case of progressive aphasia. *Brain and Language*, **60**: 55–8.

Moss, H. E. and Tyler, L. K. (2000). A progressive category-specific semantic deficit for non-living things. *Neuropsychologia*, **38**: 60–82.

Moss, H. E., Tyler, L. K., and Devlin, J. (2002). The emergence of category specific deficits in a distributed semantic system. In E. Forde and G. W. Humphreys (eds.), *Category-Specificity in Brain and Mind*. Sussex: Psychology Press, pp. 115–48.

Moss, H. E., Tyler, L. K., Durrant-Peatfield, M., and Bunn, E. M. (1998). "Two eyes of a see-through": Impaired and intact semantic knowledge in a case of selective deficit for living things. *Neurocase*, **4**: 291–310.

Moss, H. E., Tyler, L. K., and Jennings, F. (1997). When leopards lose their spots: Knowledge of visual properties in category-specific deficits for living things. *Cognitive Neuropsychology*, **14**: 901–50.

Mummery, C. J., Patterson, K., Hodges, J. R., and Wise, R. J. (1996). Generating "tiger" as an animal name or a word beginning with T: differences in brain activation. *Proceedings of the Royal Society, London B. Biological Science*, **263**: pp. 989–95.

Mummery, C. J., Patterson, K., Wise, R. J. S., Vandenbergh, R., Price, C. J., and Hodges, J. R. (1999). Disrupted temporal lobe connections in semantic dementia. *Brain*, **122**: 61–73.

Murray, E. A. and Bussey, T. J. (1999). Perceptual–mnemonic functions of the perirhinal cortex. *Trends in Cognitive Sciences*, **3**: 142–51.

Murray, E. A., Bussey, T. J., Hampton, R. R., and Saksida, L. M. (2000). The parahippocampal region and object identification. *Annals of the New York Academy of Sciences*, **911**: 166–74.

Murray, E. A., Malkova, L., and Goulet, S. (1998). Crossmodal associations, intramodal associations, and object identification in macaque monkeys. In A. D. Milner (ed.), *Comparative Neuropsychology*. Oxford: Oxford University Press, pp. 51–69.

Murray, E. A. and Richmond, B. J. (2001). Role of perirhinal cortex in object perception, memory, and associations. *Current Opinion in Neurobiology*, **11**: 188–93.

Parker, A. and Gaffan, D. (1998). Lesions of the primate rhinal cortex cause deficits in flavour–visual associative memory. *Behavioral Brain Research*, **93**: 99–105.

Perani, D., Cappa, S., Bettinardi, V., Bressi, S., Gorno-Tempini, M.-L., Matarrese, M., and Fazio, F. (1995). Different neural systems for the recognition of animals and man-made tools. *NeuroReport*, **6**: 1637–41.

Pexman, P. M., Lupker, S. J., and Hino, Y. (2002). The impact of feedback semantics in visual word recognition: number-of-features effects in lexical decision and naming tasks. *Psychonomic Bulletin & Review*, **9**: 542–9.

Pexman, P. M., Holyk, G. G., and Monfils, M. H. (2003). Number-of-features effects and semantic processing. *Memory and Cognition*, **31**: 842–55.

Phillips, J. A., Noppeney, U., Humphreys, G. W., and Price, C. J. (2002). Can segregation within the semantic system account for category-specific deficits? *Brain*, **125**: 2067–80.

Pilgrim, L. K., Fadili, J., Fletcher, P., and Tyler, L. K. (2002). Overcoming confounds of stimulus blocking: an event-related fMRI design of semantic processing. *NeuroImage*, **16**: 713–23.

Plaut, D. C. and Shallice, T. (1993). Perseverative and semantic influences on visual object naming errors in optic aphasia: a connectionist account. *Journal of Cognitive Neuroscience*, **5**: 89–117.

Randall, B., Moss, H. E., Rodd, J. M., Greer, M., and Tyler, L. K. (2004). Distinctiveness and correlation in conceptual structure: behavioral and computational studies. *Journal of Experimental Psychology: Learning, Memory, and Cognition*, **30**: 393–406.

Raposo, A., Stamatakis, E. A., Moss, H. E., and Tyler, L. K. (2004). Interactions between processing demands and conceptual structure in object recognition: an event-related fMRI study. *Journal of Cognitive Neruoscience*, **16**: Suppl.: B82.

Rogers, T. T., Hocking, J., Mechelli, A., Patterson, K., and Price, C. (2005). Fusiform activation to animals is driven by the process, not the stimulus. *Journal of Cognitive Neuroscience*, **17**: 434–45.

Rosch, E. (1978). Principles of categorization. In E. Rosch and B. B. Lloyd, (eds.), *Cognition and Categorization*. Hillsdale, NJ: Erlbaum, pp. 27–48.

Sacchett, C. and Humphreys, G. W. (1992). Calling a squirrel a squirrel but a canoe a wigwam: a category-specific deficit for artefactual objects and body parts. *Cognitive Neuropsychology*, **9**: 73–86.

Sakai, K. and Miyashita, Y. (1991). Neural organization for the long-term memory of paired associates. *Nature*, **354**: 152–5.

Sartori, G. and Job, R. (1988). The oyster with four legs: a neuropsychological study on the interaction of visual and semantic information. *Cognitive Neuropsychology*, **5**: 105–32.

Sartori, G., Job, R., Miozzo, M., Zago, S., and Marchiori, G. (1993). Category-specific form knowledge in a patient with herpes simplex virus encephalitis. *Journal of Clinical and Experimental Neuropsychology*, **15**: 280–99.

Sheridan, J. and Humphreys, J. W. (1993). A verbal semantic category-specific recognition deficit. *Cognitive Neuropsychology*, **10**: 143–84.

Sigala, N. and Logothetis, N. K. (2002). Visual categorization shapes feature selectivity in the primate temporal cortex. *Nature*, **415**: 318–20.

Simmons, W. K. and Barsalou, L. W. (2003). The similarity-in-topography principle: reconciling theories of conceptual deficits. *Cognitive Neuropsychology*, **20**: 451–86.

Squire, L. R., Stark, C. E. L., and Clark, R. E. (2004). The medial temporal lobe. *Annual Review of Neuroscience*, **27**: 279–306.

Suzuki, W. A. and Amaral, D. G. (1994). Perirhinal and parahippocampal cortices of the macaque monkey: cortical afferents. *The Journal of Comparative Neurology*, **350**: 497–533.

Tanaka, K. (1993). Neuronal mechanisms of object recognition. *Science*, **262**: 685–8.

Tanaka, K. (1996). Inferotemporal cortex and object vision. *Annual Review of Neuroscience*, **19**: 109–39.

Taylor, K. I., Moss, H., Randall, B., and Tyler, L. K. (2004). The interplay between distinctiveness and intercorrelation in the automatic activation of word meaning (abstract). *Abstracts of the Psychonomic Society*, **9**: 109.

Taylor, K. I., Moss, H. E., Stamatakis, E., and Tyler, L. K. (2006). Binding crossmodal object features in perirhinal cortex. *Proceedings of the National Academy of Sciences*, USA, **103(21)**, 8239–44.

Tranel, D., Damasio, H., and Damasio, A. R. (1997). A neural basis for the retrieval of conceptual knowledge. *Neuropsychologia*, **35**: 1319–27.

Tsunoda, K., Yamane, Y., Nishizaki, M., and Tanifuji, M. (2001). Complex objects are represented in macaque inferotemporal cortex by the combination of feature columns. *Nature Neuroscience*, **4**: 832–8.

Tyler, L. K. and Moss, H. E. (2001). Towards a distributed account of conceptual knowledge. *Trends in Cognitive Sciences*, **5**: 244–52.

Tyler, L. K., Moss, H. E., Durrant-Peatfield, M. R., and Levy, J. P. (2000a). Conceptual structure and the structure of concepts: a distributed account of category-specific deficits. *Brain and Language*, **75**: 195–231.

Tyler, L. K., Voice, J. K., and Moss, H. E. (2000b). The interaction of meaning and sound in spoken word recognition. *Psychological Bulletin & Review*, **7**: 320–6.

Tyler, L. K., Bright, P., Dick, E., Tavares, P., Pilgrim, L., Fletcher, P., Greer, M., and Moss, H. (2003a). Do semantic categories activate distinct cortical regions? Evidence for a distributed neural semantic system. *Cognitive Neuropsychology*, **20**: 54–61.

Tyler, L. K., Stamatakis, E. A., Dick, E., Bright, P., Fletcher, P., and Moss, H. (2003b). Objects and their actions: evidence for a neurally distrubuted semantic system. *NeuroImage*, **18**: 542–57.

Tyler, L. K., Stamatakis, E. A., Bright, P., Acres, K., Abdallah, S., Rodd, J. M., and Moss, H. E. (2004). Processing objects at different levels of specificity. *Journal of Cognitive Neuroscience*, **16**: 351–62.

Tyler, L. K., Marslen-Wilson, W. D., and Stamatakis, E. A. (2005). Differentiating lexical form, meaning and structure in the neural language system. *Proceedings of the National Academy of Sciences*, **102**: 8375–80.

Ungerleider, L. G. and Mishkin, M. (1982). Two cortical visual systems. In D. J. Ingle, M. A. Goodale, and R. J. W. Mansfield (eds.), *Analysis of Visual Behavior*. Cambridge, MA: MIT Press, pp. 549–86.

Warrington, E. K. and McCarthy, R. (1983). Category specific access dysphasia. *Brain*, **106**: 859–78.

Warrington, E. K. and McCarthy, R. (1987). Categories of knowledge: further fractionations and an attempted integration. *Brain*, **110**: 1273–96.

Warrington, E. K. and Shallice, T. (1984). Category-specific semantic impairment. *Brain*, **107**: 829–53.

Wise, R., Chollet, F., Hadar, U., Friston, K., Hoffner, E., and Frackowiak, R. (1991). Distribution of cortical neural networks involved in word comprehension and word retrieval. *Brain*, **114**: 1803–17.

Zannino, G. D., Perri, R., Carlesimo, G. A., Pasqualettin, P., and Caltagirone, C. (2002). Category-specific impairment in patients with Alzheimer's disease as a function of disease severity: a cross-sectional investigation. *Neuropsychologia*, **40**: 2268–79.

Zeki, S., Watson, J. D., Lueck, C. J., Fristn, K. J., Kennard, C., and Frackowiak, R. S. (1991). A direct demonstration of functional specialization in human visual cortex. *Journal of Neuroscience*, **11**: 641–9.

Neural foundations for conceptual representations: Evidence from functional brain imaging

Alex Martin

National Institute of Mental Health

12.1 Overview

Semantic memory refers to a major division of declarative memory that includes knowledge of the meaning of objects and words. This chapter will focus on one aspect of the functional neuroanatomy of semantic memory: the representation of the meaning of concrete objects and object properties. The initial motivation for our work on this topic was reports of patients with so-called category-specific knowledge disorders – specifically, patients with relatively selective impaired knowledge about animals and other animate objects, and those with relatively selective impairments for man-made, inanimate objects such as tools. Since the publication of the seminal case studies by Warrington and colleagues (Warrington & McCarthy, 1983; Warrington & Shallice, 1984), well over 100 patients have been reported with a category-specific deficit for biological categories (living things, especially four-legged animals), relative to inanimate objects (especially tools and other artifacts), and more than 25 cases with the opposite pattern of deficit (Capitani *et al.*, 2003). Our work has been motivated by an appreciation of the importance of these clinical cases for understanding the organization of conceptual knowledge, object recognition, and storage of long-term memories. In this chapter I shall outline a model of how conceptual knowledge about concrete entities (objects) is organized in the brain based on functional brain imaging studies of normal, intact individuals. From a theoretical perspective, the model attempts to incorporate the main features of property-based models that have dominated thinking about category-specific disorders for over one hundred years, and the challenge to this view from the

Many thanks to the members of my laboratory whose work I have described here: Michael Beauchamp, Linda Chao, Miranda van Turennout, Jill Weisberg, Thalia Wheatley, and Cheri Wiggs. This work was supported by the Intramural Research Program of the NIMH.

Domain Specific theory (Caramazza & Shelton, 1998; for an overview of recent theories of the organization of conceptual knowledge in the brain see Caramazza, 1998; Martin & Caramazza, 2003). The model I will outline, The Sensory—Motor Property Model for Representing Domain-Specific Information — which I shall refer to simply as the sensory—motor model — is consistent with recent attempts to accommodate the functional brain imaging and neuropsychological evidence (Caramazza & Mahon, 2003). I shall concentrate on the two broad domains of knowledge, the first is the representation of animate agents — living things that move on their own; the second is 'tools' — man-made manipulable objects for which there is a direct relationship between how an object is manipulated and its function. However, the model is relevant for understanding other object domains as well, such as place (Epstein & Kanwisher, 1998), food (Crutch & Warrington, 2003; Simmons *et al.*, 2005), and number (Dehaene *et al.*, 1999).

12.2   The expression and representation of knowledge

Before proceeding, a number of preliminary issues need to be addressed. First is the issue of knowledge expression. There is no need for any organism to acquire information unless that information can be expressed. Organisms learn, and the evidence for that learning is demonstrated by a change in behavior. What is represented (stored) in the brain is information. What is expressed is knowledge. How this knowledge is expressed is of fundamental importance for understanding how information is represented. For humans, a primary, and arguably *the* primary, mode of expression is via the language system. Questions designed to probe knowledge about a specific entity are posed orally or in written form and subjects respond verbally. Occasionally, a manual response may be required (e.g. show me how you would use a hammer) either by actually manipulating the object or via pantomime. However, regardless of whether the response is verbal or manual, knowledge is expressed explicitly. This explicit knowledge is typically referred to as associative knowledge or encyclopedic knowledge, and it is this level of knowledge representation that is typically probed in both normal and brain-damaged individuals. Associative or encyclopedic knowledge has three main characteristics. First, as noted above, retrieval is explicit. Second, there is no intrinsic limitation on the amount of information that can be stored and retrieved. For a specific category of objects (e.g. *dogs*), we may know lots of things. We know they are living things, have four legs, are smaller than a car, like to take walks, like to play fetch, are considered pets in many parts of the world, show up on the menu in other parts of the world, and so on, and so on. Moreover, it does not matter whether the information is true. If you believe that dogs can fly, then that information is part of your semantic knowledge about dogs and represented somewhere in the brain. Finally, this level of knowledge is idiosyncratic. Some people know lots about dogs, while others know very little.

This explicitly expressed knowledge about objects can be contrasted with a different level of object concept representation referred to as core properties or "semantic primitives" (Martin, 1998). In contrast to encyclopedic knowledge, semantic primitives are accessed implicitly and automatically in the service of comprehension, are highly constrained in number, and are universal. This level of representation allows us to quickly and efficiently identify objects and understand words, and forms the foundation for our vast stores of encyclopedic knowledge about objects. While the model to be described here does not address the organization of encyclopedic knowledge, it makes strong claims about the organization of semantic primitives with regard to both their representational content and organization in the brain.

In the sensory–motor model, the concept of an object is composed of semantic primitives that represent those properties of the object that allow for fast and efficient recognition. For example, the properties associated with common tools include stored representations of what they look like, how they move when used, and how they are manipulated. These primitives are stored within the same neural systems active when we learned about those properties. Specifically, they are stored within visual processing systems for perceiving object form and object motion, and action systems responsible for visuomotor transformations and for grasping and manipulating objects.

12.3   What we have learned from functional brain imaging about the representation of object properties and categories

First, I'll provide a brief overview of findings from functional brain imaging studies. Many of these findings have been reviewed in detail previously (e.g. Martin, 2001; Martin & Chao, 2001; Joseph, 2001; Bookheimer, 2002; Thompson-Schill, 2003).

1. *Conceptual processing of objects, as represented by pictures or words, is associated with activity in a widely distributed network.* The most commonly activated regions are bilateral ventral occipitotemporal and lateral temporal cortices, and left posterior parietal (especially the intraparietal sulcus), ventral premotor, and lateral prefrontal cortices.

2. *Activity within these regions is modulated by category.* Objects belonging to different conceptual categories produce different patterns of activity in these regions. The exception is left lateral prefrontal cortex, which has been

mostly strongly linked to selecting, retrieving, and manipulating semantic information assumed to be stored elsewhere (e.g. Gabrieli *et al.*, 1998; Badre *et al.*, 2005).

3. *All object categories tested to date show differential patterns of activity in ventral occipitotemporal cortex.* The most studied objects have been human faces, houses, animals, and tools (e.g. Chao *et al.*, 1999a; Yovel & Kanwisher, 2004). However, distinct object category-related patterns of activity have been reliably discriminated among relatively large sets of object categories (seven by Haxby *et al.*, 2001; seven by Spiridon & Kanwisher, 2002; ten by Cox & Savoy, 2003).

4. *Lateral temporal cortex responds to a more limited number of object categories than does ventral temporal cortex.* The most common finding has been activation of the superior temporal sulcus (STS) in response to faces and animals (typically stronger in the right than left hemisphere), and activation of the middle temporal gyrus (MTG) in response to tools (typically stronger in the left than right hemisphere). Objects shown moving in their characteristic fashion produce enhanced, category-related activity in these regions (Beauchamp *et al.*, 2002, 2003).

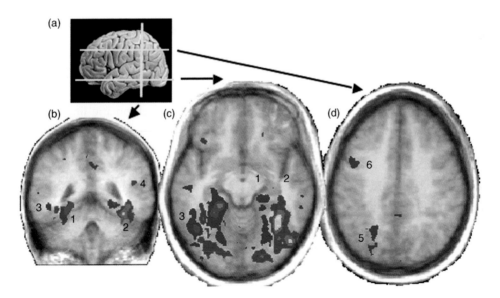

Figure 12.1. Group fMRI activation map showing the location of hemodynamic activity associated with naming pictures of animals (red–yellow spectrum) and pictures of tools (blue–green spectrum). Yellow lines on lateral view of the brain (A) indicate location of the coronal (B) and axial (C, D) slices. 1. Medial region of the fusiform gyrus. 2. Lateral region of the fusiform gyrus. 3. Left middle temporal gyrus, MTG. 4. Superior temporal sulcus, STS. 5. Left intraparietal sulcus. 6. Left ventral premotor cortex. Adapted from Chao *et al.* (2002).

5. *Activation of the intraparietal and ventral premotor cortices has been strongest to tools and other manipulable objects.* This activity is nearly always confined to the left hemisphere (e.g. Chao & Martin, 2000).

Based on these findings and the studies to be reviewed below, two conclusions can be drawn. First, the regions discussed above are involved in both perceiving and representing (storing) information about different object properties such as form (ventral occipitotemporal cortex), motion (lateral temporal cortex), and object use (intraparietal and ventral premotor regions). Second, at least some of these purported object-property regions appear to be organized by superordinate category, as well. This seems most clear for posterior regions of the temporal cortex. In the fusiform gyrus, stimuli depicting animate agents (humans and animals) produce more activity in the lateral portion than manipulable artifacts, while in the medial portion of the fusiform gyrus the opposite bias is found. In lateral temporal cortex, STS responds more to animate objects than to artifacts, while MTG responds more to manipulable artifacts than animate beings (see Figure 12.1 for the location of these regions).

12.4   Retrieving information about object properties: the representation of object-associated motion and object-associated color

In 1995 we reported findings from two experiments using positron emission tomography (PET) (Martin *et al.*, 1995). The paradigm was modeled after the now-classic verb generation paradigm developed by Petersen and colleagues (Petersen *et al.*, 1988). Subjects were presented with achromatic line drawing of objects (in one experiment) or the written names of objects (in the other experiment). In the critical conditions, subjects generated a word denoting an action associated with the object (e.g. "pull" in response to a child's wagon), and in another condition they generated a word denoting a color associated with the object ("red" for the child's wagon). One important outcome of this study was that in both experiments activity in posterior temporal cortex was modulated by the type of information subjects retrieved. Relative to color word generation, action words elicited heightened activity in several brain regions, including a posterior region of the left lateral temporal cortex, just anterior to the primary visual motion processing area, MT. It was the location of this activity near MT that initially motivated us to suggest that information about object motion may be stored in this region of the brain.

There are now well over two dozen experiments reporting an association between verb generation and activation of the posterior region of the left lateral temporal cortex, typically centering on MTG. These studies include wide variation in stimuli, mode of response, and experimental design. In addition, studies have been done in nine different native languages, thus attesting to the robustness and generality of the finding (reviewed in Martin, 2001; and see Shapiro *et al.*, 2006 for a recent functional magnetic resonance imaging (fMRI) study).

In contrast to action word generation, generating color words elicited heightened activity in ventral temporal cortex, centered on the fusiform gyrus, anterior to regions that respond to object form and color, regardless of whether the object is meaningful or not (Malach *et al.*, 1995; Martin *et al.*, 1996, Kanwisher *et al.*, 1997). Using the same logic applied to the action word generation results, we suggested that information about object color may be stored in the region of the fusiform showing greater activity during color than action word generation.

Although color word generation has not received the same attention in the literature as has action word generation, we have replicated this finding in two other studies. The first study sought to identify regions differentially engaged by semantic and episodic memory retrieval (Wiggs *et al.*, 1999). Patterns of activity associated with retrieving information about an object's typical color (the semantic memory task; e.g. responding "brown" to an achromatic drawing of a football) were contrasted with a condition in which subjects retrieved recently learned, novel color–object associations (the episodic memory task; e.g. responding "purple" to a picture of a football). These two memory retrieval conditions were equated for the stimuli used to cue retrieval (object pictures), information retrieved (color words), and accuracy of performance. Each retrieval task was found to be associated with distinct, albeit overlapping, networks. Most relevant for the present discussion, generating words denoting an object's typical color was associated with activity in the same region of the left ventral temporal cortex as identified in our initial studies.

In a second follow-up study, color word generation was evaluated in relation to color naming and color perception (Chao & Martin, 1999). During different PET scans, subjects viewed colored Mondrians and equiluminant, gray-scale versions of those Mondrians to identify color-responsive areas. During other scans subjects were presented with achromatic line drawings of objects embedded in gray-scale Mondrians and appropriately colored line drawings of objects embedded in colored Mondrians, to identify areas associated with object naming, color naming, and color word generation. The main finding was that color word generation activated the same site in left posterior ventral temporal cortex as found in our previous reports. However, retrieving color information did not activate sites in occipital cortex that were active when viewing the colored Mondrians (lingual gyrus).

This later finding was consistent with a study of color–word synethestes who experience vivid color imagery when hearing words (Paulesu *et al.*, 1995), and with a study of color perception and color imagery in normal subjects (Howard *et al.*, 1998). In both of those studies, color imagery was associated with activation of sites in the ventral temporal lobe nearly identical to those found in our color word generation studies, but not in occipital sites active during color perception (e.g. Zeki *et al.*, 1991). These findings, coupled with clinical reports of a double dissociation between color perception and color imagery in brain-damaged patients (De Vreese, 1991; Shuren *et al.*, 1996), suggest that information about object color is stored in ventral temporal cortex, and that the critical site is close to, but does not include, sites in occipital cortex that selectively respond to the presence of color.

This claim appears to be at odds with the assertion that the same neural systems are involved, at least in part, in perceiving and knowing about specific object attributes. However, in our study (Chao & Martin, 1999), relative to naming colored objects, naming the color of colored objects elicited activity in occipital regions active when passively viewing colored Mondrians, as well as in the more anterior site in the fusiform gyrus of the temporal lobe active during the color word generation task. Thus, when forced to attend to the specific color of an object, more anterior regions of the temporal lobe are active. This finding is consistent with the notion that the same system may be active during perceiving and knowing about a specific object feature or attribute.

Recent fMRI evidence has provided direct evidence for this claim. Beauchamp and colleagues (1999) replicated previous studies showing that activity is limited to the occipital lobes when color perception was tested by passive viewing. However, when a more attention-demanding color perception task was used, modeled after a standard clinical color perception test (Farnsworth–Munsell Color Perception Task), activity associated with perceiving color now extended from occipital cortex into ventral temporal cortex and the fusiform gyrus. Using Beauchamp's adaptation of the Farnsworth–Munsell Color Perception Task, Simmons and colleagues have now shown that retrieving information about object color – but not object motion – does in fact activate the same region in the fusiform gyrus active when color is perceived (Simmons *et al.*, 2006). Thus these data provide strong evidence that information about a particular object property like its typical color is stored in the same neural system active when colors are actively perceived.

I shall now discuss studies that suggest a relationship between these property-based systems and object categories.

12.5   Property-based neural circuits for representing object categories

In 1996 we reported findings from two PET experiments on the neural systems
associated with naming objects from two different semantic categories (animals
and tools; Martin *et al.*, 1996). Subjects named line drawings of objects in
one study, and object silhouettes in the other study. Both studies yielded similar
results. The main findings were that both animal and tool naming elicited bilateral
activity in the posterior region of ventral temporal cortex (centered on the
fusiform gyrus). In addition, relative to naming tools, naming animals showed
heightened activity in the medial region of the occipital cortex. In contrast, relative
to naming animals, naming tools yielded heightened activity in the posterior
region of the left MTG — overlapping with the activity associated with action
word generation — and in left premotor cortex. To account for these findings,
we suggested that this activity may reflect the fact that identifying tools is
dependent on access to information about how these objects move (left MTG) and
how they are manipulated (left ventral premotor cortex).

12.6   Distributed representations for animals, tools, faces, and houses

A surprising and problematic finding from our PET study was that the medial
region of the occipital cortex was the only site more active for naming animals than
tools. To explain this finding we suggested that it might reflect top–down
modulation of early visual areas when access to knowledge about subtle differences
in visual properties is needed to distinguish one category member (dog) from
another (cat). We rejected the argument that the medial occipital activity was due
to greater visual complexity of the animal compared to the tool stimuli based on
the findings from the silhouette study (and see Martin, 2001 for a review of studies
showing greater occipital lobe activity for animals than tools using words, as well
as pictures). The occipital finding, however, was problematic for two reasons.
First, if medial occipital activity was driven top–down, then from where did this
activity originate? Second, although cases have been reported with impaired
knowledge of animals resulting from an occipital lesion (Nielsen, 1958;
Tranel *et al.*, 1997), most cases have had lesions of the temporal lobe (Capitani
et al., 2003). Thus we turned to fMRI to see if the increased spatial resolution
afforded by this imaging modality over PET might reveal more fine-grained
category-related differences in patterns of activity. Our first report (Chao *et al.*,
1999a) concentrated on occipitotemporal cortex. Two of the experiments
evaluated category-related activity during viewing and delayed match-to-sample
with photographs of animals, tools, faces, and houses. Two other experiments
evaluated category-related activity by covert naming of photographs of animals

and tools, and by a property verification task using written words to probe knowledge about animals and tools. The main findings were that, in addition to replicating greater occipital lobe activity for animals than tools, category-related differences were noted in the temporal lobes. Specifically, animals (as well as faces) showed heightened, bilateral activity in the lateral region of the fusiform gyrus, while tools (and houses) showed heightened bilateral activity in the medial region of the fusiform gyrus. Recent investigations from a number of other laboratories have shown a similar distinction between the lateral and medial fusiform gyrus for animate and manipulable objects, respectively. For example, Whatmough *et al.* (2002) reported greater activation in the medial fusiform for naming tools than animals, Price *et al.* (2003) reported greater activation of the lateral fusiform for animal pictures relative to tools, and Devlin *et al.* (2005) confirmed the distinction between lateral and medial fusiform for animals and tools using words, rather than pictures, as stimuli. In addition, as in our PET study, we found greater activity in the posterior region of the left MTG for tools than for animals. In contrast, greater activity for animals (and for faces) was found in STS, especially in the right hemisphere.

In the fusiform gyrus there was substantial overlap in the patterns of activity between animals and faces, and between tools and houses. Nevertheless, direct comparison of these categories revealed differences between them, as well. Specifically, animals activated more cortex than faces, and the strongest activity associated with viewing tools was lateral to those associated with houses (see Chao *et al.*, 1999a, for details). These findings suggested that object categories are represented by more elaborate, distributed, and fine-grained networks than revealed by PET. These networks include category-related patterns of activity in both ventral (fusiform gyrus) and lateral (STS, MTG) regions of the posterior temporal cortex.

The regions of posterior temporal cortex that responded more to animals than tools were in areas previously identified as part of the face processing system. Specifically, the lateral occipital gyrus, the lateral region of the fusiform gyrus (the fusiform face area; FFA), and the STS. Activation of the lateral region of the fusiform gyrus in response to human faces relative to other object categories has probably been replicated more times than any other finding in functional brain imaging (for a recent series of elegant studies on faces processing and domain-specificity see Yovel & Kanwisher, 2004). One explanation for this commonality is that the response to animals was not about animals, per se, but rather reflected perceptual processing of the animal faces. We directly addressed this issue by contrasting activity during a delayed match-to-sample task with pictures of animals with their faces completely obscured by a white circle, unobscured animals, human faces, and houses (Chao *et al.*, 1999b). The main finding was that animals with faces and animals without faces showed increased activation in the same lateral fusiform region that showed a greater response to human faces than houses. Moreover, in this region (and in STS) activity associated with animals and faceless animals did not differ. Our results strongly suggest that the response to animals in the lateral fusiform gyrus and STS was not driven by perceptual processes unique to face perception. A similar finding has been reported by Cox *et al.*, who showed that the FFA was active even when human faces were completely occluded (Cox *et al.*, 2004; although see Kanwisher *et al.*, 1999 for contrary evidence).

12.7   The representation of motion properties in the posterior, lateral temporal cortex (MTG, STS)

One of the main assumptions of the sensory–motor account is that activity in lateral temporal cortex reflects properties of motion associated with specific categories of objects. Previous data from studies of monkeys (e.g. Oram & Perrett, 1994) and many functional brain imaging studies of humans (e.g. Puce *et al.*, 1998; Grossman & Blake, 2001) have shown that STS is particularly responsive to biological motion. As noted previously, we have suggested that motion-related information needed to identify manipulable objects is represented in the cortex inferior to STS, specifically in the left MTG and adjoining inferior temporal sulcus. Consistent with this speculation, Tranel and colleagues found that patients with lesions in left MTG (or left intraparietal, or left premotor regions) have selective difficulty naming and retrieving information about tools and their associated actions (Tranel *et al.*, 1997, 2003). However, whether MTG is sensitive to motion, and whether it is differentially sensitive to motion characteristic of non-biological objects, had not been determined. Thus, to directly address this issue, we carried out a series of experiments to test the hypothesis that lateral temporal cortex is differentially sensitive to the motion properties of different object categories.

In the first series of studies, we examined hemodynamic responses to low- and high-contrast moving gratings (used to identify primary motion processing region MT), to biological motion (human figures), and to motion of manipulable objects (tools) (Beauchamp *et al.*, 2002). Three regions in posterior lateral temporal cortex – area MT, STS and MTG – responded to the motion stimuli, and all three areas preferred human and tool motion to moving gratings. As expected, area MT did not show a category bias, with responses here being equally strong for human and tool-related motion. However, anterior and superior to MT in STS, a larger response was observed for human compared with tool motion, while anterior and inferior to MT in MTG, a larger response was observed for tool motion compared with human motion. Thus these regions showed a strong category-related effect.

We then sought to demonstrate that activity in STS and MTG was related to object-associated motion, rather than simply reflecting the category-related responses observed for static stimuli as found in our previous studies. Subjects performed tasks with both static and moving images. As in the studies reviewed previously, different patterns of category-related activity were noted in the fusiform gyrus, with the lateral portion more responsive to human figures, and the medial portion more responsive to tools. Most importantly, these regions of ventral temporal cortex responded similarly to moving and static objects, even though the moving stimuli were more visually complex and interesting than the static images. Thus ventral temporal cortex showed strong category effects, but these effects were not modulated by motion. In contrast, in addition to a category effect, lateral temporal areas responded much more strongly to moving than static stimuli, supporting the hypothesis that lateral temporal cortex is the cortical locus of complex motion processing (Figure 12.2). These findings also suggest the possibility that these motion sensitive regions have a category-based organization.

In a third experiment, we explored the visual properties underlying the differential sensitivity of STS and MTG to human and tool motion. When humans move, different body parts typically move with complex motion trajectories connected by articulated joints, while tools typically move with simple motion trajectories and few degrees of articulation. We reasoned that if STS prefers flexible, articulated motion, then STS should respond more to humans moving with articulated motion (as during a jumping jack) than to humans moving with unarticulated motion (moving up and down like a hammer). Similarly, if MTG prefers the rigid, unarticulated motion characteristic of tools, it should respond more to unarticulated human motion than to articulated human motion. We constructed stimuli containing humans and tools moving with artificial motion trajectories consisting of simple translation and rotation with no articulation. As predicted, STS preferred humans moving with many degrees of articulation to humans moving with unarticulated motion vectors, while MTG responded more strongly to unarticulated human movements than to articulated human movements. This suggests that the category preferences in STS and MTG may be related to, or emerge from, preferences for different types or patterns of motion (Beauchamp *et al.*, 2002; Beauchamp & Martin, in press).

To follow up on these findings, we created stimuli for which information about object category was dependent on an analysis of motion by using point-light

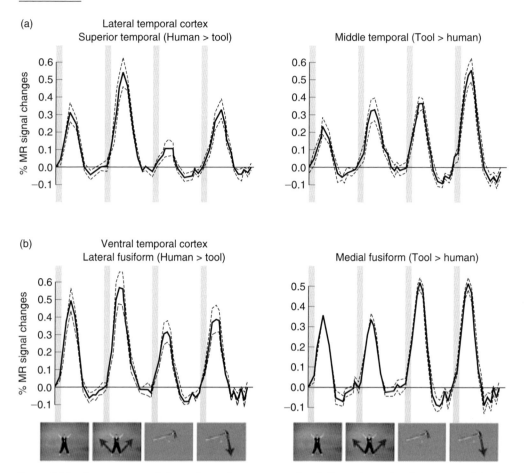

Figure 12.2. Group averaged hemodynamic responses to static and moving humans and tools in (A) lateral and (B) ventral temporal cortices. Vertical gray bars indicate stimulus presentation (2 s). Dashed lines indicate ± 1 SEM. Adapted from Beauchamp *et al.* (2002).

displays (moving dots that are readily interpreted as a single, complex object in motion; Beauchamp *et al.*, 2003). While previous neuroimaging studies examined cortical responses to human point-light displays (e.g. Grossman & Blake 2001, 2002), none compared point-light displays of human motion to point-light displays of tool motion.

Subjects viewed short movies of real objects and point light displays and decided if they depicted a human or a tool. Consistent with our previous studies, real-object and point-light displays of humans elicited stronger activity in the lateral fusiform gyrus and STS than tool stimuli. In contrast, real-object and point-light displays of tools elicited stronger activity in the medial fusiform gyrus, MTG (as well as in left parietal and ventral premotor cortices) relative to human stimuli. Importantly, regions in ventral (lateral and medial fusiform regions) and lateral

(STS and MTG) temporal cortex showed differential responses to human and tool point-light displays. In lateral temporal regions, the responses were nearly equivalent to real-object and point-light displays, suggesting that visual motion, not color or form, is a key determinant of activity in lateral temporal cortex. In contrast, in ventral temporal cortex, the response to the point-light displays was significantly reduced relative to real-object videos (Beauchamp *et al.*, 2003).

Taken together with the previously described studies, these data add to a growing body of evidence on the different response properties of ventral and lateral temporal cortex. Both ventral and lateral cortex responded in a category-related manner (lateral fusiform and STS showing a greater response to human figures than tools, medial fusiform and MTG showing the opposite response pattern). Adding motion had little effect on the responses in fusiform regions, but markedly increased responses in lateral temporal cortex (Beauchamp *et al.*, 2002). Eliminating form and color (point-light displays) had little effect on lateral temporal regions, but markedly reduced the response in ventral temporal cortex (Beauchamp *et al.*, 2003).

12.8 Beyond the temporal lobes: premotor and intraparietal regions associated with grasping objects are active when viewing and naming tools

The relationship between activity in the dorsal stream − particularly in left intraparietal sulcus and left ventral premotor cortex − and the representation of man-made, manipulable objects, has been an very active field of investigation (for review see Johnson-Frey, 2004). Naming photographs of tools, or even simply viewing these pictures, has been shown to elicit enhanced activity for tools in left ventral premotor cortex and in left parietal cortex centered on the intraparietal sulcus, relative to viewing animals, houses, and faces, and relative to naming pictures of animals (Chao & Martin, 2000). These findings are consistent with data from monkey neurophysiology showing that ventral premotor and intraparietal regions contain neurons that respond when the monkey grasps objects and also when seeing objects that they have had experience manipulating ("canonical neuron"; Jeannerod *et al.*, 1995). In the human brain, information about how objects are used may be stored in these regions. As in other regions of the network (medial region of the fusiform gyrus, left MTG), this information may be automatically activated whenever an object is identified (for a recent replication an extension of these findings using words, see Noppeney *et al.*, 2006).

12.9   What do the overlapping patterns of cortical activity mean? Learning-dependent modulation of object category-related activity

All of the fMRI studies from our laboratory and others have shown that regions showing category-related activity respond to many different categories of objects. That is, a region responding maximally to one object category (e.g. preferring tools over animals or faces) is not silent to the "non-preferred" categories (animals, faces). Rather, the response is simply less robust to these other categories. Nevertheless, the activations elicited by these non-preferred categories are significantly above a non-object baseline (see Figure 12.2). There are two views on these weaker activations. In one view they are considered non-specific responses to the presence of any complex visual form. Thus, in this view, weaker activations carry no information about these object categories. This is a necessary assumption if one wants to label a region as face-selective, or tool-selective, etc. (Spiridon & Kanwisher, 2002). The alternative view is that the weaker activations are meaningful in the sense that they carry information about the non-preferred object category. In this view, object categories are associated with widespread, and overlapping, patterns of activity (given the spatial resolution of fMRI; Haxby *et al.*, 2001). A category of objects is represented by the entire pattern of activity, not just by the activity in the region showing a stronger response to this category versus others. We reasoned that an experimental manipulation that modulates the strength of activation should allow us to differentiate between these interpretations.

It has been well established that prior experience with an object results in more efficient processing (i.e. repetition priming), and a reduced hemodynamic response — typically referred to as repetition suppression — when that object is encountered at a latter time (see Grill-Spector *et al.*, 2006, for recent review of neural models of repetition suppression). Recent studies have documented the usefulness of using repetition paradigms — also referred to as adaptation paradigms — for evaluating the processing characteristics of select brain regions (Grill-Spector & Malach, 2001). Within a region, if the responses to both the preferred and non-preferred category are informative, then both responses should be reduced with repetition. If the response to only the preferred category is informative, then a repetition-related reduction in hemodynamic response should be found for only the preferred category.

To evaluate these possibilities, subjects were given experience in naming and performing other tasks with sets of animal and tool pictures. Four days later they were scanned while silently naming these pictures and pictures of animals and tools they had not previously seen (Chao *et al.*, 2002). The results provided evidence that both views may be correct, depending on region and category.

Within the ventral object processing stream, responses to both preferred and non-preferred categories were reduced with experience. The lateral region of the fusiform gyrus, defined by a greater response to naming animals than tools, showed a reduced response to previously named animals and tools, relative to those not seen before. The medial region of the fusiform gyrus, defined by a greater response to naming tools than animals, showed an experience-related reduction in response to both object categories, as well (see Avidan *et al.*, 2002 for similar findings).

In contrast, other regions (right STS, left MTG, left intraparietal, and ventral premotor cortices) showed reduced hemodynamic responses only to the preferred category. For example, as in our previous studies, naming tools elicited a stronger response in ventral premotor cortex than naming animals. Although the response to naming animal pictures was significantly above baseline, this response was equivalent for both new and old animal pictures (i.e. no repetition suppression effect). This result was interpreted as consistent with the sensory–motor account of concept organization. If information about how objects are used is represented in parietal and premotor areas, then responses in these regions should be associated only with objects that are typically manipulated (i.e. tools, not animals). A major implication of these findings is that the presence of a significant hemodynamic response does not, in and of itself, indicate whether that response is meaningful. In each case, evidence will be needed to show that the response can be experimentally modulated in a predictable fashion.

Given these findings, I shall now discuss a series of studies aimed at addressing particular questions and concerns about the organization of conceptual knowledge in the brain as revealed by functional brain imaging.

12.10   Is activity in the fusiform gyrus related to conceptual processing?

I have suggested that category-related activity in the fusiform gyrus and elsewhere in ventral object processing stream reflects, in part, the automatic retrieval of stored information about object form properties necessary to identify objects quickly and efficiently. Furthermore, I have argued that this information is accessed regardless of the physical nature of the stimulus used to represent the object. Support for this notion comes from studies that have presented objects in the form of their written names, rather than as pictures. Alternatively, it could be argued that these activations do not reflect conceptual processing, per se, but rather the explicit retrieval of visual object imagery that accompanies task performance. Thus one could argue that the words in these tasks triggered visual imagery, which then recruited ventral occipitotemporal cortex indirectly, rather than this area doing any conceptual work. Indeed, fusiform gyrus activity has been associated with object imagery (Ishai *et al.*, 2000; O'Craven & Kanwisher, 2000), word imageability (Wise *et al.*, 2000), imagery associated with property verification tasks (Kan *et al.*, 2003) and with the generation of mental images from spoken words relative to passive listening (D'Esposito *et al.*, 1997).

As noted previously, repetition suppression effects can be used to evaluate learning-related changes in specific regions of the cortex. To address this important concern about explicit visual image generation we sought to determine if automatic semantic priming is associated with a repetition suppression. In an automatic semantic priming paradigm, word pairs are presented using a short stimulus–onset asynchrony (SOA, the time from the onset of the first word in a pair to the onset of the second word). We reasoned that modulations associated with automatic semantic priming would occur too quickly to be reasonably ascribed to explicit visual image generation. Thus finding repetition suppression effects due to reading semantically related word pairs would add considerable weight to the claim that these regions are involved in conceptual representation. In our study, we presented word pairs consisting of the names of unrelated (apple–lion), semantically related (chair–bed), and identical (dog–dog) objects. The duration of the word pairs was 400 ms (150 ms per word with a blank 100 ms inter-stimulus interval (ISI), yielding a 250 ms SOA). We identified all of the brain regions that were active when subjects read the word pairs, and then investigated the pattern of activity in these regions associated with the different word pair types (unrelated, semantically related, identical). Repetition-related reductions in hemodynamic responses (i.e. repetition suppression) was observed in several regions, prominently including the fusiform gyrus. Activity in the fusiform gyrus was greatest for unrelated pairs, less for semantically related pairs, and least for the same-word repetitions, mirroring the pattern of behavioral performance based on reading times for the second word in each pair (slowest for unrelated, faster for related, and fastest for identical words; Wheatley *et al.*, 2005) (Figure 12.3). Thus the fusiform gyrus, and other regions (left prefrontal cortex) were sensitive to object meaning, even when neither explicit selection nor retrieval of semantic information was required. Moreover, because of the extremely short duration between word pairs, these data seem to rule out the possibility that fusiform activity was due to the explicit generation of visual object images.

It is important to stress that I am not suggesting that visual imagery (i.e. retrieving stored information about what an object looks like) played no part in producing the pattern of results we observed in this and other studies. To the contrary, I would argue that it was the retrieval of visual information about the objects that was primarily responsible for the activations we observed in the fusiform gyrus. However, it is assumed that this visual object information

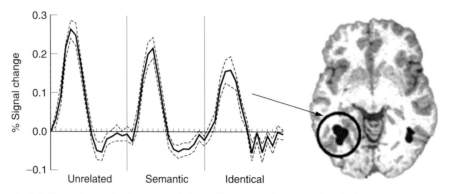

Figure 12.3. Modulation of neural activity associated with automatic semantic priming. Group averaged hemodynamic response from the region of left fusiform gyrus identified by comparing all word pair conditions to visual fixation. Dashed lines indicate ± 1 SEM. Axial slice shows location of the activation. Adapted from Wheatley *et al.* (2005).

is automatically retrieved as an unconscious and obligatory byproduct of normal reading of concrete nouns. In that case, automatic, implicit generation of an object image would be the mechanism by which we access an important property underlying the meaning of words denoting concrete entities (i.e. information about what the object looks like). In this sense, implicit visual imagery would be an obligatory component of reading for meaning. The main point here is that these data argue against the idea that activation of the fusiform gyrus during conceptual processing tasks can be readily explained by the non-obligatory, explicit generation of visual object images that occurred after the word's meaning had been determined (and see Gold *et al.*, in press, for a recent replication of repetition suppression in the fusiform gyrus by automatic semantic priming).

12.11 Are these neural circuits involved in learning about object property information?

Within the context of the sensory–motor model outlined here, differential activation of the medial fusiform gyrus, left MTG, intraparietal, and ventral premotor regions represent automatic retrieval of information about form, motion, and use-associated motor skills, respectively, of man-made manipulable objects such as common tools. It is further assumed that this information is necessary for the rapid and efficient identification of objects from this superordinate category. If so, then it should be possible, in principle, to elicit activity in these regions, *de novo*, as a result of experience with novel objects.

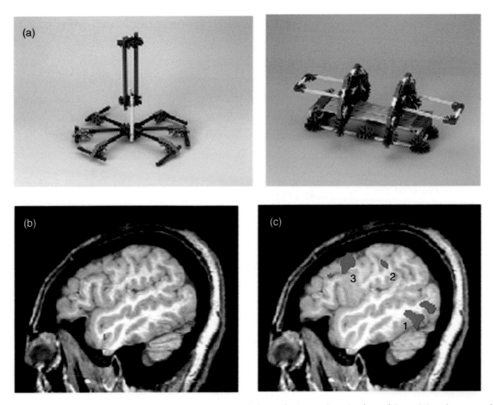

Figure 12.4. (A) Examples of novel objects. Left lateral view of a single subject (A) prior to training, and (B) after extensive training to use the novel objects to perform specific functional tasks. 1. MTG; 2. intraparietal sulcus. 3. ventral premotor cortex. Adapted from Weisberg *et al.* (in press).

To address this possibility, we created a set of 32 novel objects (Figure 12.4) (Weisberg *et al.*, in press). Although they do not look like tools, each object could be used to perform a specific, tool-like task. Subjects were given extensive experience performing functional tasks with 16 of these objects (three 90-minute sessions, over a 10-day period). Subjects were scanned, prior to and after training, while performing a simple visual matching task with pictures of the objects taken from different views, and with phase-scrambled images of the objects.

The critical question was: how did the pattern of activity associated with viewing these objects change after subjects had received extensive experience using them as tools? Prior to training, performing the simple visual matching task elicited activity in the posterior ventral cortex, consistent with previous reports on viewing non-meaningful objects (e.g. van Turennout *et al.*, 2000). However, after training, a very different picture remerged. First, activations in ventral cortex became more focal. Specifically, whereas prior to training, activity was widespread in the fusiform gyrus, after training activity was markedly reduced in the more lateral parts of the fusiform (i.e. regions preferring biological, animate objects such as animals and people, and faces), and markedly increased in the medial portion of the fusiform associated with known tools. In addition, after training, new activations emerged in the network of left-hemisphere regions previously linked to naming and retrieving information about tools. Specifically, training-related, heightened activity was now seen in the left MTG, left intraparietal sulcus, and left premotor cortex (Figure 12.4).

Thus, in contrast to repetition suppression, we observed repetition enhancements (Desimone, 1996; Henson, 2003). Moreover, these enhancements occurred in regions linked to perceiving and knowing about common tools. Previous studies have suggested that repetition enhancement occurs when there is a qualitative difference in the way an object is perceived from one repetition to the next. For example, repetition of ambiguous, degraded objects led to increased ventral temporal activity when subjects were exposed to intact, unambiguous versions of the objects interspersed between repetitions (Dolan et al., 1997). In a similar fashion, hands-on experience with the objects in our study may have augmented their representations with detailed information about their appearance (medial portion of the fusiform gyrus), and with information about the motion (middle temporal gyrus) and motor-related properties (parietal and premotor cortices) associated with their use. As a result, objects perceived as meaningless during the first scanning session were now perceived as objects with distinct functional properties. Thus the training interspersed between scanning sessions transformed the representation of these objects, leading to heightened activity from one scanning session to the next. Moreover, this heightened activity occurred in circumscribed regions associated with tools and their use, each of which is presumed to store information about perceptual or functional object properties.

These findings are consistent with the idea that we possess specialized neural circuitry for learning about specific sensory- and motor-related properties associated with an object's appearance and use (Santos et al., 2003). Furthermore, the fact that this network was automatically engaged when perceiving the novel objects following training suggests that one role of these specialized systems may be to allow the organism to acquire information about the properties critical for identifying a category of objects, and to use this information in order to discriminate among them quickly and efficiently (Mahon & Caramazza, 2003). Moreover, our findings show that the locus of learning-related cortical plasticity appears to be highly constrained by both the nature of the information to be learned, and how it is acquired.

12.12   Can object category-related neural systems be active in a purely top–down fashion?

A central question related to the functional neuroanatomy of object category-related activity is the extent to which patterns of activity in posterior regions of temporal cortex (especially in the fusiform gyrus) reflect top–down versus bottom–up processes. If, for example, the activations in lateral and medial regions of the fusiform gyrus reflect, at least in part, stored information about the shapes of animate objects (animal, faces, humans) and tools, respectively, then it should be possible to elicit these category-related patterns of activity when the same visual objects are used to represent animate entities and artifacts. This would eliminate the concern that these category-related activations were solely due to bottom–up processing of visual differences in the shape or color of the stimuli used to represent them.

To address this question, we developed a set of animations composed of simple geometric forms in motion (Martin & Weisberg, 2003). The study was modeled after the now-classic demonstration by Heider and Simmel (1944) that simple geometric forms in motion can be interpreted, with little effort, as depicting animate beings with specific goals and intentions. Subjects were shown animated vignettes designed to elicit concepts related to social interactions (e.g. children playing baseball, sharing ice cream) or mechanical devices (a factory conveyor belt, a pin-ball machine). The same geometric forms were shown in random motion and in static displays for control conditions. The results showed the same dissociation in ventral and lateral temporal cortices as seen for animate objects and artifacts (Figure 12.5). In ventral temporal cortex, vignettes interpreted as conveying social interactions elicited heightened activity in the lateral fusiform gyrus, while the mechanical vignettes led to heightened activity in the medial fusiform gyrus. In lateral temporal cortex, the social vignettes elicited bilateral activation of STS (stronger in the right than left hemisphere), as typically seen with animate objects, whereas the mechanical vignettes elicited activity in left MTG, as typically seen for tools. Because the same geometric forms were used in both the social and mechanical animations, these results cannot be due to bottom–up processing of the visual stimuli. They must reflect top–down influences.

Interpreting the social vignettes also elicited activity in several regions associated with social and affective processes (e.g. Adolphs, 2001). Specifically, greater activity for social than mechanical vignettes was found in anterior regions of STS, the amygdala, and in ventromedial prefrontal cortex, all strongly lateralized to the right hemisphere (Figure 12.5). Thus these regions can be activated by stimuli that, in and of themselves, have neither affective valence nor

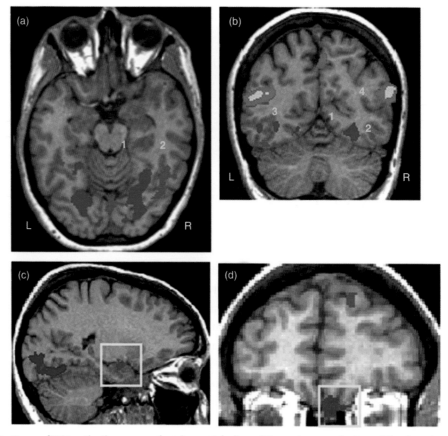

Figure 12.5. Group fMRI activation map showing axial view (A), and coronal view (B) of regions with greater activity associated with social (red) and mechanical (blue) interpretations of moving geometric forms. 1. Medial fusiform gyrus; 2. Lateral fusiform gyrus; 3. MTG, 4. STS. (compare to Figure 12.1). Yellow squares indicate right amygdala (C) and ventromedial prefrontal region (D) more active for social than mechanical vignettes. Adapted from Martin and Weisberg (2003).

social significance. The findings associated with the social vignettes closely replicated and extended the findings reported by Castelli and colleagues (Castelli *et al.*, 2000) and Shultz and colleagues (Schultz *et al.*, 2003) using a different set of animations that more closely resemble the original Heider and Simmel stimuli. By including the mechanical condition in our study, we were able to distinguish between regions associated with specific conceptual domains (social, mechanical) from those involved in the more general-purpose, problem-solving aspects of the tasks. These findings suggest that a higher-order concept like "animacy" may be represented in a network of regions composed of areas that store knowledge of what animate objects look like (lateral fusiform gyrus), how they move (STS), coupled with areas for representing and modulating affect (amygdala and ventromedial frontal cortex). In this way, a property-based framework can provide the foundation or building blocks for realizing a large variety of basic object, as well as higher-order conceptual representations. A network dedicated to processing within the social domain is consistent with a domain-specific account, as well. Specifically, the data are consistent with the argument that natural selection has equipped us with a dedicated neural system for quick and efficient problem solving within the social domain.

12.13   Concluding comments

The evidence reviewed in this chapter suggests that we have dedicated neural circuitry for perceiving and knowing about animate agents and common tools. For animate agents, this circuitry includes two regions in posterior temporal cortex: the lateral portion of the fusiform gyrus and the STS. In addition, evidence is mounting that the amygdala also plays a prominent role in this circuitry, perhaps as a means of alerting the organism to a potentially threatening predator or prey (Yang *et al.*, 2005). Other regions, such as medial prefrontal cortex, may also be prominently involved when retrieving information about others (e.g. Mitchell *et al.*, 2002). For common tools, the neural circuitry includes the medial portion of the fusiform gyrus, as well as MTG, intraparietal sulcus, and premotor cortex, all within the left hemisphere.

In addition to the studies and evidence discussed in this chapter, findings from a large number of laboratories have provided evidence for other examples of domain-specificity in this region of the brain. This work includes studies showing that a region of the parahippocampal cortex is particularly responsive to depictions of places (outdoor scenes, buildings) and, on a more conceptual level, to objects strongly associated with spatial contexts (Bar & Aminoff, 2003). In addition, consistent with the idea that visual form is represented in ventral temporal cortex, there is mounting evidence for a region specialized for processing letter strings (the visual word form area, VWFA; Polk & Farah, 1998; Cohen *et al.*, 2000). Thus, rather than being a homogeneous, general object processing system, ventral occipital–temporal cortex has a distinct organization. Moreover, and perhaps most surprisingly, the spatial layout of these category-related regions is highly consistent from one subject to another. How to account for this consistency is a particularly challenging problem for future investigations. On the one hand, this consistently suggests the operation of strong, and perhaps genetically determined, constraints. On the other hand, the existence of a visual word form area provides equally strong argument against genetic influences. After all, how could we be predisposed to develop a brain region specialized to accomplish a task — reading — that was only invented about 5500 years ago? One solution to this difficult problem is to suppose that the VWFA performs a visual processing function that predisposed it to being co-opted for reading. On this view, all of the so-called "category-related regions" discussed in this chapter presumably perform some as yet unspecified visual processing function that made them particularly well suited to process and store information associated with different object categories. The suggestion here is that the origin of these processing biases may be related to bottom–up features of the visual processing system (e.g. retinotopic organization; Malach *et al.*, 2002), and/or physical features of the stimuli themselves (e.g. spatial frequency, curvy versus angular forms, etc.). Top–down influences also likely play a prominent role in the form of predetermined connections between regions of occipitotemporal cortex and other brain areas. For example, the lateral regions of the fusiform gyrus may have developed its role in perceiving and storing information about animate objects due to privileged access to information from the amygdala (see Freese & Amaral, 2005, for evidence for direct feedback connections in the monkey from the amygdala to posterior regions of temporal and occipital cortex). In a similar fashion, the medial parts of the fusiform gyrus may receive privileged access to information about object manipulation from intraparietal and premotor regions, the parahippocampal area may received privileged access from parietal regions concerned with spatial vision, and the VWFA may have developed its role in reading due, in part, to privileged access to information originating in frontal and temporal regions that support language. Thus the possibility that different regions of ventral occipitotemporal cortex receive privileged bottom–up and top–down inputs may provide important clues to understanding the organization, and development, of object category-related regions in ventral temporal cortex.

Many questions remain to be resolved about the organization of neural systems supporting the expression of conceptual knowledge. Prominently included in that list will be a better understanding of how the nodes of the neural systems described in this chapter are bound together (e.g. Damasio, 1989), and how activity within the network is coordinated in the service of conceptual processing (Kraut *et al.*, 2002). An understanding of how category-related information links with lexical information and with other brain regions involved in supporting more general conceptual and semantic processes (e.g. left anterior temporal and inferior frontal cortices) is also lacking. Equally important will be to identify the neural systems that house the encyclopedic and associative object knowledge mentioned at the beginning of this chapter. In this regard, it is assumed that the neural systems discussed here provide the foundation or scaffolding that allowed this information to be acquired in a fast and efficient manner.

One great advantage of functional imaging studies of the human brain is that it provides a means of not only identifying regions involved in performing a particular task, but also designing studies to probe the processing characteristics of each of those regions (e.g. testing hypotheses about the sensitivity of different regions of lateral temporal cortex to different types of object-associated motion; Beauchamp *et al.*, 2002, 2003). Nevertheless, it is important to note that the labels I've applied to the regions discussed in this chapter should be viewed only as place holders awaiting a much more precise and useful description of the role that these regions play in perceptual and conceptual information processing and storage. Future studies using high-resolution brain imaging and electrophysiological recordings in human and nonhuman primates offer the promise that this goal may be in reach.

REFERENCES

Adolphs, R. (2001). The neurobiology of social cognition. *Current Opinion in Neurobiology*, **11**: 231–9.

Avidan, G., Hasson, U., Hendler, T., Zohary, E., and Malach, R. (2002). Analysis of the neuronal selectivity underlying low fMRI signals. *Current Biology*, **12**: 964–72.

Badre, D., Poldrack, R. A., Pare-Blagoev, E. J., Insler, R. Z., and Wagner, A. D. (2005). Dissociable controlled retrieval and generalized selection mechanisms in ventrolateral prefrontal cortex. *Neuron*, **47**: 907–18.

Bar, M. and Aminoff, E. (2003). Cortical analysis of visual context. *Neuron*, **38**: 347–58.

Beauchamp, M. S., Haxby, J. V., Jennings, J. E., and DeYoe, E. A. (1999). An fMRI version of the Farnsworth–Munsell 100-Hue test reveals multiple color-selective areas in human ventral occipitotemporal cortex. *Cerebral Cortex*, **9**: 257–63.

Beauchamp, M. S. and Martin, A. (in press). Grounding object concepts in perception and action: evidence from fMRI studies of tools. *Cortex*.

Beauchamp, M. S., Lee, K. E., Haxby, J. V., and Martin, A. (2002). Parallel visual motion processing streams for manipulable objects and human movements. *Neuron*, **34**: 149–59.

Beauchamp, M. S., Lee, K. E., Haxby, J. V., and Martin, A. (2003). fMRI responses to video and point-light displays of moving humans and manipulable objects. *Journal of Cognitive Neuroscience*, **15**: 991–1001.

Bookheimer, S. (2002). Functional MRI of language: new approaches to understanding the cortical organization of semantic processing. *Annual Review of Neuroscience*, **25**: 151–88.

Capitani, E., Laiacona, M., Mahon, B., and Caramazza, A. (2003). What are the facts of semantic category-specific deficits? A critical review of the clinical evidence. *Cognitive Neuropsychology*, **20**: 213–61.

Caramazza, A. (1998). The interpretation of semantic category-specific deficits: what do they reveal about the organization of conceptual knowledge in the brain? Introduction. *Neurocase*, **4**: 265−72.

Caramazza, A. and Mahon, B. Z. (2003). The organization of conceptual knowledge: the evidence from category-specific semantic deficits. *Trends in Cognitive Sciences*, **7**: 354−61.

Caramazza, A. and Shelton, J. R. (1998). Domain-specific knowledge systems in the brain the animate−inanimate distinction. *Journal of Cognitive Neuroscience*, **10**: 1−34.

Castelli, F., Happe, F., Frith, U., and Frith, C. (2000). Movement and mind: a functional imaging study of perception and interpretation of complex intentional movement patterns. *NeuroImage*, **12**: 314−25.

Chao, L. L. and Martin, A. (1999). Cortical representation of perception, naming, and knowledge of color. *Journal of Cognitive Neuroscience*, **11**: 25−35.

Chao, L. L. and Martin, A. (2000). Representation of manipulable man-made objects in the dorsal stream. *NeuroImage*, **12**: 478−84.

Chao, L. L., Haxby, J. V., and Martin, A. (1999a). Attribute-based neural substrates in temporal cortex for perceiving and knowing about objects. *Nature Neuroscience*, **2**: 913−19.

Chao, L. L., Martin, A., and Haxby, J. V. (1999b). Are face-responsive regions selective only for faces? *Neuroreport*, **10**: 2945−50.

Chao, L. L., Weisberg, J., and Martin, A. (2002). Experience-dependent modulation of category-related cortical activity. *Cerebral Cortex*, **12**: 545−51.

Cohen L., Dehaene, S., Naccache, L., Lehericy, S., Dehaene-Lambertz, G., Henaff, M. A., and Michel, F. (2000). The visual word form area − spatial and temporal characterization of an initial stage of reading in normal subjects and posterior split-brain patients. *Brain*, **123**: 291−307.

Cox, D. D. and Savoy, R. L. (2003). Functional magnetic resonance imaging (fMRI) "brain reading": detecting and classifying distributed patterns of fMRI activity in human visual cortex. *Neuroimage*, **19**: 261−70.

Cox, D. D., Meyers, E., and Sinha, P. (2004). Contextually evoked object-specific responses in human visual cortex. *Science*, **304**: 115−17.

Crutch, S. J. and Warrington, E.K. (2003). The selective impairment of fruit and vegetable knowledge: A multiple processing channels account of fine-grain category specificity. *Cognitive Neuropsychology*, **20**: 355−72.

Damasio, A. R. (1989). Time-locked multiregional retroactivation: a systems-level proposal for the neural substrates of recall and recognition. *Cognition*, **33**: 25−62.

De Vreese, L. P. (1991). Two systems for colour-naming defects: verbal disconnection vs colour imagery disorder. *Neuropsychologia*, **29**: 1−18.

Dehaene, S., Spelke, E., Pinel, P., Stanescu, R., and Tsivkin, S., (1999). Sources of mathematical thinking: behavioral and brain-imaging evidence. *Science*, **284**: 970−4.

Desimone, R. (1996). Neural mechanisms for visual memory and their role in attention. *Proceedings of the National Academy of Sciences USA*, **93**: 13494−9.

D'Esposito, M., Detre, J. A., Aguire, G. K., Stallcup, M., Alsop, D. C., Tippet, L. J., and Farah, M. J. (1997). A functional MRI study of mental image generation. *Neuropsychologia*, **35**: 725−30.

Devlin, J. T., Rushworth, M. F. S., and Matthews, P. M. (2005). Category-related activation for written words in the posterior fusiform is task specific. *Neuropsychologia*, **43**: 69–74.

Dolan, R. J., Fink, G. R., Rolls, E., Booth, M., Holmes, A., Frackowiak, R. S. J., and Friston, K. J. (1997). How the brain learns to see objects and faces in an impoverished context. *Nature*, **389**: 596–9.

Epstein, R. and Kanwisher, N. (1998). A cortical representation of the local visual environment. *Nature*, **392**: 598–601.

Freese, J. L. and Amaral, D. G. (2005). The organization of projections from the amygdala to visual cortical areas TE and V1 in the macaque monkey. *Journal of Comparative Neurology*, **486**: 295–317.

Gabrieli, J. D., Poldrack, R. A., and Desmond, J. E. (1998). The role of left prefrontal cortex in language and memory. *Proceedings of the National Academy of Sciences USA*, **95**: 906–13.

Gold, B. T., Balota, D. A., Jones, S. A., Powell, D. K., Smith, C. D., and Andersen, A. H. (2006). Dissociation of automatic and strategic lexical–semantics: fMRI evidence for differing roles of mid-IT and multiple frontal regions. *Journal of Neuroscience*, **26**, 6523–32.

Grill-Spector, K. and Malach, R. (2001). fMR-adaptation: a tool for studying the functional properties of human cortical neurons. *Acta Psychologica*, **107**: 293–321.

Grill-Spector, K., Henson, R., and Martin, A. (2006). Repetition and the brain: Neural models of stimulus-specific effects. *Trends in Cognitive Science*, **10**: 14–23.

Grossman, E. D. and Blake, R. (2001). Brain activity evoked by inverted and imagined biological motion. *Vision Research*, **41**: 1475–82.

Grossman, E. D. and Blake, R. (2002). Brain areas active during visual perception of biological motion. *Neuron*, **35**: 1167–75.

Haxby, J. V., Gobbini, M. I., Furey, M. L., Ishai, A., Schouten, J. L., and Pietrini, P. (2001). Distributed and overlapping representations of faces and objects in ventral temporal cortex. *Science*, **293**: 2425–30.

Heider, F. and Simmel, M. (1944). An experimental study of apparent behavior. *American Journal of Psychology*, **57**: 243–9.

Henson, R. N. A. (2003). Neuroimaging studies of priming. *Progress in Neurobiology*, **70**: 53–81.

Howard, R. J., ffytche, D. H., Barnes, J., McKeefry, D., Ha, Y., Woodruff, P. W., Bullmore, E. T., Simmons, A., Williams, S. C. R., David, A. S., and Brammer, M. (1998). The functional anatomy of imagining and perceiving colour. *Neuroreport*, **9**: 1019–23.

Ishai, A., Ungerleider, L. G., and Haxby, J. V. (2000). Distributed neural systems for the generation of visual images. *Neuron*, **28**: 979–90.

Jeannerod, M., Arbib, M. A., Rizzolatti, G., and Sakata, H. (1995). Grasping objects: the cortical mechanisms of visuomotor transformation. *Trends in Neurosciences*, **18**: 314–20.

Johnson-Frey, S. H. (2004). The neural bases of complex tool use in humans. *Trends in Cognitive Sciences*, **8**: 71–8.

Joseph, J. E. (2001). Functional neuroimaging studies of category specificity in object recognition: A critical review and meta-analysis. *Cognitive, Affective, & Behavioral Neuroscience*, **1**: 119–36.

Kan, I. P., Barsalou, L. W., Solomon, K. O., Minor, J. K., and Thompson-Schill, S. L. (2003). Role of mental imagery in a property verification task: fMRI evidence for perceptual representations of conceptual knowledge. *Cognitive Neuropsychology*, **20**: 525−40.

Kanwisher, N., Stanley, D., and Harris, A. (1999). The fusiform face area is selective for faces not animals. *Neuroreport*, **10**: 183−7.

Kanwisher, N., Woods, R. P., Iacoboni, M., and Mazziotta, J. C. (1997). A locus in human extrastriate cortex for visual shape analysis. *Journal of Cognitive Neuroscience*, **9**: 133−42.

Kraut, M. A., Kremen, S., Segal, J. B., Calhoun, V., Moo, L. R., and Hart, J. (2002). Object activation from features in the semantic system. *Journal of Cognitive Neuroscience*, **14**: 24−36.

Mahon, B. Z. and Caramazza, A. (2003). Constraining questions about the organisation and representation of conceptual knowledge. *Cognitive Neuropsychology*, **20**: 433−50.

Malach, R., Levy, I., and Hasson, U. (2002). The topography of high-order human object areas. *Trends in Cognitive Science*, **6**: 176−84.

Malach, R., Reppas, J. B., Benson, R. R., Kwong, K. K., Jiang, H., Kennedy, W. A., Ledden, P. J., Brady, T. J., Rosen, B. R., and Tootell, R. B. (1995). Object-related activity revealed by functional magnetic resonance imaging in human occipital cortex. *Proceedings of the National Academy of Sciences USA*, **92**: 8135−9.

Martin, A. (1998). The organization of semantic knowledge and the origin of words in the brain. In N. Jablonski and L. Aiello (eds.), *The Origins and Diversification of Language*. San Francisco: California Academy of Sciences, pp. 69−98.

Martin, A. (2001). Functional neuroimaging of semantic memory. In R. Cabeza and A. Kingstone (eds.), *Handbook of Functional NeuroImaging of Cognition*. Cambridge: MIT Press, pp. 153−86.

Martin, A. and Caramazza, A. (2003). Neuropsychological and neuroimaging perspectives on conceptual knowledge: an introduction. *Cognitive Neuropsychology*, **20**: 195−212.

Martin, A. and Chao, L. L. (2001). Semantic memory and the brain: structure and processes. *Current Opinion in Neurobiology*, **11**: 194−201.

Martin, A. and Weisberg, J. (2003). Neural foundations for understanding social and mechanical concepts. *Cognitive Neuropsychology*, **20**: 575−87.

Martin, A., Haxby, J. V., Lalonde, F. M., Wiggs, C. L., and Ungerleider, L. G. (1995). Discrete cortical regions associated with knowledge of color and knowledge of action. *Science*, **270**: 102−5.

Martin, A., Wiggs, C. L., Ungerleider, L. G., and Haxby, J. V. (1996). Neural correlates of category-specific knowledge. *Nature*, **379**: 649−52.

Mitchell, J. P., Heatherton, T. F., and Macrae, C. N. (2002). Distinct neural systems subserve person and object knowledge. *Proceedings of the National Academy of Sciences USA*, **99**: 15238−43.

Nielsen, J. M. (1958). *Memory and Amnesia*. Los Angeles: San Lucas Press.

Noppeney, U., Price, C. J., Penny, W. D., and Friston, K. J. (2006). Two distinct neural mechanisms for category-selective responses. *Cerebral Cortex*, **16**: 437−45.

O'Craven, K. M. and Kanwisher, N. (2000). Mental imagery of faces and places activates corresponding stimulus-specific brain regions. *Journal of Cognitive Neuroscience*, **12**: 1013−23.

Oram, M. W. and Perrett, D. I. (1994). Responses of anterior superior temporal polysensory (STPa) neurons to "biological motion" stimuli. *Journal of Cognitive Neuroscience*, **6**: 99–116.

Paulesu, E., Harrison, J., Baron-Cohen, S., Watson, J. D., Goldstein, L., Heather, J., Frackowiak, R. S., and Frith, C. D. (1995). The physiology of coloured hearing. A PET activation study of colour–word synaesthesia. *Brain*, **118**: 661–76.

Petersen, S. E., Fox, P. T., Posner, M. I., Mintun, M., and Raichle, M. E. (1988). Positron emission tomographic studies of the cortical anatomy of single-word processing. *Nature*, **331**: 585–9.

Polk, T. A. and Farah, M. J. (1998). The neural development and organization of letter recognition: evidence from functional neuroimaging, computational modeling, and behavioral studies. *Proceedings of the National Academy of Science USA*, **95**: 847–52.

Price, C. J., Noppeney, U., Phillips, J., and Devlin, J.T. (2003). How is the fusiform gyrus related to category-specificity? *Cognitive Neuropsychology*, **20**: 561–74.

Puce, A., Allison, T., Bentin, S., Gore, J. C., and McCarthy, G. (1998). Temporal cortex activation in humans viewing eye and mouth movements. *Journal of Neuroscience*, **18**: 2188–99.

Santos, L. R., Miller, C. T., and Hauser, M. D. (2003). Representing tools: how two non-human primate species distinguish between the functionally relevant and irrelevant features of a tool. *Animal Cognition*, **6**: 269–81.

Schultz, R. T., Grelotti, D. J., Klin, A., Kleinman, J., Van der Gaag, C., Marois, R., and Skudlarski, P. (2003). The role of the fusiform face area in social cognition: implications for the pathobiology of autism. *Philosophical Transactions of the Royal Society of London Series B – Biological Sciences*, **358**: 415–27.

Shapiro, K. A., Moo, L. R., and Caramazza, A. (2006). Cortical signatures of noun and verb production. *Proceedings of the National Academy of Sciences USA*, **103**: 1644–9.

Shuren, J. E., Brott, T. G., Schefft, B. K., and Houston, W. (1996). Preserved color imagery in an achromatopsic. *Neuropsychologia*, **34**: 485–9.

Simmons, W. K., Martin, A., and Barsalou, L. W. (2005). Pictures of appetizing foods activate gustatory cortices for taste and reward. *Cerebral Cortex*, **15**: 1602–8.

Simmons, W. K., Ramjee, V., Beauchamp, M. S., McRae, K., Martin, A., and Barsalou, L. W. (2006). A common neural substrate for perceiving and knowing about color. *Neuropsychologia*, in press.

Spiridon, M. and Kanwisher, N. (2002). How distributed is visual category information in human occipito-temporal cortex? An fMRI study. *Neuron*, **35**: 1157–65.

Thompson-Schill, S. L. (2003). Neuroimaging studies of semantic memory: inferring "how" from "where". *Neuropsychologia*, **41**: 280–92.

Tranel, D., Damasio, H., and Damasio, A. R. (1997). A neural basis for the retrieval of conceptual knowledge. *Neuropsychologia*, **35**: 1319–27.

Tranel, D., Kemmerer, D., Adolphs, R., Damasio, H., and Damasio, A. R. (2003). Neural correlates of conceptual knowledge for actions. *Cognitive Neuropsychology*, **20**: 409–32.

van Turennout, M., Ellmore, T., and Martin, A. (2000). Long-lasting cortical plasticity in the object naming system. *Nature Neuroscience*, **3**: 1329–34.

Warrington, E. K. and McCarthy, R. (1983). Category specific access dysphasia. *Brain*, **106**: 859−78.

Warrington, E. K. and Shallice, T. (1984). Category specific semantic impairments. *Brain*, **107**: 829−54.

Weisberg, J., van Turrennout, M., and Martin, A. (in press). A neural system for learning about object function. *Cerebral Cortex*, published on-line March 31, 2006, **doi: 10.1093/ cercor/bhj 176**.

Whatmough, C., Chertkow, H., Murtha, S., and Hanratty, K. (2002). Dissociable brain regions process object meaning and object structure during picture naming. *Neuropsychologia*, **40**: 174−86.

Wheatley, T., Weisberg, J., Beauchamp, M. S., and Martin, A. (2005). Automatic priming of semantically related words reduces activity in the fusiform gyrus. *Journal of Cognitive Neuroscience*, **17**: 1871−85.

Wiggs, C. L., Weisberg, J., and Martin, A. (1999). Neural correlates of semantic and episodic memory retrieval. *Neuropsychologia*, **37**: 103−18.

Wise, R. J. S., Howard, D., Mummery, C. J., Fletcher, P., Leff, A., Büchel, C., and Scott, S. K. (2000). Noun imageability and the temporal lobes. *Neuropsychologia*, **38**: 985−94.

Yang, J. J., Francis, N., Bellgowan, P. S. F., and Martin, A, (2005). Object concepts and the human amygdala: Enhanced activity for identifying animals independent of input modality and stimulus format. Presented at Cognitive Neuroscience Society Annual Meeting, New York.

Yovel, G. and Kanwisher, N. (2004). Face perception: domain specific, not process specific. *Neuron*, **44**: 889−98.

Zeki, S., Watson, J. D., Lueck, C. J., Friston, K. J., Kennard, C., and Frackowiak, R. S. (1991). A direct demonstration of functional specialization in human visual cortex. *Journal of Neuroscience*, **11**: 641−9.

13

Neural hybrid model of semantic object memory (version 1.1)

John Hart, Jr.[1] and Michael A. Kraut[2]

[1]University of Texas at Dallas
[2]The Johns Hopkins University School of Medicine

Delineating the neural bases of semantic memory, even for single entities (objects, features of objects, categories, actions, etc.) has been fraught with numerous difficulties, including variable definitions of semantic terms and several different models of the functional organization of semantic memory (see previous chapters). The development of new investigative techniques has been a major asset in detecting regions associated with semantic memory, but has not led to a consensus on semantic organization, since the results from these studies have frequently been discordant. For example, the results of activation studies (positron emission tomography, functional magnetic resonance imaging event-related potential – PET, fMRI, ERP, etc.), which demonstrate regions likely "involved" in performing a task, have yet to be fully integrated with the results of lesion-based studies that show regions "essential" for performing a task.

Historically, attempts at delineating the anatomic substrates of semantic memory have been guided by one of two general models or classes of models: parallel distributed representation (McClelland & Rumelhart, 1985 and Hinton, 1981) and center processing (Geschwind, 1965). It is clear, however, that neither of these models in their pure form explains adequately the growing body of data from anatomic and functional studies. In other words, the brain comprises neither a homogeneous network of equivalent neuronal elements that encode every aspect of a memory, nor circumscribed processing centers that encode all memory elements. Also, it is unlikely that the actual neural mechanisms by which semantic

We would like to thank Laura, Jack, Charlie, Naomi, Jennie, Sarah, and Rebecca for their continued love and support.
We would also like to thank Sarah Kremen, Lauren Moo, Jeff Pitcock, and Scott Slotnick for their invaluable contributions to this project. We would also like to acknowledge Dr. D. T'ib for his critical comments on previous versions of this manuscript and express our good wishes to him and his family and wish him a speedy recovery from his extended illness.

memory is accessed can be delineated neurophysiologically by either a homogeneous network of neurons/units with weighted connections or neuronal firing delimited to circumscribed processing centers. It was evident to us that semantic memory, even delimited to accessing just objects, was best accounted for by a hybrid of several different neural models, leading to the following, evolving, model of semantic object recall.

13.1   Neural hybrid model of semantic memory (version 1.1)

The general framework of the model is based on several concepts previously described in relation to semantic object memory. With the intended goal of the model to account for semantic memory storage and processing at a neurophysiological level, the present version represents a mechanistic account of semantic memory given the evidence available, with the limitations of current investigative techniques, their inherent assumptions, and shortcomings. As findings are proposed or techniques advanced to further clarify the model, it will evolve to provide a clearer (e.g. neurotransmitter, molecular, etc.) explanation for semantic memory and is thus referred to as version 1.1. (see version 1.0 in Hart *et al.*, 2002 and Kraut *et al.*, 2003). One aspect of this model was that it posited that there were cortical regions that likely encode for representations associated with objects in sensorimotor and higher-order cognitive systems (e.g. lexical–semantic, etc.). Based on our and others' work, we have proposed both feature- (see Hart & Gordon, 1992; Haxby *et al.*, 2001; Miceli *et al.*, 2001 for further description of featural organization) and category-based neural representations for several of these sensorimotor/cognitive domains. The following further describes these aspects of the model.

13.1.1   Semantic memory subsystems

One proposed schema for storing of components of object memory is that elements specific to a certain sensorimotor system are stored in that system (e.g. visual memory of the shape of an apple is stored in the visual memory system, etc.; Hart *et al.*, 2002). This scheme extends to the multiple sensorimotor systems (Johnson & Hsaio, 1992; Haxby *et al.*, 1991; Kraut *et al.*, 2003; Grafton *et al.*, 1997; Downing *et al.*, 2006) as well as the emotional and lexical–semantic systems, which hereafter will be referred to as systems. These systems are those that have been identified thus far, but the list will almost certainly be expanded over time.

In terms of generalized brain/behavioral organization principles, certain common attributes of object memory have emerged to some degree across these systems. The organization appears to reflect responsiveness of neural ensembles at both feature and category levels, with variable expression of this general organization across and within each system. This variability depends on a variety of factors, not the least of which is the sensitivity of present investigative techniques to detect their presence. In addition, the specific, individual features and categories may vary between systems, typically reflecting the parameters along which that system is organized in the physical world. For example, the features encoded in the visual system are based on visual parameters by which the visual system acquires (e.g. via the rods and cones in the retina) and processes (rudimentary through more complex visual shapes, color, texture, motion) visual data.

The lexical–semantic was first imputed to have a categorical organization by Nielsen (1946), with the double dissociation between the ability to name living things and nonliving things (with opposite patterns of preservation or impairment across different patients). Since then, there have been many individual and group reports of such dissociations (Semenza & Zettin, 1988, 1989; Goodglass *et al.*, 1966, 1986; Funnell & Sheridan, 1992; Hillis & Caramazza, 1991; Farah *et al.*, 1991, 1996; Silveri *et al.*, 1991; Damasio *et al.*, 1990; Farah & Wallace, 1992; Temple, 1986; Warrington & Shallice, 1984; Rapcsak *et al.*, 1989, 1993; McCarthy & Warrington, 1988; Berndt, 1988; Humphreys & Riddoch, 1987; Damasio, 1990; Silveri & Gainotti, 1988; Warrington & McCarthy, 1983; Sartori *et al.*, 1993; Robinson *et al.*, 1996; Gainotti *et al.*, 1995; Mauri *et al.*, 1994; Tippett *et al.*, 1996; Sartori & Job, 1988; Sacchett & Humphreys, 1992; Lyons *et al.*, 2002c; della Rocchetta & Cipolotti, 2004; Vitali *et al.*, 2005; see Grossman *et al.*, 1998 for similar issues in degenerative conditions). The living–nonliving distinction, broadly characterized, has been the one reported most often (Damasio *et al.*, 1996; Cappa *et al.*, 1998; Garrard *et al.*, 1998; Ferreira *et al.*, 1997). It should be noted, however, that the specific categories that have most often been studied are animals (representing living things) and tools (representing nonliving artifacts). These categories seem to have the greatest contrasts in terms of their features (e.g. tools such as hammers and saws are typically hard, smooth, straight-edged, dry, devoid of their own intention, and put to use by humans; animals are almost the exact opposite). In addition, there are enough familiar items that fall under the categories of "animals" and "tools" to make them useful and convenient for experimentation. So, for a combination of theoretical and practical reasons, these are the categories of items most studied in patient populations and neuroimaging studies.

From an anatomical basis, it must be noted that at least a substantial plurality, if not a majority, of these category-specific deficits follow from herpes simplex encephalitis (HSE). There are several difficulties with interpreting these lesion data. Most importantly, it is not clear that imaging of HSE lesions on MRI is adequate to assess the damage from HSE, which spreads throughout the central nervous system via two mechanisms: contiguous and trans-synaptic dissemination. Neuroimaging techniques can capture pathology of the contiguous spread as long as the size of the area of pathologic change is within the resolution of MRI. However, trans-synaptic spread of the virus is on a microscopic level, typically below the resolution of standard imaging techniques, and can extend well beyond the boundary of the primary imageable lesion. For example, in the case of semantic memory, this can lead to "false localization." One proposed explanation of categorical organization is via a hierarchical ordering of objects and features under an anatomically distinct categorical node. Thus trans-synaptic spread to a neuron or group of neurons encoding a hierarchical node, or mediating a critical input to a node, could both impair a specific category and not be detected on MRI.

With these caveats in mind, the key anatomical findings that are cited across these lesion studies are that impairment of animal-specific semantic knowledge in particular, and possibly all animate items, are generally associated with left temporal lobe pathology. There are few cases of patients with inanimate object deficits. Some have inferred, based on the association of impaired verb naming and lesions in the left premotor area (Damasio & Tranel, 1993), that semantic knowledge of inanimate objects, with their associated motor actions, are related to disruption in this area. Functional neuroimaging studies have also shown evidence for category-level differences, including detailed anatomical accounts for categorical localization. The animals versus tools distinction has been examined in normal subjects, using PET and most recently fMRI. The picture naming task was used by both Martin *et al.* (1996) and Damasio *et al.* (1996) in PET studies to explore category-level differences. Both groups of investigators found that the different categories elicited different regions of metabolic increase, many of which were in left temporal lobe. In this respect, these studies agreed with the data from patients with focal lesions and degenerative conditions reviewed above. However, the specific regions found by the two groups were not in agreement. Martin *et al.* (1996) found that both types of stimuli led to activation of both ventral temporal lobes, and of Broca's area. Animals, in the Martin *et al.* (1996) study, selectively activated the left medial occipital lobe. Tools selectively activated the left middle temporal gyrus and the left premotor region. (They also pointed out that the two areas selectively activated by tools were the same regions selectively activated by generation of action words and by imagined hand movements, respectively.) In contrast, Damasio *et al.* (1996) found that naming animals was associated with activation of the left third (inferior) and fourth temporal gyri, while naming of tools was associated with activation of the left middle and inferior temporal gyri. Spitzer *et al.* (1995) also used naming of pictures to explore differences in category representation, but used fMRI, with its intrinsically higher spatial resolution than PET. The objects in the Spitzer study represented the categories of animals, tools, furniture, and fruit. Spitzer reported finding activations for all categories that were generally within left superior temporal, left medial temporal, and left lateral frontal regions. This helps corroborate both the other functional imaging studies reviewed above, and the conclusions from focal lesions and degenerative cases. But perhaps the most interesting aspect of the Spitzer report was that, within these regions, they found different specific loci of activation for items from different categories. These results were interpreted as evidence for differences in the spatial representation of different categories of information in the dominant temporal lobe; however, they did not localize these differences between left temporal and frontal lobe as other studies had.

What can be concluded at this point is that in the lexical–semantic system there is behavioral evidence from patients of categorical distinctions. The lesion-based evidence for discrete anatomical regions associated with specific categories is not conclusive and the evidence for localizations associated with neuroimaging has been forthcoming, but partially contradictory.

In addition to the lack of consistency for anatomical localizations for specific categories, there is inconsistency in the assignment of function to these anatomical regions. Some investigators impute the role of lexical access or knowledge stores to circumscribed, localized groups of neuronal populations. However, it has not been specified at a physiological level how these populations of neurons mediate these functions of lexical access nor how these same populations store category-specific memory, especially since lesions to the region typically do not have corresponding loss of memory stores. The role that these regions presumably assume in the neural hybrid model will be outlined below.

The visual memory system is one of the most extensively studied for object memory organization, starting with the delineation of the bilateral ventral temporo-occipital "what" system for objects (Ungerleider & Haxby, 1994; Kraut et al., 1997). As was noted above, there have been many studies demonstrating that the visual memory system is organized by visual features. In addition, numerous studies have suggested that the "what" system is organized by distinct categories of items, access to which is mediated by specific anatomic regions in these ventral temporo-occipital regions. Among the classes of stimuli for which dedicated neural processing substrates have been imputed are faces, objects, scenes, bodies, and houses (Spiridon & Kanwisher, 2002; Downing et al., 2006). Other investigators have contended that these localizations are not fixed, and may reflect individual subjects' expertise, as well as the level of categorization (Tarr & Gauthier, 2000) imposed by the experimental paradigms. In an in-depth study of categorical organization in the visual object semantic memory system, it was suggested that as opposed to categories, objects were encoded based on their visual features which are encoded as overlapping and widely distributed neural substrates (Haxby *et al.*, 2001; but see also Gerlach *et al.*, 2004).

The existence of visual perceptual featural organization in lexical–semantic memory for objects has been detailed previously (see Hart & Gordon, 1992; Haxby *et al.*, 2001; Sim & Kiefer, 2005; Miceli *et al.*, 2001 for further description). In terms of semantic memory for objects in the motor system, Martin *et al.* (1996) showed that pictures of tools yielded focal signal changes in the left middle temporal gyrus and the left premotor region. Damasio *et al.* (1996), using comparable stimuli and task, showed left middle and inferior temporal gyri activation for tools. In addition to the difference in location of activation, Damasio *et al.* (1996) claimed that their activation patterns represented regions related to lexical access, as opposed to Martin *et al.*'s contention that theirs indicated semantic knowledge. In either account, it is not clear that these regions play a role specific to category-level processing. For example, one alternative explanation for the observed differences is that the differential activation for tools in the left premotor region could be attributable to different cognitive operations thought to be engaged in tool naming (Grafton *et al.*, 1997). Signal changes in this premotor region may reflect the motor system's general processing of features associated with certain items. For example, items (irrespective of their category membership) that engage motor representations, likely related to hand movements and/or the manipulability of the items as a salient feature, will activate this common motor processing region. This is conceptually analogous to motor cortical representations being organized by basic movement patterns; some of the same hand and wrist movements used to manipulate a screwdriver, for example, are used to peel or to eat a fruit.

We postulated that if the motor memory system were organized by categories, then access to category-level information regarding fruit and vegetables would be located in one region, and tools in another. However, if the motor system were organized by the motor feature of manipulability, then both would be located in the same region, which we proposed would be the premotor region. We studied normal controls with fMRI using a category judgment task with word pairs as stimuli. Detection of word pairs that were both tools and both fruits & vegetables activated the same premotor regions in the left BA 6/44 junction (Kraut *et al.*, 2002c), suggesting that this region may detect features of motor manipulability common to items from both of these categories. The lack of signal changes in left inferior frontal area for word pairs from the animal category suggests that the property of manipulability, or perhaps some other property common to fruits & vegetables and tools but not animals, is processed in this region. The signal changes with the fruits & vegetables stimulus pairs were contained within the areas of activation detected with the tool pairs (see Figure 13.1). That the activation pattern in frontal areas for fruits & vegetables is a completely contained subset of

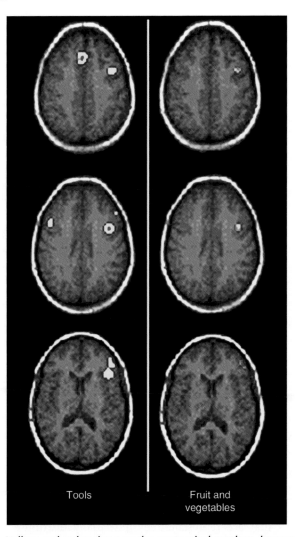

Figure 13.1. Yellow and red regions on the anatomical overlays demonstrate signal changes associated with deciding that a pair of words represented items from the same category, without categories ever being designated in the experiment. These signal changes represent "implicit" activation of items from the categories tools and fruit & vegetables. The signal changes in the left premotor regions in Brodmann area 6/44 junction for fruit & vegetables is a completely contained subset of that for tools. This supports our contention that the left premotor region activations described in numerous studies reflect motor manipulability features (e.g. that we hold and manually manipulate items in these groups with our hands) common to the items from both of these categories (adapted from Kraut *et al.*, 2002c).

that for tools supports our contention that these are not category-specific regions, but specific to the motor manipulability features common to the items from both of these categories. Thus, for the motor system, we propose that a plausible organization is based on common features shared by various items, irrespective of their category membership. Our data showed that as subjects determine category membership, the signal change patterns more closely reflect the items' features in the motor system than the specific categories to which the items belong.

In the case of the motor system, the common feature proposed for tools and fruits & vegetables is of the typical experience of holding items from those categories in their hand. Some have suggested the importance of motor memories representing a semantic concept such as "manipulability." Alternatively, this circumscribed region in the premotor area could represent a neuronal population that facilitates access to specific motor memory for specific objects, independent of properties such as manipulability. The individual motor memories may consist of patterns of neural population firing, with the neurons all contained within the node, with different motor memories consisting of different neuronal firing patterns. If this region is actually encoding aspects of the motor memory itself, then there are obviously other brain regions (motor strip, basal ganglia, etc.) that are connected to and plausibly contributing to some aspects of the motor memory of the objects and execution of that memory. This organizational scheme seems somewhat unlikely, however, as it suggests that damage to a relatively small brain region would affect efficient access to semantic information about all manipulable items, regardless of their more "natural" categories (tools, food). There are few if any lesion data to support this contention.

Another possible role for the nodes is that they mediate access to individual motor memories that are not necessarily encoded for by neurons residing entirely in the node. In this case, the node may facilitate access to individual motor memory encodings that are represented by a spatially distributed pattern of neuronal firing of neurons not located in the node. To date, no one has reported data that strongly support this idea, possibly because of the technical difficulties associated with detecting the presence of these spatially distributed neuronal firing patterns.

Yet another concept of the neurophysiological function of these nodes is a detector of the presence of a particular semantic memory trait, feature, category, etc. In this conceptualization, the neuronal population in the node would have a distinct firing pattern if a stimulus input to it has a specific semantic quality. Experimental verification of nodes functioning in this way depends upon being able to show that a specific node is only active when a specific stimulus property is present. We have reported such nodes that appear to function as seman-tic detectors for stimuli in the "animal" category, and having the feature of "threatening" when these two distinct regions receive nonverbal sound input. We studied normal control subjects with fMRI using a task of deciding if a nonverbal sound presented was one that they had heard before from an object. There were four groups of nonverbal sound targets: animal/nonthreatening, animal/threatening, object/nonthreatening, and object/threatening. We also presented scrambled versions of each "real" sound as foils. Each real sound was scrambled to form a nonsound with the same acoustic perceptual qualities (all sounds had a ceiling on loudness amplitude to eliminate this as a threatening feature). Two distinct anatomical foci were detected in the right superior temporal gyrus when subjects identified sounds representing either animals or threatening items. Both of these foci were outside of regions typically attributed to including primary auditory cortex, but in relatively close proximity to that region (see Figure 13.2). Stimuli

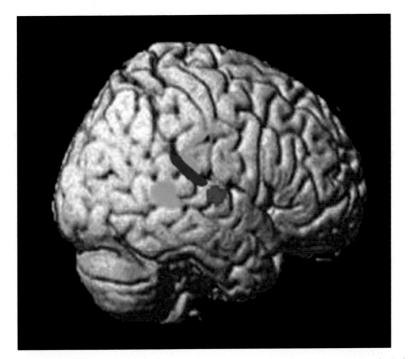

Figure 13.2. The neural semantic detector model for nonverbal sound of objects/animals (adapted from Kraut *et al.*, in press). The figure focuses on the regions engaged in early extraction of meaning following perceptual analysis that occurs in primary auditory cortex (blue region drawn from data presented by Rademacher *et al.*, 2001). The two other distinct anatomical foci are regions in the right superior temporal gyrus when subjects identified sounds representing either animals (red) or threatening items (green). Both of these foci are close to, but not within primary auditory cortex. Threatening animal stimuli activated both the red and green regions, demonstrating that in the nonverbal sound system, categorical and featural-level information is encoded in a spatially distributed system.

that represented threatening animals, and thus having both the animal categorical designation and threatening featural attribute, activated both the right superior temporal gyrus foci, suggesting a distributed neural representation. The object stimuli did not activate the animal node and the nonthreatening stimuli did not activate the threatening node to a significant degree, suggesting that these nodes were specific to the stimuli reported. Given the specificity of these nodes and their proximity to primary sensory cortices, these category- and feature-specific nodes most likely engage in the earliest extraction of semantic memory information from these sounds. The serial and transient nature by which auditory stimuli are momentarily present mandates rapid, online identification of the objects/items producing those sounds. Accomplishing this efficient, rapid processing can be expeditiously mediated with close proximity between regions that perform the early stages of auditory perceptual processing and those regions that perform higher-order operations, such as evaluating perceptual constructs in auditory memory in the context of the object identification process.

We proposed from these findings a model of auditory sound object memory referred to as the neural semantic detector model. The two right superior temporal loci of fMRI signal change represent nodes or detectors that are engaged in early auditory semantic memory processing, and which respond differentially to the animal category and the threatening feature of sound stimuli (Kronbichler et al., 2004). If several of these attributes are present in a sound, then several of these detectors will be activated simultaneously, and the summated and contemporaneous co-activation of the detectors will facilitate object recall. Thus there is clearly an interaction in threatening animal sound of both the categorical and featural organization for the same items in the auditory semantic system. We predict that as future detectors are identified, many will reside in neighboring regions to the ones presently identified, in order to minimize the temporal delay incurred by transmission of data between brain regions. As a consequence, these detectors that mediate access to the auditory semantic memory system will likely be organized concentrically surrounding the posterior aspects of the right superior temporal gyrus (Figure 13.2).

That these represent detector nodes extends from the experimental design of the study: (1) the task of choosing real sounds from nonsounds, as opposed to being required to make explicit category/feature judgments about the stimuli, indicates that these regions are operating in an online continuous, or at least phasic, manner, to extract semantic information from the auditory environment, regardless of the subject's focus; (2) the nonsound stimuli in the task contained the same auditory perceptual information as the real sounds, virtually eliminating low-level acoustic properties of the stimuli as the determinant of the differential signal changes we detected; and (3) the contrasts employed for detection of differential signal changes in our data analysis dovetailed with the task we employed; that is, we asked the subjects to make a fairly basic judgment about the stimuli, but we analyzed the patterns of signal change with a view towards detecting patterns of signal change related to semantic categorical or featural properties of the sounds being presented. In this proposed framework, there are likely many of these detectors to mediate efficient processing of the wide variety of semantic features, objects, or categories almost certainly to be encountered, and perhaps other detectors encoding for features that are not specifically semantic, but that may represent intrinsic attributes of certain classes of stimuli, such as motion. Thus, if several of these attributes are present in a sound, then several of these detectors will be activated simultaneously, and the summated and contemporaneous co-activation of the detectors will facilitate object recall. Co-activation of multiple detectors could itself represent the integrated auditory object memory, may elicit the memory by evoking or amplifying a synchronizing cortical gamma rhythm (Kraut *et al.*, 2003; Pulvermüller *et al.*, 1999), access some spatially distributed representation of this integrated memory, or might result in the activation of some as-yet-unidentified unimodal synthesis region or store (Hart *et al.*, 2002). These detectors, which are located in auditory association cortices, are connected to regions external to auditory-related cortex which are presumably further along in the semantic memory processing chain, which can be engaged by the entire set of stimuli in the group, and which may include other neural systems dedicated to multimodal semantic processing (e.g. inferior parietal—posterior temporal region that is located posterior to these foci (Beauchamp *et al.*, 2004; Hart & Gordon, 1990) or retrieval of a multimodal semantic conceptual representation (see thalamic synchronization as a mechanism of semantic object recall (Kraut *et al.*, 2003).

Neural regions selective for threatening/unpleasant sounds are similar to those of nonhuman primates, demonstrating that semantic memory organization for basic biological/survival primitives is present across species (Gil-de-Costa *et al.*, 2004). In addition, previous authors have posited that there is an evolutionary significance for information being stored in a categorical organization and for which specific categories are represented distinctly (Caramazza & Shelton, 1998). Caramazza and Shelton (1998) noted on review of the cases in the literature that those describing category-specific deficits are not best accounted for selective damage to featural subsystems. These authors argued that disruption of a categorical-based organization in the brain best explains the reported findings, and that this supports the existence of domain-specific knowledge systems that are typically based on evolutionarily essential items. We would suggest that with the addition of further recent studies (Gil-de-Costa *et al.*, 2004; Kraut *et al.*, in press), there may well be an evolutionary significance for categorical and/or feature organization or at least a preference for item groups that have attributes/features that are essential for survival purposes, considering that these represent dangerous stimuli and would likely initiate a sensorimotor (flight/fight) response. Attribute-specific neural substrates are also teleologically appealing for auditory sound stimuli due to the need for rapid analysis of auditory stimuli in general, reflecting the transient nature of the auditory stimulus input, and especially the need for rapid detection of threats to an organism's life. Thus we have proposed a model of conceptual knowledge that extends from, but is intermediate to, models that posit concepts are stored in multiple modalities of a featural organization (Barsalou *et al.*, 2003) and the domain-specific hypothesis supporting evolutionarily driven, amodal semantic knowledge representations. *We posit that object memory is organized on a category-based and/or feature-based framework, depending upon the specific semantic memory system (lexical–semantic, visual, sensorimotor, etc.). A clear example of the coexistence of these schemata are the separable feature and category neural representations existing in the nonverbal sound system as described above.*

13.1.2   Semantic processing, irrespective of stimulus type

In addition to delineating the organization of memory representations in specific semantic memory subsystems, there have been focal regions isolated that are associated with semantic processes, irrespective of the stimuli subtypes involved. Efforts at differentiating the neural substrates primarily concerned with processing of semantic inputs from those that instantiate a representation of a semantic entity have not been successful. Distributed parallel distributed processing models would suggest that both from a functional and anatomical basis, there is no differentiation between representation and processing (Tyler *et al.*, 2000). From a behavioral perspective, our claim that there are anatomical regions that subserve semantic processing, and not necessarily semantic representations, stems from findings of lesions to circumscribed brain regions that disrupt or at least impede specific semantic processes/operations, but do not interrupt access to specific groups or qualities of the items studied (e.g. not specific to any feature or category type).

Even assuming that there are separate mechanisms that underlie semantic processes and semantic access, the neuronal operations through which either is accomplished is unknown. Activity within a node could plausibly mediate communication between brain regions that encode for different aspects of a semantic representation through the elaboration and propagation of synchronizing rhythms (see Pulvermüller *et al.*, 1999). This "link" at a neural level is unclear at present but we can propose several plausible mechanisms. Amongst the semantic "links" that could be mediated by neural activity in these nodes are

(1) intramodal semantic relationships (e.g. that a feature [wing] is part of an object [bird]) within a specific semantic memory subsystem (e.g. lexical semantic for the words for wing and bird), (2) a multimodal semantic relationship between semantic entities from different semantic memory subsystems (e.g. the visual memory of a tail and the word dog) (Hart & Gordon, 1990; Beauchamp *et al.*, 2004), and/or it may determine if there is a pre-existing specific semantic association between two entities in semantic memory, for example if the semantic entity of a dog is associated with the category animal. Further investigation with more sensitive investigative techniques will help to clarify these options and potentially introduce other mechanisms.

Within neuroscientific investigations into the underpinnings of semantic memory, one specific operation that has been investigated extensively has been categorization of objects. A major difficulty in trying to synthesize results from many of the investigations into categorization is the wide variety of specific tasks and stimulus modalities used to probe the underlying mechanisms. Perani *et al.* (1995) had their subjects push a button if the two pictured items were from the same basic category (e.g. on being shown pictures of individual dogs, push the button if they were both pictures of "dogs"). They used pictures of both animals and artifacts. Categorization of animals in this fashion activated the inferior temporal regions bilaterally. Categorization of artifacts activated the left dorsolateral frontal region. Mummery *et al.* (1998) used printed words rather than pictures. The task they gave subjects was considerably different than that used in the Perani *et al.* study, in that subjects not only had to make similarity judgments, but also had to consider either the color of the items, or whether items were found in specific locations. Compared to a control condition (judgments of the number of syllables), Mummery *et al.* found that similarity judgments activated the temporoparietal–occipital (TPO) junction, the posterior mid-temporal gyrus, the inferomedial and inferolateral temporal lobe, and the inferior frontal lobe, all on the left. Selection by the color attribute activated the left anteromedial temporal lobe and the left caudate nucleus. Selection by location, in contrast, activated the left TPO junction, the left medial parietal lobe, and the posterior cingulate. The multiple regions activated during categorization tasks likely reflects to a substantial degree differences in task and stimulus details, and thus leaves unclear which of the regions noted above are engaged in the fundamental categorization process itself.

Lesion studies have been helpful in localizing regions involved in semantic processing and its associated correlates. In a study of 18 aphasics (Hart & Gordon, 1990), three demonstrated isolated deficits in generalized semantic processing for multiple modalities of stimuli. All three patients were impaired, compared to the other aphasics, in category, property, and synonym judgment and in naming to definition, with multiple modalities of stimulus presentation. In all three patients, the lesion was in the left inferior parietal–superior temporal region, which is anatomically ideally located to integrate auditory and visually based semantic knowledge. This was supported by a later activation study showing the same region (posterior superior temporal sulcus and middle temporal gyrus) to be a multimodal semantic processing center (Beauchamp *et al.*, 2004). Other studies investigating specific semantic tasks and operations have shown engagement of this same region (Grossman *et al.*, 2002).

This superior temporal–inferior parietal region (Figure 13.3) thus appears to be associated with semantic processing in general, with the likely major function of the region being multimodal integration. Some clarification as to how this region performs its imputed operations may derive from invasive electrophysiologic studies in nonhuman primates, as posterior parietal–temporoparietal junction regions have been shown to participate in multimodal integration studies in nonhuman species.

Another brain region has been identified as a likely multimodal integration region for semantic processing, using the technique of direct electrical cortical

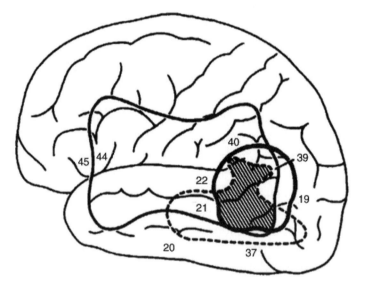

Figure 13.3. Lateral view of the left hemisphere. The circles are lateral projections of strokes that affected cortical regions in patients who were assessed for multiple semantic processes. The striped region in the left superior temporal–inferior parietal region was common to all of the patients with deficits that affected multiple semantic processes involving stimuli from multiple modalities, suggesting that this region is engaged in multimodal integration.

interference (Hart *et al.*, 1998). This technique is used in patients who have had placement of subdural electrodes for monitoring of electrical seizure activity and functional mapping of regions associated with cognition. By passing electrical current between pairs of electrodes, a temporary, reversible deactivation of cortical regions underlying the electrodes is produced. Administration of cognitive tasks when there is and again when there is not electrical interference administered at a given electrode site allows for a given patient to act as their own control. Electrical interference at a pair of electrodes overlying the left fusiform gyrus resulted in impairment on multiple semantic object processing tasks (categorization, synonym judgment, feature–object agreement, naming to definition) in both the auditory and visual modalities, without impairment in input and output processes, thus identifying another region that appears to play an important role in general semantic processing.

The dorsolateral prefrontal cortex (DLPFC), an admittedly large and poorly defined region, also appears to play a role in general semantic processing. Since Posner *et al.* (1988) first reported the DLPFC involvement with the process of producing a semantically associated verb for a presented noun, that area has been associated with a variety of cognitive tasks in general, and semantic tasks in particular (Posner *et al.*, 1988; Petersen *et al.*, 1988, 1990; Demb *et al.*, 1995; Kapur *et al.*, 1994; Demonet *et al.*, 1992; Binder *et al.*, 1996; Fiez, 1997; Ricci *et al.*, 1999). Thompson-Schill *et al.* (1997) have tried to specifically delineate which semantic operations or functions are associated with the DLPFC. Using sets of semantic judgment tasks that differed in the number of possible correct choices, they suggested that the inferior frontal gyrus was involved in the selection of semantic knowledge amongst alternative choices. This selection role is likely a component in the manipulations necessary to perform in a variety of semantic tasks (Thompson-Schill *et al.*, 1997, 1998), explaining its involvement during various activation studies. Data gathered in patients with focal lesions (Kemmerer & Tranel, 2000; Thompson-Schill *et al.*, 1998) corroborated the critical role that the left inferior frontal gyrus plays in verb generation, as have the data from cortical stimulation studies (Ojemann *et al.*, 2002). However, the region may not be specific to just semantic processing and may represent a general cognitive processing region.

The previous regions identified have been associated with multiple semantic processes, and in addition, processing stimuli from multiple input modalities. Regions have also been identified that appear to represent semantic processing zones, but are specific either to certain semantic processes or modalities. For example, the posterior aspect of the left middle temporal gyrus was found by using direct cortical electrical interference (Hart, Lesser, & Gordon, 1992) to be important in judging the size of an object that was specified by a verbal question.

Electrical stimulation at that site produced no interference with other feature judgments such as color, shape, orientation, movement, and texture, and there was no impairment when stimuli were presented as pictures (including size-matched pictures). Thus a reversible lesion to a 1 cm circumscribed region in the left posterior middle temporal gyrus resulted in selective impairment in the semantic process of making the feature judgment about the size of an object in the verbal domain, without any loss of size representations in the verbal domain.

In a series of studies, we have assessed semantic object memory processing in a variety of fMRI studies. In each task, we used either one word, sound, or picture, two words, or a picture and a word for the subject to make a semantic decision. These decisions ranged from whether the stimuli were from the same category, resulted in recall of a specific object or action, and/or were semantically associated. In every case, there was significant signal change in the medial Brodmann area 6 region bilaterally (see Figure 13.4). While this meta-analysis is not a direct assessment of whether medial BA6 is selective to semantic processing, the studies support such a claim. The onset of signal changes for each region engaged by the semantic object recall from featural input task (Kraut et al., 2003) showed that BA6 was the first region to be activated in the course of processing in the task. Given these and other studies in the literature (Crosson et al., 1999), we agree with the proposal by Crosson et al. (1999) that the dorsomedial frontal lobes are engaged in forming the framework for the object to be searched for in semantic memory (Kraut et al., 2003). Thus this region supports a specific semantic process that can engage (and perhaps elicit and evaluate) input from multiple modalities.

In addition to the regions most consistently associated with semantic processing (DLPFC, left inferior parietal–posterior temporal lobe, left fusiform gyrus, dorsomedial BA6), the left inferior frontal gyrus has been implicated in semantic working memory (Martin & Chao, 2001). Other regions have been suggested and with further investigations will expand this list.

The present proposal advances the notion of multiple or single semantic processes being encoded by circumscribed anatomical regions. The semantic processing supported by these regions has been clearly demonstrated to support input stimuli from multiple modalities (auditory word, auditory sound, visual word, visual picture, etc.). While there is not clear evidence at present, we would propose that processing units that support only a single modality of input will eventually be detected, with the development of more sophisticated investigative techniques. The neural mechanism by which these regions mediate semantic processing has only been speculated upon. Pulvermüller et al. (1999) have suggested that local 30 Hz synchronizing rhythms may mediate the processing, but

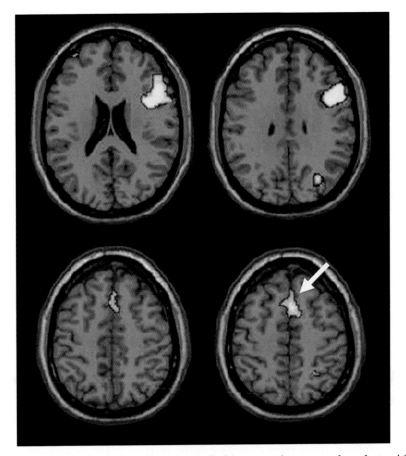

Figure 13.4. Areas activated when an object is recalled in semantic memory from featural inputs. The medial aspects of Brodmann Area 6 bilaterally (arrow, lower right image) have also been found to be activated in multiple other tasks of semantic object memory, including those with input stimuli being either one word, sound, or picture, two words, or a picture and a word for the subject to make a semantic decision. Given these and other studies (Crosson *et al.*, 1999), we agree with Crosson *et al.* that this region is engaged in forming the framework for the object to be searched for in semantic memory (Kraut *et al.*, 2003).

while coordination of activity among multiple brain regions may be critically important to the performance of semantic operations, and interregional neural communications more generally, how these regions actually do what they do, either individually or in concert, has yet to be worked out. Another plausible alternative that we propose is that these regions can detect specific input from multiple modalities and, following this detection, function as nodes to activate/ access other semantic representation (see above as to plausible encodings) or association that has been formed through previous learning (e.g. category membership) or co-occurrence in time and space that creates a semantic relationship (e.g. continually encoding that birds have wings as part of them). While these purported neural mechanisms are proposed at present, other possible mechanistic approaches need to be further explored as to how these regions mediate semantic processing.

13.1.3 Connections across and within systems

The applications of our object-activation-from-featural input task (Kraut *et al.*, 2002a) demonstrated that the trials resulting in object recall showed signal changes in BA6/pre-SMA, bilateral ventral temporal lobe, and the left thalamus. To determine whether this finding of thalamic involvement was specific to the stimuli that were used, a task analogous to the word–word feature binding task was developed using a picture–word pair (e.g. the picture of a candle and the word "icing" for the object cake). Functional MRI studies with these stimuli using the same instructions as the word–word feature binding task revealed the same pattern of activation except that there were additional signal changes in the right thalamus and the cortical and subcortical motor system (Kraut *et al.*, 2002b). The additional right thalamic activation may be related to the presence of picture stimuli, as a previous object activation task using only word stimuli did not show its involvement. This is consistent with studies showing left hemisphere processing for word stimuli and additional right hemisphere involvement for picture–word stimuli (Underwood & Whitfield, 1985). These findings in the somatomotor system, both cortically and subcortically, raise the possibility that feature stimuli from multiple modalities elicit a more extensive activation of the multiple semantic memory representations of the objects, including somatomotor activation. It is unlikely that the individual features themselves or the objects induced resulted in this somatomotor activation, as our stimuli did not explicitly encode motor activity; nor did the lexical labels for the stimuli evoke actions.

That the thalamus was engaged in a process of binding together two features that resulted in the recall of an object in semantic memory had several important neuroanatomical and neurophysiological implications. The thalamus has two major anatomical and physiological features as part of its "relay station" role: (1) the thalamocortical and corticothalamic connections to all of the cortical regions associated with semantic memory stores in multiple sensorimotor and cognitive domains, and (2) elaboration and modulation of multiple synchronizing, oscillating electrophysiological rhythms that coordinate cortical activity between different brain regions (Singer, 1993).

Our fMRI results motivated a study by Slotnick *et al.* (2002), in which we attempted to more directly assess the role of the thalamus in feature binding and object recall. A patient was receiving implanted bilateral thalamic depth electrodes for electrical stimulation treatment of intractable epilepsy. Prior to starting the stimulation, the word—word feature binding and the control association task were presented to the subject while recording electroencephalogram (EEG) from both the thalamic electrodes and a limited number of surface electrodes. The findings demonstrated that during all trials of the feature binding task there was a global decrease in alpha band EEG power, which was followed by an increase in spatially specific gamma band EEG power in the thalamus and occipital scalp electrodes for only those trials where feature binding resulted in semantic object recall. Slotnick *et al.* proposed that the generalized low-frequency (alpha band) power rhythm decreases were likely driven by inhibitory (e.g. GABAergic) projections from the thalamic reticular nucleus to thalamocortical cells in other thalamic nuclei, which mediate cyclic activity (Klimesch, 1996, 1999; Klimesch *et al.*, 1993, 1999; Schier, 2000). The high-frequency (gamma) rhythms were felt to reflect spatially specific, oligosynaptic excitatory (e.g. glutaminergic) corticothalamocortical pathways. Based upon these proposals and the framework of this semantic object recall task, the early reduction in low-frequency EEG power could reflect a cortical process whereby cortical regions are readied for synchronizing inputs. Further, the spatially specific fast rhythm burst (gamma) may facilitate feature binding during recall via the synchronization of neural regions associated with feature representations in semantic memory systems of the object to be recalled (Singer, 1993; Joliot *et al.*, 1994; Singer & Gray, 1995; Klimesch, 1996; Steriade, 2000).

This latter study provided a plausible mechanism for semantic object recall via synchronizing rhythms modulated by the thalamus. However, the role that the other brain regions — particularly BA6 — played in feature binding was not clear, and given the lack of electrode coverage over most of the head, their possible contributions to performance of the task could not be assessed. We were thus motivated to study the word—word feature binding task using event-related fMRI. With this fMRI technique, one can detect the relative time or sequence of activation of the specific brain regions associated with the task investigated (Kraut *et al.*, 2003). The findings of this study extended the previous results (Kraut *et al.*, 2002a; 2002b; Slotnick *et al.*, 2002) in two important ways. First, they demonstrated two distinct loci of thalamic signal change, one in the dorsomedial region, and the other more posteriorly, in the pulvinar. Second, analysis of the regionally specific signal change waveform shapes demonstrated distinct patterns that are likely, at least in part, reflective of different time courses of neural activity in different brain regions. The data showed that the signal changes in BA6 had a steep climb towards an early peak and an early drop-off. The signal changes detected in the dorsomedial thalamus increased and peaked in a comparable fashion to BA6, and then decreased more slowly than BA6.

Given its numerous anatomical connections, the dorsomedial nucleus (DM) activity more likely is involved in setting the search criteria, or performing the actual search, perhaps in conjunction with BA6, to which it has direct connections (Ilinsky *et al.*, 1985; Inase *et al.*, 1996). The DM may interact with or trigger the pulvinar via corticothalamic feedback connections, since sectors of prefrontal cortex interconnect with both DM and the pulvinar (Gutierrez *et al.*, 2000; Preuss & Goldman-Rakic, 1987; Yeterian & Pandya, 1988), and/or via direct intrathalamic communication. Finally, DM may be engaged in the process of decreasing the alpha rhythm power throughout the cortex in order to engage regions that encode semantic memory of features that are stored or accessed in different sensorimotor/cognitive modalities.

There are several possibilities as regards the role of the pre-SMA region (BA6). Crosson *et al.* (1999) showed that this region is active during word generation. Kraut *et al.* (2002a, 2002b) suggested that this activation is likely associated with a search strategy, which may be semantic or language related, while others have suggested that its function is more simply in preparedness to make a motor response (Thompson-Schill *et al.*, 1997). However, the absence of its activation in very similar tasks that also require a motor response suggests either: (1) semantic or generic search strategy or (2) generation of an object concept framework from featural input. Nadeau and Crosson (1997) have suggested that the frontal lobe, via the inferior thalamic peduncle, reticular nucleus, and centromedian thalamic nuclear complex, selectively engages portions of a network of regions necessary to represent an object or concept. We suggest that BA6, along with its dorsomedial nucleus connections, is most likely involved in the process of generating a target object concept from featural input stimuli via initially engaging the network of brain regions (including regions encoding featural representations) involved in representing an object which could be mediated via the decrease in alpha power in cortical regions.

The signal changes in the pulvinar exhibit distinctly slower signal increase and decrease phases than any of the other regions in which we evaluated the signal change dynamics. The findings suggested that the pulvinar region engages later in this object recall process and is thus likely the mediator/modulator of the selective gamma burst rhythm that we propose binds or unites the features in this instance of object recall. The prolonged fMRI response suggests that the pulvinar is more likely engaged after the semantic fields of each feature have been searched and a common object is detected. From the previous studies, the gamma synchronizing rhythm is most readily detected when an actual object is recalled and thus is unlikely to reflect the search for the object. However, whether the gamma rhythm heralds the detection of the target object or unites the features to represent the object is unclear and cannot be determined from the present studies. Medial portions of the pulvinar connect with inferotemporal visual cortex as well as somatosensory cortex of the insula and with the amygdala (for review, see Gutierrez *et al.*, 2000). Thus the pulvinar with its wide array of cortical areas is ideally situated to be involved in modulating connections in the semantic object recall network.

13.1.4 Integrated object concept in semantic memory

We have proposed that the co-activation of all of the features, and likely other factors such as associates and category membership, for example, bound together via neuronal firing synchronized with a 30 Hz gamma rhythm in itself represents the integrated object concept in semantic memory (see Figure 13.5). We caution that this should be considered as only one plausible mechanism of semantic object

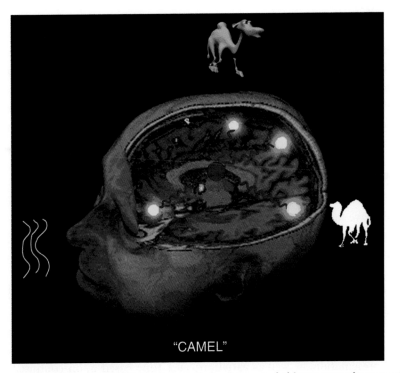

Figure 13.5. A proposed neural mechanism for recall of an integrated object concept in semantic memory. In this instantiation, an object memory consists of the synchronized neural firing of the regions that encode for the features and related attributes of the object. These co-activated features and related associates are bound together via neuronal firing synchronized with a 30 Hz gamma rhythm (blue waves) that is mediated by the pulvinar nucleus in the thalamus (blue solid circle), and this integrated neural activation itself represents the integrated object concept in semantic memory. (Solid yellow circles represent cortical featural representations in multiple semantic memory systems in different modalities including smell, motion, and visual features of the object/item "camel.")

recall to an integrated concept. We do not exclude that there are other models to account for the integrated object concept. What does appear to be the case, though, is that this model of 30 Hz synchronization is consistent with the other models of semantic representation in semantic memory, including those proposed by other contributors to this book. In addition, we think that it is important to note that recall of an object does not necessitate that an integrated, multimodal object concept be fully activated in the brain. Based upon the task and/or needs at the time, the semantic memory representations of the object, the input stimulus, there may be no need to activate an integrated object representation to a significant degree to perform a task. (We acknowledge that local or thalamically mediated distant 30 Hz synchronization may be engaged in other semantic operations where different elements in semantic memory are united, see Assaf et al., 2006.)

We propose that the object concept consists of semantic elements that are integrated via 30 Hz synchronization. These elements include but may not be limited to features and category assignment, with various weightings of the values for each of these elements. The overall strength of the semantic memory reflects the frequency and presumably the contexts in which the object, its constituent features, or its superordinate category, have been encountered. The more often an object is experienced, the increased number of times the neurons encoding that object were co-activated, thus strengthening that memory and the familiarity effect.

Within this framework, not every sensorimotor/cognitive domain will necessarily have featural information about an object, nor will all features have the same strength of association to a given object (see Sartori & Lombardi, 2004). The varying strength of association for each cognitive domain's featural component of semantic memory for a given object is likely based on the individual's encoding process in addition to experience with that object over time, thus allowing for different weights of saliency for features to an object and for individual variability. The network of feature representations for each object thus will vary by object and reflect varying weights and saliency of each feature to that object's overall representation, as well as variations over time based upon continual changes in exposure to objects and features and new entities being experienced.

Some of the ideas we have advanced can clearly be tested in animal models, wherein detection of electrical evidence for spatially distributed brain activity can be followed up using invasive intracortical or intrathalamic/intrastriatal electrical recordings. Absent some future development of techniques that can interrogate noninvasively the behaviors of neural ensembles, direct electrical recordings appear to be an optimal method to obtain details of what directs the object recall process, discerning the mechanisms by which the thalamocortical rhythms are modulated, and processes underlying the influences of the thalamocortical rhythms upon intracortical computational processes.

In conclusion, the neural hybrid model advocates the concept of distinct neural encodings for category-based and/or feature-based semantic knowledge representations that exist in separate systems in various sensory, motor, lexical—semantic, and limbic domains. There are also circumscribed neural regions (e.g. IP—ST) that are engaged in mediating semantic processes (e.g. categorization, multimodal integration). We have proposed a neural mechanism by which components of an object (features, category membership) from multiple modalities represented at separated sites within the brain can be bound to form an integrated object memory. This synchronous co-activation is mediated by the thalamus via 30 Hz oscillating rhythms.

REFERENCES

Assaf, M., Calhoun, V., Kuzu, C., Kraut, M., Rivkin, P., Hart, J., and Pearlson, G. (2006). Neural correlates of the object recall process in semantic memory. *Psychiatry Research: Neuroimaging*, Oct 30; 147 (2–3): 115–26.

Barsalou, L. W., Kyle Simmons, W., Barbey, A. K., and Wilson, C. D. (2003). Grounding conceptual knowledge in modality-specific systems. *Trends in Cognitive Science*, 7: 84–91.

Beauchamp, M. S., Lee, K. E., Argall, B. D., and Martin, A. (2004). Integration of auditory and visual information about objects in superior temporal sulcus. *Neuron*, **41**: 809–23.

Berndt, R. S. (1988). Category-specific deficits in aphasia. *Aphasiology*, **2**: 237–40.

Binder, J. R., Swanson, S. J., Hammeke, T., Morris, G., Mueller, W., Fischer, M., Benbadis, S., Frost, J., Rao, S., and Haughton, V. (1996). Determination of language dominance using functional MRI: a comparison with the Wada test. *Neurology*, **46**: 978–84.

Cappa, S. F., Frugoni, M., Pasquali, P., Perani, D., and Zorat, F. (1998). Category-specific naming impairment for artefacts: a new case. *Neurocase*, **4/5**: 391–8.

Caramazza, A. and Shelton, J. R. (1998). Domain-specific knowledge systems in the brain the animate—inanimate distinction. *Journal of Cognitive Neuroscience*, **10**: 1–34.

Crosson, B., Sadek, J. R., Bobholz, J. A., Gokcay, D., Mohr, C., Leonard, C., Maron, L., Auerbach, E., Browd, S., Freeman, A., and Briggs, R. (1999). Activity in the paracingulate and cingulate sulci during word generation: An fMRI study of functional anatomy. *Cerebral Cortex*, **9**: 307–16.

Damasio, A. R. (1990). Category-related recognition defects as a clue to the neural substrates of knowledge. *Trends in Neuroscience*, **13**: 95–8.

Damasio, A. R. and Tranel, D. (1993). Nouns and verbs are retrieved with differently distributed neural systems. *Proceedings of the National Academy of Sciences USA*, **90**: 4957–60.

Damasio, H., Grabowski, T. J., Tranel, D., Hichwa, R. D., and Damasio, A. R. (1996). A neural basis for lexical retrieval. *Nature*, **380**: 499–505.

della Rocchetta, A. I. and Cipolotti, L. (2004). Preserved knowledge of maps of countries: Implications for the organization of semantic memory. *Neurocase*, **10**: 249–64.

Demb, J. B., Desmond, J. E., Wagner, A. D., Vaidya, C. J., Glover, G. H., and Gabrieli, J. D. (1995). Semantic encoding and retrieval in the left inferior prefrontal cortex: a functional MRI study of task difficulty and process specificity. *Journal of Neuroscience*, **15**: 5870–8.

Demonet, J. F., Chollet, F., Ramsay, S., Cardebat, D., Nespoulous, J., Wise, R., Rascol, A., and Frackowiak, R. (1992). The anatomy of phonological and semantic processing in normal subjects. *Brain*, **115**: 1753–68.

Downing, P. E., Chan, A. W., Peelen, M. V., Dodds, C. M., and Kanwisher, N. (2006). Domain specificity in visual cortex. *Cerebral Cortex*, **16**: 1453–61.

Farah, M. J., McMullen, P., and Meyer, M. (1991). Can recognition of living things be selectively impaired? *Neuropsychologia*, **29**: 185–93.

Farah, M. J., Meyer, M. M., and McMullen, P. A. (1996). The living/nonliving dissociation is not an artifact: giving an a priori implausible hypothesis a strong test. *Cognitive Neuropsychology*, **13**: 137–54.

Farah, M. J. and Wallace, M. A. (1992). Semantically-bounded anomia: implications for the neural implementation of naming. *Neuropsychologia*, **30**: 609–22.

Ferreira, C. T., Giusiano, B., and Poncet, M. (1997). Category-specific anomia: implication of different neural networks in naming. *Neuroreport*, **8**: 1595–602.

Fiez, J. A. (1997). Phonology, semantics, and the role of the left inferior prefrontal cortex. *Human Brain Mapping*, **5**: 79–83.

Funnell, E. and Sheridan, J. (1992). Categories of knowledge? Unfamiliar aspects of living and nonliving things. *Cognitive Neuropsychology*, **9**: 135–53.

Gainotti, G., Silveri, M., Daniele, A., and Giustolisi, L. (1995). Neuroanatomical correlates of category-specific semantic disorders: a critical survey. *Memory*, **3/4**: 247–64.

Garrard, P., Patterson, K., Watson, P. C., and Hodges, J. R. (1998). Category-specific semantic loss in dementia of Alzheimer's type: functional–anatomical correlations form cross-sectional analyses. *Brain*, **121**: 633–46.

Gerlach, C., Law, I., and Paulson, O. B. (2004). Structural similarity and category-specificity: a refined account. *Neuropsychologia*, **42**: 1543–53.

Geschwind, N. (1965). Disconnexion syndromes in animals and man. *Brain*, **88**: 237–97, 585–644.

Gil-da-Costa, R., Braun, A., Lopes, M., Hauser, M. D., Carson, R. E., Herscovitch, P., and Martin, A. (2004). Toward an evolutionary perspective on conceptual representation: species-specific calls activate visual and affective processing systems in the macaque. *Proceedings of the National Academy of Sciences USA*, **101**: 17516–21.

Goodglass, H., Klein, B., Carey, P., and Jones, K. (1966). Specific semantic word categories in aphasia. *Cortex*, **2**: 74–89.

Goodglass, H., Wingfield, A., Hyde, M., and Theurkauf, J. C. (1986). Category specific dissociations in naming and recognition by aphasic patients. *Cortex*, **22**: 87–102.

Grafton, S. T., Fadiga, L., Arbib, M. A., and Rizzolatti, G. (1997). Premotor cortex activation during observation and naming of familiar tools. *NeuroImage*, **6**: 231–6.

Grossman, M., Robinson, K., Biassou, N., White-Devine, T., and D'Esposito, M. (1998). Semantic memory in Alzheimer's disease: representativeness, ontologic category, and material. *Neuropsychology*, **12**: 34–42.

Grossman, M., Smith, E. E., Koenig, P., Glosser, G., DeVita, C., Moore, P., and McMillan, C. (2002). The neural basis for categorization in semantic memory. *NeuroImage*, **17**: 1549–61.

Gutierrez, C., Cola, M. G., Seltzer, B., and Cusick, C. (2000). Neurochemical and connectional organization of the dorsal pulvinar complex in monkeys. *Journal of Comparative Neurology*, **419**: 61–86.

Hart, J. and Gordon, B. (1990). Delineation of single-word semantic comprehension deficits in aphasia, with anatomical correlation. *Annals of Neurology*, **27**: 226–31.

Hart, J. and Gordon, B. (1992). Neural subsystems for object knowledge. *Nature*, **359**: 60–4.

Hart, J., Lesser, R. P., and Gordon, B. (1992). Selective interference with the representation of size the human by direct cortical stimulation. *Journal of Cognitive Neuroscience*, **4**: 337–44.

Hart, J., Crone, N. E., Lesser, R. P., Sieracki, J., Miglioretti, D. L., Hall, C., Sherman, D., and Gordon, B. (1998). Temporal dynamics of verbal object comprehension. *Proceedings of the National Academy of Sciences USA*, **95**: 6498–503.

Hart, J., Moo, L., Segal, J. B., Adkins, E., and Kraut, M. (2002). Neural substrates of semantics. In A. Hillis (ed.), *Handbook of Language Disorders*. Philadelphia: Psychology Press, pp. 207–27.

Haxby, J. V., Grady, C. L., Horwitz, B., Ungerleider, L. G., Mishkin, M., Carson, R. E., Herscovitch, P., Schapiro, M. B., and Rapoport, S. I. (1991). Dissociation of object and spatial visual processing pathways in human extrastriate cortex. *Proceedings of the National Academy of Sciences USA*, **88**: 1621–5.

Haxby, J., Gobbini, M. I., Furey, M. L., Ishai, A., Schouten, J. L., and Pietrini, P. (2001). Distributed and overlapping representations of faces and objects in ventral temporal cortex. *Science*, **293**: 2405–7.

Hillis, A. and Caramazza, A. (1991). Category-specific naming and comprehension impairment: a double dissociation. *Brain*, **114**: 2081–94.

Hinton, G. E. (1981). Implementing semantic networks in parallel hardware. In G. E. Hinton and J. A. Anderson (eds.), *Parallel Models of Associative Memory*. Hillsdale, NJ: Erlbaum, pp. 161–87.

Humphreys, G. W. and Riddoch, M. J. (1987). On telling your fruits from your vegetables: a consideration of category-specific deficits after brain damage. *Trends in Neuroscience*, **10**: 145–8.

Ilinsky, I. A., Jouandet, M. L., and Goldman-Rakic, P. S. (1985). Organization of the nigrothalamocortical system in the rhesus monkey. *Journal of Comparative Neurology*, **236**: 315–30.

Inase, M., Tokuno, H., Nambu, A., Akazawa, T., and Takada, M. (1996). Origin of thalamocortical projections to the presupplementary motor area (pre-SMA) in the macaque. *Neuroscience Research*, **25**: 217–27.

Johnson, K. O. and Hsiao, S. S. (1992). Neural mechanisms of tactile form and texture perception. *Annual Review of Neuroscience*, **15**: 227–50.

Joliot, M., Ribary, U., and Llinas, R. (1994). Human oscillatory brain activity near 40 Hz coexists with cognitive temporal binding. *Proceedings of the National Academy of Sciences USA*, **91**: 11748–51.

Kapur, S., Rose, R., Liddle, P. F., Zipursky, R. B., Brown, G. M., Stuss, D., Houle, S., and Tulving, E. (1994). The role of the left prefrontal cortex in verbal processing: semantic processing or willed action? *Neuroreport*, **5**: 2193–6.

Kemmerer, D. and Tranel, D. (2000). Verb retrieval in brain-damaged subjects: 1. Analysis of stimulus, lexical, and conceptual factors. *Brain and Language*, **73**: 347–92.

Klimesch, W. (1996). Memory processes, brain oscillations and EEG synchronization. *International Journal of Psychophysiology*, **24**: 61–100.

Klimesch, W. (1999). EEG alpha and theta oscillations reflect cognitive and memory performance: a review and analysis. *Brain Research: Brain Research Reviews*, **29**: 169–95.

Klimesch, W., Doppelmayr, M., Schwaiger, J., Auinger, P., and Winkler, T. (1999). "Paradoxical" alpha synchronization in a memory task. *Brain Research: Cognitive Brain Research*, **7**: 493–501.

Klimesch, W., Schimke, H., and Pfurtscheller, G. (1993). Alpha frequency, cognitive load and memory performance. *Brain Topograpy*, **5**: 241–51.

Kraut, M., Hart, J., Soher, B. J., and Gordon, B. (1997). Object shape processing in the visual system evaluated using functional MRI. *Neurology*, **48**: 1416–20.

Kraut, M. A., Kremen, S., Segal, J. B., Calhoun, V., Moo, L., and Hart, J. (2002a). Object activation from features in the semantic system. *Journal of Cognitive Neuroscience*, **14**: 24–36.

Kraut, M. A., Kremen, S., Moo, L. R., Segal, J., Calhoun, V., and Hart, J. (2002b). Object activation in semantic memory from visual multimodal feature input. *Journal of Cognitive Neuroscience*, **14**: 37–47.

Kraut, M., Moo, L., Segal, J., and Hart, J. (2002c). Neural activation during an explicit categorization task: category- or feature-specific effects? *Brain Research: Cognitive Brain Research*, **13**: 213–20.

Kraut, M., Calhoun, V., Pitcock, J. A., Cusick, C., and Hart, J. (2003). Neural hybrid model of semantic object memory: Implications from event-related timing using fMRI. *Journal of the International Neuropsychological Society*, **9**: 1031–40.

Kraut, M., Pitcock, J., Calhoun, V., Li, J., and Hart, J. (in press). Neuroanatomic organization of sound memory in humans. *Journal of Cognitive Neuroscience*.

Kronbichler, M., Hutzler, F., Wimmer, H., Mair, A., Staffen, W., and Ladurner, G. (2004). The visual word form area and the frequency with which words are encountered: evidence from a parametric fMRI study. *NeuroImage*, **21**: 946–53.

Lyons, F., Hanley, J. R., and Kay, J. (2002). Anomia for common names and geographical names with preserved retrieval of names of people: a semantic memory disorder. *Cortex*, **38**: 23–35.

Martin, A., Wiggs, C. L., Ungerleider, L. G., and Haxby, J. V. (1996). Neural correlates of category-specific knowledge. *Nature*, **379**: 649–52.

Martin, A. and Chao, L. L. (2001). Semantic memory and the brain: structure and processes. *Current Opinion in Neurobiology*, **11**: 194–201.

Mauri, A., Daum, I., Sartori, G., Riesch, G., and Birbaumer, N. (1994). Category-specific semantic impairment in Alzheimer's disease and temporal lobe dysfunction: a comparative study. *Journal of Clinical and Experimental Neuropsychology*, **16**: 689–701.

McCarthy, R. A. and Warrington, E. K. (1988). Evidence for modality-specific meaning systems in the brain. *Nature*, **334**: 428–30.

McClelland, J. L. and Rumelhart, D. E. (1985). Distributed memory and the representation of general and specific information. *Journal of Experimental Psychology: General*, **114**: 159–88.

Miceli, G., Fouch, E., Capasso, R., Shelton, J., Tomaiuolo, F., and Caramazza, A. (2001). The dissociation of color from form and function knowledge. *Nature Neuroscience*, **4**: 662–7.

Mummery, C. J., Patterson, K., Hodges, J. R., and Price, C. J. (1998). Functional neuroanatomy of the semantic system: divisible by what? *Journal of Cognitive Neuroscience*, **10**: 766–77.

Nadeau, S. E. and Crosson, B. (1997). Subcortical aphasia. *Brain and Language*, **58**: 355–402.

Nielsen, J. M. (1946). *Agnosia, apraxia, aphasia: their value in cerebral localization*, 2nd edn. New York: Paul B. Hoeber.

Ojemann, J., Ojemann, G., and Lettich, E. (2002). Cortical stimulation mapping of language cortex by using a verb generation task: effects of learning and comparison to mapping based on object naming. *Journal of Neurosurgery*, **97**: 33–8.

Perani, D., Cappa, S., Bettinardi, V., Bressi, S., Gorno-Tempini, M., Matarrese, M., and Fazio, F. (1995). Different neural systems for the recognition of animals and man-made tools. *Neuroreport*, **6**: 1637–9.

Petersen, S. E., Fox, P. T., Posner, M. I., Mintun, M., and Raichle, M. E. (1988). Positron emission tomographic studies of the cortical anatomy of single-word processing. *Nature*, **331**: 585–9.

Petersen, S. E., Fox, P. T., Snyder, A. Z., and Raichle, M. E. (1990). Specific extrastriate and frontal cortical areas are activated by visual words and word-like stimuli. *Science*, **249**: 1041–4.

Posner, M. I., Petersen, S. E., Fox, P. T., and Raichle, M. E. (1988). Localization of cognitive operations in the human brain. *Science*, **240**: 1627–31.

Preuss, T. M. and Goldman-Rakic, P. S. (1987). Crossed corticothalamic and thalamocortical connections of macaque prefrontal cortex. *Journal of Comparative Neurology*, **257**: 269–81.

Pulvermüller, F., Lutzenberger, W., and Preissl, H. (1999). Nouns and verbs in the intact brain: evidence from event-related potentials and high-frequency cortical responses. *Cerebral Cortex*, **9**: 497–506.

Rademacher, J., Morosan, P., Schormann, T., Schleicher, A., Werner, C., Freund, H. J., and Zilles, K. (2001). Probabilistic mapping and volume measurement of human primary auditory cortex. *NeuroImage*, **13**: 669–83.

Rapcsak, S. Z., Comer, J. F., and Rubens, A. B. (1993). Anomia for facial expressions: neuropsychological mechanisms and anatomical correlates. *Brain and Language*, **45**: 233–52.

Rapcsak, S. Z., Kaszniak, A. W., and Rubens, A. B. (1989). Anomia for facial expressions: evidence for a category specific visual–verbal disconnection syndrome. *Neuropsychologia*, **27**: 1031–41.

Ricci, P. T., Zelkowicz, B. J., Nebes, R. D., Meltzer, C. C., Mintun, M. A., and Becker, J. T. (1999). Functional neuroanatomy of semantic memory: recognition of semantic associations. *NeuroImage*, **9**: 88–96.

Robinson, K. M., Grossman, M., White-Devine, T., and D'Esposito, M. (1996). Category-specific difficulty naming with verbs in Alzheimer's disease. *Neurology*, **47**: 178–82.

Sacchett, C. and Humphreys, G. W. (1992). Calling a squirrel a squirrel but a canoe a wigwam: a category-specific deficit for artefactual objects and body parts. *Cognitive Neuropsychology*, **9**: 73–86.

Sartori, G. and Job, R. (1988). The oyster with four legs: a neuropsychological study on the interaction of visual and semantic information. *Cognitive Neuropsychology*, **5**: 105–32.

Sartori, G. and Lombardi, L. (2004). Semantic relevance and semantic disorders. *Journal of Cognitive Neuroscience*, **16**: 439–52.

Sartori, G., Job, R., Miozzo, M., Zago, S., and Marchiori, G. (1993). Category-specific form–knowledge deficit in a patient with herpes simplex virus encephalitis. *Journal of Clinical and Experimental Neuropsychology*, **15**: 280–99.

Schier, M. A. (2000). Changes in EEG alpha power during simulated driving: a demonstration. *International Journal of Psychophysiology*, **37**: 155–62.

Semenza, C. and Zettin, M. (1988). Generating proper names: a case of selective inability. *Cognitive Neuropsychology*, **5**: 711–21.

Semenza, C. and Zettin, M. (1989). Evidence from aphasia for the role of proper names as pure referring expressions. *Nature*, **342**: 678–9.

Silveri, M. C. and Gainotti, G. (1988). Interaction between vision and language in category-specific semantic impairment. *Cognitive Neuropsychology*, **5**: 677–709.

Silveri, M. C., Daniele, A., Giustolisi, L., and Gainotti, G. (1991). Dissociation between knowledge of living and nonliving things in dementia of the Alzheimer type. *Neurology*, **41**: 545–6.

Sim, E. J. and Kiefer, M. (2005). Category-related brain activity to natural categories is associated with the retrieval of visual features: evidence from repetition effects during visual and functional judgments. *Brain Research Cognitive Brain Research*, **24**: 260–73.

Singer, W. (1993). Synchronization of cortical activity and its putative role in information processing and learning. *Annual Review of Physiology*, **55**: 349–74.

Singer, W. and Gray, C. M. (1995). Visual feature integration and the temporal correlation hypothesis. *Annual Review of Neuroscience*, **18**: 555–86.

Slotnick, S., Moo, L., Kraut, M., Lesser, R., and Hart, J. (2002). Thalamic modulation of cortical rhythms during semantic memory recall in humans. *Proceedings of the National Academy of Sciences USA*, **99**: 6440–3.

Spiridon, M. and Kanwisher, N. (2002). How distributed is visual category information in human occipito-temporal cortex? An fMRI study. *Neuron*, **35**: 1157–65.

Spitzer, M., Kwong, K. K., Kennedy, W., Rosen, B. R., and Bellivean, J. W. (1995). Category-specific brain activation in fMRI during picture naming. *Neuroreport*, **6**: 2109–12.

Steriade, M. (2000). Corticothalamic resonance, states of vigilance and mentation. *Neuroscience*, **101**: 243–76.

Tarr, M. J. and Gauthier, I. (2000). FFA: a flexible fusiform area for subordinate-level visual processing automatized by expertise. *Nature Neuroscience*, **3**: 764–9.

Temple, C. (1986). Anomia for animals in a child. *Brain*, **109**: 1225–42.

Thompson-Schill, S., D'Esposito, M., Aguirre, G., and Farah, M. (1997). Role of left inferior prefrontal cortex in retrieval of semantic knowledge: A reevaluation. *Proceedings of the National Academy of Sciences USA*, **94**: 14792–7.

Thompson-Schill, S., Swick, D., Farah, M., D'Esposito, M., Kan, I., and Knight, R. (1998). Verb generation in patients with focal frontal lesions: A neuropsychological test of neuroimaging findings. *Proceedings of the National Academy of Sciences USA*, **95**: 15855–60.

Tippett, L. J., Glosser, G., and Farah, M. J. (1996). A category-specific naming impairment after temporal lobectomy. *Neuropsychologia*, **34**: 139–46.

Tyler, L. K., Moss, H. E., Durrant-Peatfield, M. R., and Levy, J. P. (2000). Conceptual structure and the structure of concepts: a distributed account of category-specific deficits. *Brain and Language*, **75**: 195–231.

Underwood, G. and Whitfield, A. (1985). Right hemisphere interactions in picture–word processing. *Brain and Cognition*, **4**: 273–86.

Ungerleider, L. G. and Haxby, J. V. (1994). "What" and "where" in the human brain. *Current Opinion in Neurobiology*, **4**: 157–65.

Vitali, P., Abutalebi, J., Tettamanti, M., Rowe, J., Scifo, P., Fazio, F., Cappa, S. F., and Perani, D. (2005). Generating animal and tool names: an fMRI study of effective connectivity. *Brain and Language*, **93**: 32–45.

Warrington, E. K. and McCarthy, R. A. (1983). Category specific access dysphasia. *Brain*, **106**: 859–78.

Warrington, E. K. and McCarthy, R. A. (1987). Categories of knowledge: further fractionation and an attempted integration. *Brain*, **110**: 1273–96.

Warrington, E. K. and Shallice, T. (1984). Category specific semantic impairments. *Brain*, **107**: 829–54.

Yeterian, E. H. and Pandya, D. N. (1988). Corticothalamic connections of paralimbic regions in the rhesus monkey. *Journal of Comparative Neurology*, **269**: 130–46.

Index

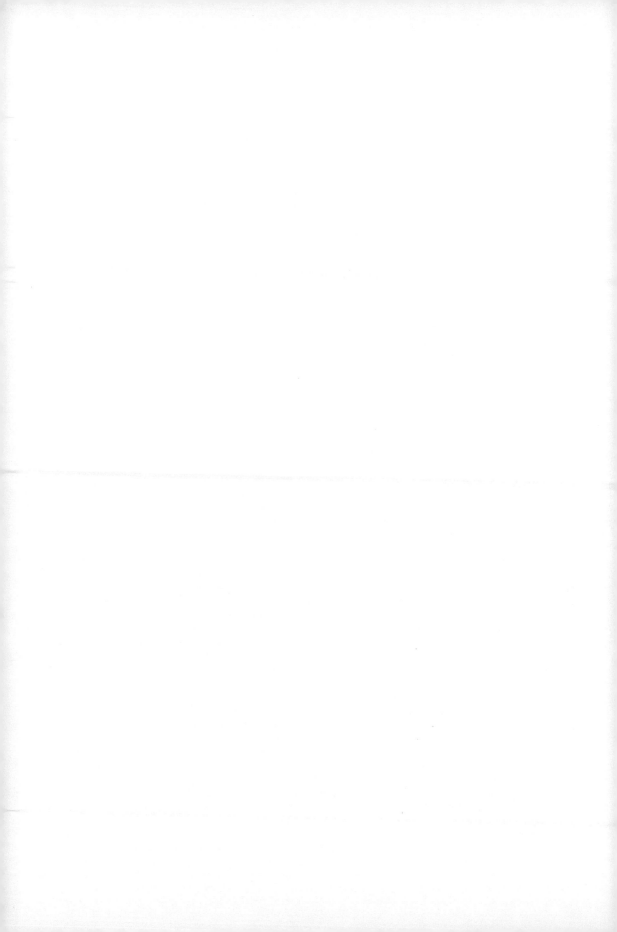